Emergency Surgery and Critical Care

A COMPANION TO SPECIALIST SURGICAL PRACTICE

Series editors

Sir David C. Carter
O. James Garden
Simon Paterson-Brown

Emergency Surgery and Critical Care

Edited by

Simon Paterson-Brown

Consultant General and Upper Gastrointestinal Surgeon
University Department of Surgery
Royal Infirmary
Edinburgh

W B Saunders Company Limited
London · Philadelphia · Toronto · Sydney · Tokyo

W. B. Saunders Company Ltd 24–28 Oval Road
London NW1 7DX

The Curtis Center
Independence Square West
Philadelphia, PA 19106-3399, USA

Harcourt Brace & Company
55 Horner Avenue
Toronto, Ontario M8Z 4X6, Canada

Harcourt Brace & Company, Australia
30–52 Smidmore Street
Marrickville, NSW 2204, Australia

Harcourt Brace & Company, Japan
Ichibancho Central Building, 22-1 Ichibancho
Chiyoda-ku, Tokyo 102, Japan

A catalogue record for this book is available from the British Library

ISBN 0-7020-2140-7

Typeset by Florencetype Ltd, Stoodleigh, Devon
Printed in Great Britain by The Bath Press, Bath

Contents

Contents

Contributors

Iain D. Anderson *BSc FRCS MD FRCS(Gen)*
Senior Lecturer in Surgery and Honorary Consultant Surgeon, University Department of Surgery, Hope Hospital, Salford, Manchester, UK

Ian Bailey *MS FRCS*
Senior Surgical Registrar, Royal United Hospital, Bath, UK

Kenneth L. Campbell *MD FRCS*
Lecturer, Department of Surgery, University of Aberdeen, Foresterhill, Aberdeen, UK

Oleg Eremin *MD FRACS FRCS(Ed)*
Regius Professor of Surgery, University of Aberdeen and Honorary Consultant Surgeon, Aberdeen Royal Hospitals NHS Trust, Aberdeen, UK

Nicholas J. Everitt *MD FRCS(Eng)*
Senior Registrar in Surgery, Doncaster Royal Infirmary, Sheffield, UK

Roger Grace *FRCS*
Professor of Colorectal Surgery, Coloproctology Research Unit, New Cross Hospital, Wolverhampton, UK

Steven D. Heys *MD PhD FRCS(Glas)*
Reader in Surgery, Director of the Surgical Nutrition and Metabolism Unit, University of Aberdeen and Honorary Consultant Surgeon, Aberdeen Royal Hospitals NHS Trust, Aberdeen, UK

Alexander Munro *ChM FRCS(Ed)*
Consultant Surgeon, Raigmore Hospital, Inverness, UK

Simon Paterson-Brown *MS MPhil FRCS(Ed) FRCS(Eng) FCSHK*
Consultant General and Upper Gastrointestinal Surgeon, University Department of Surgery, Royal Infirmary, Edinburgh, UK

Brian J. Rowlands *MD FRCS FACS*
Professor of Surgery, Institute of Clinical Science, Queens University of Belfast, Belfast, UK

William G. Simpson *MRCPath*
Senior Registrar in Clinical Biochemistry, Aberdeen Royal Hospitals NHS Trust, Honorary Lecturer, University of Aberdeen, UK

Lewis Spitz *PhD FRCS*
Nuffield Professor of Paediatric Surgery, Institute of Child Health, University of London, Consultant Paediatric Surgeon, Great Ormond Street Hospital for Children, London, UK

Robert J. C. Steele *BSc MD FRCS*
Professor of Surgery, Department of Surgery, Ninewells Hospital, Dundee, UK

Jeremy J. T. Tate *MS FRCS*
Consultant Surgeon, Department of Surgery, Royal United Hospital, Bath, UK

William E. G. Thomas *BSc MS FRCS(Eng)*
Consultant Surgeon, Royal Hallamshire Hospital, Glossop Road, Sheffield, UK

Jeremy N. Thompson *MChir FRCS*
Consultant Gastrointestinal Surgeon, Department of Surgery, Chelsea & Westminster & The Royal Marsden Hospitals, London, UK

Foreword

General surgery defies easy definition. Indeed, there are those who claim that it is dying, if not yet dead – a corpse being picked clean by the vulturine proclivities of the other specialties of surgery. Unfortunately for those who subscribe to this view, general surgery is not lying down, indeed it is rejoicing in a new enhanced vigour, as this new series demonstrates.

The general surgeon is the specialist who, along with his other colleagues, provides a 24-hour, 7-day, emergency surgical cover for his, or her, hospital. Also it is to general surgical clinics that patients are referred, unless their condition is manifestly related to one of the other surgical specialties e.g. urology, cardiothoracic services, etc. Moreover trainees in these specialities must, during their training, receive experience in general surgery, whose techniques underpin the whole of surgery. General surgery occupies a pivotal position in surgical training. The number of general surgeons required to serve a community, outstrips that required by any other surgical specialty.

General surgery is a specialty in its own right. Inevitably, there are those who wish to practice exclusively one of the sub-specialties of general surgery, e.g. vascular or colorectal surgery. This arrangement may be possible in a few large tertiary referral centres. Although the contribution of these surgeons to patient care and to advances in their discipline will be significant, their numbers are necessarily low. The bulk of surgical practice will be undertaken by the general surgeon who has developed a sub-specialty interest, so that, with his other colleagues in the hospital, comprehensive surgery services can be provided.

There is therefore a great need for a text which will provide comprehensively the theoretical knowledge of the entire specialty and act as a guide for the acquisition of the diagnostic and therapeutic skills required by the general surgeon. The unique contribution of this companion is that it comes as a series, each chapter fresh from the pen of a practising clinician and active surgeon. Each volume is right up to date and this is evidenced by the fact that the first volumes of the series are being published within 12 months from the start of the project. This is a series which has been tightly edited by a team from one of the foremost teaching hospitals in the United Kingdom.

Quite properly the series begins with a volume on emergency surgery and critical care – two of the greatest challenges confronting the practising surgeon. These are the areas that the examination candidate finds the greatest difficulty in acquiring theoretical knowledge and practical experience. Moreover, these are the areas in which advances are at present so rapid that they constantly test the experienced consultant surgeon.

This series not only provides both types of reader with the necessary up-to-date detail but also demonstrates that general surgery remains as challenging and vigorous as it ever has been.

Sir Robert Shields *DL, MD, DSc, FRCS(Ed, Eng, Glas, Ire),*
FRCPEd, FACS
President, Royal College of Surgeons of Edinburgh

Preface

A Companion to Specialist Surgical Practice was designed to meet the needs of the higher surgeon in training and busy practising surgeon who need access to up-to-date information on recent developments, research and data in the context of accepted surgical practice.

Many of the major surgery text books either cover the whole of what is termed 'general surgery' and therefore contain much which is not of interest to the specialist surgeon, or are very high level specialist texts which are outwith the reach of the trainee's finances, and though comprehensive are often out of date due to the lengthy writing and production times of such major works.

Each volume in this series therefore provides succinct summaries of all key topics within a specialty and concentrates on the most recent developments and current data. They are carefully constructed to be easily readable and provide key references.

A specialist surgeon, whether in training or in practice, need only purchase the volume relevant to his or her chosen specialist field plus the emergency surgery and critical care volume, if involved in emergency care.

The volumes have been written in a very short time frame, and produced equally quickly so that information is as up to date as possible. Each volume will be updated and published as a new edition at frequent intervals, to ensure that current information is always available.

We hope that our aim – of providing affordable up-to-date specialist texts – has been met and that all surgeons, in training or in practice will find the volumes to be a valuable resource.

Sir David C. Carter *MD, FRCS(Ed), FRCS(Glas), FRCS(Eng), Hon FRCS(Ire), Hon FACS, FRCP(Ed), FRS(Ed)*
Chief Medical Officer in Scotland
Formerly Regius Professor of Clinical Surgery, University Department of Surgery, Royal Infirmary, Edinburgh

O. James Garden *BSc, MB, ChB, MD, FRCS(Glas), FRCS(Ed)*
Senior Lecturer and Honorary Consultant Hepatobiliary Surgeon; Director of Organ Transplantation, University Department of Surgery, Royal Infirmary, Edinburgh

Simon Paterson-Brown *MS, MPhil, FRCS(Ed), FRCS(Eng), FCSHK*
Consultant General and Upper Gastrointestinal Surgeon, University Department of Surgery, Royal Infirmary, Edinburgh

Acknowledgements

I am indebted to all the authors who have contributed to this volume for their perseverance and expertise. I am grateful to my fellow editors for assistance and advice in the initial planning of this book. The series editors give special thanks to Rachael Stock and Linda Clark from W. B. Saunders for their initial persuasion, continuing enthusiasm and ongoing support. I am grateful to my secretary, Susan Keggie, for her expert help with the preparation and editing of the manuscripts. Finally, as always, I am indebted to my wife, Sheila, for her never-ending support in yet another academic venture.

S. PATERSON-BROWN

1 Diagnosis and investigation in the acute abdomen

Simon Paterson-Brown

Introduction

The care of emergency surgical admissions remains one of the most important aspects of general surgical practice[1] and, with the current trend of increasing emergency admissions throughout the UK in all medical specialties,[2] this responsibility will undoubtedly increase. It has been estimated that as much as 50% of all general surgical admissions are emergencies[3] and as approximately half of these are due to acute abdominal pain the workload for the general surgeon remains substantial. The increasing trend towards sub-specialization in general surgery has also had an influence on emergency surgical practice, with many hospitals and units providing emergency cover for acute admissions in sub-specialties such as vascular and hepatobiliary-pancreatic surgery. There has also been a suggestion that patients undergoing emergency colorectal surgery are less likely to have a stoma fashioned if the surgeons operating are attached to firms with a specialist interest in colorectal surgery as compared to those without a special interest.[4] More recently other reports have confirmed similar differences between specialists and non-specialists in relation to leak rate after colorectal resections,[5] but as yet data are not available on outcome. If these reports are substantiated by long-term follow-up, they would have major implications on the provision of acute surgical services. What does appear to be clear at the present time, and the Confidential Enquiry into Post-Operative Deaths has confirmed this,[6] is that outcome for patients requiring emergency surgery is improved when senior surgical staff are involved, not only in the preoperative decision-making, but also in the surgery.

Many changes have occurred over the last decade in the assessment and management of patients with acute abdominal pain and surgeons who take responsibility for the care of emergency surgical patients must be aware of these changes in order to ensure that their patients are receiving the best possible care, not just in the choice of surgical procedure, but, perhaps of even greater importance, in the initial assessment, diagnosis and clinical decision-making process. For the purposes of most studies looking at abdominal pain, the broad definition is taken as: 'abdominal pain of less than one week's duration requiring admission to hospital, which has not been previously treated or investigated'. However, this must be accepted as a fairly loose definition.

Conditions presenting as acute abdominal pain

Many studies have looked at the spectrum of patients who are admitted to hospital with acute abdominal pain and the approximate percentage represented by each condition is now well understood and figures from one study[7] appear to be fairly representative (Table 1.1). In this study the 30-day mortality in 1190 emergency admissions was 4%, with a perioperative mortality of 8%. Not surprisingly the mortality rate was age related, with the perioperative mortality in patients below 60 years being 2%, rising to 12% between 60 and 69 years and reaching 20% in patients over the age of 80 years. Laparotomy for irresectable disease was the most common cause of perioperative mortality (28%), with ruptured abdominal aortic aneurysm (23%), perforated peptic ulcer (16%) and colonic resections (14%) all being associated with a significant perioperative mortality.

Table 1.1 *Conditions which may present with acute abdominal pain (after Irvin[7])*

Condition	%
Non-specific abdominal pain (NSAP)	35
Acute appendicitis	17
Intestinal obstruction	15
Urological causes	6
Gallstone disease	5
Colonic diverticular disease	4
Abdominal trauma	3
Abdominal malignancy	3
Perforated peptic ulcer	3
Pancreatitis	2

The following conditions contribute 1% or less:

Exacerbation of peptic ulcer
Ruptured abdominal aortic aneurysm
Gynaecological causes (these may go undetected as NSAP)
Inflammatory bowel disease
Medical conditions
Mesenteric ischaemia
Gastroenteritis
Miscellaneous

Table 1.2 *Causes of non-specific abdominal pain[8]*

Viral infections
Bacterial gastroenteritis
Worm infestation
Irritable bowel syndrome
Gynaecological causes
Psychosomatic pain
Abdominal wall pain[10]
    Iatrogenic peripheral nerve injuries
    Hernias
    Myofascial pain syndromes
    Rib tip syndrome
    Nerve root pain
    Rectus sheath haematoma

What stands out from all the studies on acute abdominal pain published over the last decade or so is the high incidence of non-specific abdominal pain (NSAP), with published figures of 40% or more.[8] NSAP usually reflects a failure of diagnosis as many of these patients do have a cause for the pain and it has been shown that further investigations, such as laparoscopy, can reduce the overall incidence of NSAP to around 27%.[9]

Some authors have examined this diagnosis of NSAP further and describe a certain number of alternative conditions which could be related (Table 1.2),[8] including abdominal wall pain,[10] and rectus nerve entrapment.[11] In some cases of NSAP, detection of abdominal wall tenderness (increased abdominal pain on tensing the abdominal wall muscles) may be a useful diagnostic test.[12] Possible causes of abdominal wall pain are also given in Table 1.2. The major problem with making a diagnosis of NSAP is in missing serious underlying disease and the late Tim de Dombal estimated that 10% of patients over the age of 50 years who were admitted to hospital with acute abdominal pain were subsequently found to have intra-abdominal malignancy.[13] Half of these patients had colonic carcinoma and the major concern was that 50% of the patients who were subsequently proved to have intra-abdominal cancer were discharged from hospital with a diagnosis of NSAP.

Another group of diagnoses which may often go under the umbrella of NSAP, simply because of a failure to take a good history, examination, or even perform a thorough pelvic examination, whether digitally, ultrasonographically or at operation, are acute gynaecological conditions such as pelvic inflammatory disease and ovarian cyst accidents. In one study from a general surgical unit, gynaecological causes represented 13% of all diagnoses in a consecutive series of all emergency admissions (both male and female) initially presumed to be 'surgical' in origin.[14] As many of these patients present with 'query appendicitis' accurate assessment is essential if unnecessary operations are to be avoided, and even then the diagnosis may remain hidden unless the surgeon examines the pelvic organs once a normal appendix has been found. With the increased use of diagnostic laparoscopy, discussed later in this chapter, these conditions are now being recognised by the emergency surgeon with much greater frequency. Early recognition and appropriate treatment of pelvic inflammatory disease may help to avoid potentially serious longer-term sequelae and must be encouraged.[15] Indeed the condition of Curtis–Fitz–Hugh syndrome, when transperitoneal spread of pelvic inflammatory disease produces right upper quadrant pain due to peri-hepatic adhesions, is now well recognised and care must be taken to differentiate this from acute biliary conditions.[16–18]

Although much is made of possible 'medical' causes of acute abdominal pain in surgical textbooks, the incidence of conditions such as myocardial infarction, lobar pneumonia and some metabolic disorders is extremely small although many still masquerade as NSAP (Table 1.1). However, the possibility of such conditions must still be borne in mind during the clinical assessment of all patients with acute abdominal pain.

History and examination (including computer aided diagnosis)

In the early 1970s de Dombal[19] in Leeds and Gunn[20] in Edinburgh developed a computer program based on Bayesian reasoning which produced a list of probable diagnoses for individual patients with acute abdominal pain. They demonstrated that the accuracy of clinical diagnosis could be improved by around 20%, and since then many other studies have confirmed this finding.[21–23] Furthermore, these studies have shown that there is a reduction in the unnecessary laparotomy rate, bad management errors (patients whose surgery is incorrectly delayed) and when used in the Accident and Emergency department there is an associated reduction in 'inappropriate' admissions.[20] However, many clinicians have remained reluctant to incorporate computer aided diagnosis (CAD) into the overall manage-ment of patients with acute abdominal pain.[24] When the reasons for the improvement in diagnostic accuracy associated with the use of CAD are examined there appears to be three main factors involved: firstly peer review and audit which is invariably associated with improved results in most aspects of medical management;[25,26] secondly an educational factor related to feedback;[27] and thirdly, probably of greatest significance, the use of structured data sheets onto which the history and examination findings are documented. One study demon-strated that the diagnostic accuracy of junior doctors improved by nearly 20% when they used structured data sheets alone, without going on to use the CAD program.[28] The same study also demon-strated that medical students assessing patients with the structured data sheets and then using the CAD program reached similar levels of diagnostic accuracy. Other studies have since confirmed similar improvements in clinical decision-making following the introduction of these data sheets.[29] The message is clear – a good history and examination remain essential for both diagnostic accuracy and good clinical decision-making, and the use of a structured data sheet helps the clinician to achieve this objective. In one of his studies de Dombal demonstrated that in over 50% of cases clinicians did not even ask the most appropriate questions, such as aggravation of pain by movement.[30]

The aim of both the history and examination is to determine a diagnosis and clinical decision. There are undoubtedly specific features associated with all acute abdominal conditions which are well established; however, it remains the ability to identify the presence or absence of peritoneal inflammation which probably has the greatest influence on the final surgical decision. In other words the presence or absence of guarding and rebound tenderness, and a recent study has demonstrated that a history of pain on coughing correlates well with the presence of peritonitis.[31] There has always been great store taken from tenderness elicited on rectal examination during the assessment of patients with suspected acute appendicitis. However, when rebound tenderness is detected in the lower abdomen, as evident by pain on gentle percussion, further examination by rectal examination has been shown to provide no new information.[32] Rectal examination can, therefore, be avoided in such cases, and reserved for those patients without rebound tenderness, or where specific pelvic disease needs to be excluded. Measurement of temperature has also been shown to be relatively non-discriminatory in the early assessment of the acute abdomen.[33]

Early management of patients with acute abdominal pain

After the initial assessment (history and examination) of patients with acute abdominal pain, steps should be taken towards resuscitation, pain relief and further diagnostic tests as required. There is now good evidence to support the early administration of opiate analgesia in patients with acute abdominal pain.[34] This has been clearly shown to have no detrimental effect on subsequent clinical assessment, but, on the contrary, because the patient becomes more comfortable, further assessment may actually be facilitated. The cruel practice of withholding analgesia until the emergency surgeon has examined the patient with acute abdominal pain must be condemned.[35]

Once the initial assessment has been completed the surgeon will reach a differential diagnosis, but, perhaps more importantly, a clinical decision – early operation definitely required, early operation definitely not required or need for early operation uncertain. Clearly further investigations in the first category are unlikely to influence management, with the exception of a serum amylase level, which may reveal acute pancreatitis.[36] Further investigations in the group in which the surgeon considers early operation is not required can be organised on a more leisurely basis, and it is not surprising that it is the group in which the surgeon is uncertain as to whether early operation is required that most difficulty exists.[37] Most of the uncertainty relates to 'query appendicitis', particularly in the young female, but also involves patients with intestinal obstruction and the elderly in whom the diagnosis of mesenteric ischaemia must always be considered.[38] The value of 'active observation' with re-assessment after 2–3 hours by the same surgeon, repeated thereafter as necessary, in patients with equivocal signs and symptoms is well established[39] and should be routine in all units.

In the assessment of the role of subsequent investigations in the acute abdomen it is important to identify their potential influence on clinical decision-making rather than evaluating them purely on diagnostic potential.

Blood tests

Although blood tests are often useful as a baseline, their influence on the diagnosis of acute abdominal pain remains unclear, with the exception of serum amylase for acute pancreatitis.[36] Studies examining the influence of white cell concentration,[40] C-reactive protein[41] and skin temperature in the right iliac fossa[42] in patients with 'query appendicitis' have concluded that serial white cell counts are useful, as compared with a single measurement, and both C-reactive protein and measurement of skin temperature over the right iliac fossa are of little value. Thus routine measurement of the white cell count in patients with acute abdominal pain can be justified, if simply for a baseline with which to compare subsequent levels depending on clinical progress.

Liver function tests are unlikely to become available during the early assessment of the acute abdomen, but are extremely useful in confirming or refuting acute biliary disease.[43,44]

The other area which has attracted great interest in the role of blood tests for aiding diagnosis in the acute abdomen is intestinal ischaemia, whether from strangulated obstruction or mesenteric ischaemia and infarction. Estimation of acid–base status to assess the degree of metabolic acidosis is often a late change and measurement of serum phosphate, lactate, kinase, creatine, lactate dehydrogenase, alkaline phosphatase, diamine oxidase and porcine ileal peptide have all been shown to be unreliable.[38]

Radiological investigations

Plain X-rays

The role of plain radiology in the investigation of the acute abdomen has come under critical review over the last two decades. There is general consensus that the erect chest radiograph is the most appropriate investigation for the detection of free intraperitoneal gas,[45] and the lateral decubitus film can be used if either the erect chest film cannot be taken (due to the patient's condition) or is equivocal. The same view is not true of the plain abdominal radiograph. Some surgeons have claimed that the supine abdominal radiograph provides valuable information in patients with an acute abdomen which contributes to management.[46] However, more recent reports do not sustain this view with one study, which was performed by radiologists and surgeons,[47] demonstrating that across the spectrum of the 'acute abdomen' the plain abdominal radiograph altered the clinical diagnosis in only 7% of patients and actually only influenced management in 4%. This of course does not suggest that its use should be abandoned, but merely limited to circumstances when diagnostic or management uncertainty exist, such as intestinal obstruction, suspected perforation, renal colic and trauma.[48–50]

Similar controversy exists in the use of erect abdominal radiographs for the assessment of patients with suspected intestinal obstruction. The majority of radiologists consider that the supine abdominal film is sufficient,[51,52] but most surgeons still prefer both views on the basis that in a few patients the erect film can be helpful. As most radiographs taken in patients with suspected obstruction are assessed by junior surgeons, it is not unreasonable to request both the supine and erect view, unless an experienced radiologist is available to perform immediate reporting.

Contrast radiology

Although contrast radiology has been available for many years, its role in the acute abdomen has, until relatively recently, been poorly understood and as a result its use has been erratic and ill-defined, with the exception of intravenous urography for the assessment of patients with ureteric colic. It has been recognised for many years that gastrointestinal contrast studies can be used to differentiate between intestinal obstruction and postoperative ileus,[53,54] but their ability to evaluate other acute gastrointestinal conditions has only recently become more accepted.[55]

Perforated peptic ulcer

Although the erect chest radiograph is recognized as the most appropriate first line investigation for a suspected perforated peptic ulcer,[45] in approximately 50% of patients no free gas can be identified on X-ray.[56] This leaves the emergency surgeon with three options: first, to review the diagnosis – such as re-considering acute pancreatitis; secondly, to proceed to laparotomy based on the clinical findings alone; or thirdly, particularly if there are reasonable grounds for uncertainty, to arrange a water-soluble contrast study.[57] This test will confirm or refute the presence of perforation, but will not differentiate between the patient without a perforation and one in whom the perforation has sealed.[56] The addition of ultrasonography in this scenario may help by revealing free abdominal fluid in the patient whose perforation has sealed spontaneously. As has been well-understood for quite some time now, many patients with perforated peptic ulcers can be managed non-operatively,[58,59] in which knowledge the assessing surgeon has plenty of time to resuscitate the patient and make efforts to confirm or refute the diagnosis before rushing to emergency surgery. Patients who might be considered for non-operative treatment of their perforation should have a contrast meal to confirm spontaneous sealing of the perforation. This topic is discussed in more detail in Chapter 6.

Small bowel obstruction

Surgery for small bowel obstruction is performed for one of two reasons: first, there has been failure of non-operative management, or secondly, there is a clinical suspicion of impending strangulation. Although plain abdominal radiographs are useful in establishing the diagnosis of small bowel obstruction, they cannot differentiate between strangulated and non-strangulated gut. The criteria on which strangulated intestine must be suspected are well established – peritonism, fever, tachycardia and leukocytosis[60] – but even when the diagnosis is suspected the changes at operation are often irreversible and resection required. Some workers have looked at other methods, such as computers[61] and serum markers such as phosphate and lactate concentrations,[38] to help identify patients with possible strangulation in order to allow earlier surgery but unfortunately none are reliable. More recently ultrasonography has been tried with quite promising early results,[62] but the problem of detecting early ischaemic changes in small bowel obstruction remains largely unsolved. Many centres have assessed the influence of water-soluble contrast studies in patients with small bowel obstruction with the hypothesis that if those patients whose obstruction will not settle with non-operative treatment can be identified early, then these patients can undergo surgery without waiting for a 'trial' of non-operative treatment, thus reducing the number who may develop strangulation. Although small bowel contrast studies do appear to improve the diagnostic accuracy of small bowel obstruction[63] and can provide useful clinical information in more than three-quarters of patients,[64] their influence on clinical decision-making remains to be established. Suffice to say that in selected patients contrast studies can be of value in helping the surgeon reach a decision as to whether to proceed on a course of non-operative management or abandon it in favour of laparotomy,[65] particularly when the underlying cause is likely to be adhesions.[66]

More detailed information on the surgical management of small bowel obstruction is covered in Chapter 6.

Large bowel obstruction

The management of large bowel obstruction has changed greatly over the last 10–15 years both in the investigative algorithm and more recently the surgical procedures and these are discussed at length in

Chapter 5. The major change in philosophy in the investigation of patients with large bowel obstruction followed the recognition of the entity of a 'functional' obstruction which usually did not require surgery as opposed to a mechanical cause which invariably did require operative correction. As long ago as 1896 this functional obstruction was recognised and termed 'spastic ileus',[67] later refined to pseudo-obstruction,[68] which is the term recognised today. Patients with acute colonic pseudo-obstruction present with similar history and clinical signs to the patient with a mechanical obstruction, though factors which are recognised to precipitate pseudo-obstruction such as dehydration, electrolyte abnormalities, pelvic and spinal surgery, acid–base imbalance and so on, may alert the clinician as to the possible cause, but cannot confirm it without further investigation. As the treatment for one is non-operative and the other is usually operative an accurate assessment is essential. There are now enough data to support the *routine* use of water-soluble contrast enemas in all patients who present with a clinical and radiological diagnosis of large bowel obstruction. In one study[69] 35 of 99 patients thought to have a mechanical large bowel obstruction had other diagnoses following a contrast enema, of whom 11 had pseudo-obstruction. Of the 18 patients thought to have pseudo-obstruction, two were discovered to have a mechanical cause. Other studies have since confirmed these results.[70] Although colonoscopy can also differentiate the two conditions and can be therapeutic in the case of pseudo-obstruction,[71] it is less-easily arranged in the emergency setting and experienced personnel are required.

The surgical management of both large bowel obstruction and the next topic, acute diverticulitis, is covered in Chapter 5.

Acute diverticulitis

The majority of patients who present with symptoms and signs of acute diverticulitis can be managed non-operatively with the exception of those patients who have overt peritonitis from perforation. Although ultrasonography in experienced hands might identify a thickened segment of colon, perhaps with an associated paracolic collection of fluid, invariably there is too much gas for adequate assessment and quite significant collections can go unnoticed. For this reason clinicians have attempted to evaluate other modalities such as water-soluble contrast radiology and CT scanning.[72] The former has the ability to identify a 'leak', the latter a collection. Both of these pieces of information may be of use to the surgeon in reaching a decision to operate, even though the ultimate decision must be based on clinical, rather than radiological criteria. Overall, CT scanning is no more specific than a contrast enema, but does allow guided percutaneous drainage if a collection is identified.[73]

Ultrasonography

Grey-scale ultrasound scanning has been used for many years, primarily to assess the gall bladder, kidneys and pregnant uterus. However, with the development of real-time scanning over the last two decades, the role of ultrasonography in all aspects of abdominal investigation, but particularly the acute abdomen, has become increasingly popular. Accurate detection of small amounts of intraperitoneal fluid associated with conditions such as perforated peptic ulcer, acute cholecystitis, acute appendicitis, strangulated bowel and ruptured ovarian cysts can be very helpful in alerting the clinician to the possible severity of the patients' symptoms. Furthermore, reports on the accuracy of ultrasonography in the detection of specific conditions such as acute cholecystitis and appendicitis are impressive. The presence of free fluid, gallstones, a thickened gall bladder wall, and a positive ultrasonographic Murphy's sign are all good indicators of acute cholecystitis,[74] and have allowed ultrasound to replace radioisotope scanning (HIDA scanning) as the first-line investigation for acute biliary disease with a sensitivity greater than 95% for the detection of acute cholecystitis.[75] As approximately 25% of patients admitted to hospital with suspected acute cholecystitis are subsequently shown to have another, non-biliary, diagnosis[76] an accurate early diagnosis is essential if current trends in early cholecystectomy for acute cholecystitis are to continue.[77] Suspicion of acute biliary disease usually follows clinical assessment but abnormal liver function tests are additional useful markers of underlying biliary disease.[43] Discriminate analysis of patients admitted with suspected acute biliary disease has shown that abnormal liver function tests and a fever are the only reliable features[44] and so in the majority, if not all patients, ultrasonography should be performed.

The role of ultrasonography in the detection of acute appendicitis is less well defined than for acute biliary disease. One of the seminal studies on ultrasonography and acute appendicitis came from a group of radiologists and surgeons from the Netherlands who demonstrated that an acutely inflamed non-perforated appendix can be identified by ultrasonography with a sensitivity of 81% and specificity of 100%.[78] Because the technique relies on visualising a non-compressible swollen appendix, the sensitivity for perforated appendicitis was much lower (29%). Since then other studies have confirmed the high sensitivity and specificity of ultrasound in the diagnosis of acute appendicitis[79] and there is little doubt that its use has risen over the last few years. Clearly it would be inappropriate to scan everyone with suspected appendicitis, but where the diagnosis is uncertain, particularly in women, the case for ultrasound scanning is strong as many alternative diagnoses can be detected.[80]

As surgeons have begun to achieve a better understanding of ultrasonography, it was only a matter of time before they started performing the ultrasound examinations in the acute setting.[81] Early reports have been mixed, with some centres demonstrating little value for immediate scanning in all patients,[82] whereas others have found it valuable.[83] However, there does appear to be agreement that surgical trainees can reach similar levels of accuracy to radiological trainees, and the main question remaining to be answered is whether immediate bedside ultrasonography in all patients admitted with acute abdominal pain, whether performed by trainees in surgery or radiology, is better than a more selective policy performed by an experienced radiologist after a period of observation. Until such time as this question is answered, the current practice of selective ultrasonography performed by senior personnel based on clinical grounds is likely to continue. Other areas where ultrasound is specifically used to assess the acute abdomen are abdominal aortic aneurysms, renal tract disease and acute gynaecological emergencies. A recent report has suggested that ultrasound may also have a role to play in the diagnosis of strangulated small bowel obstruction, by detecting dilated non-peristaltic loops of bowel in association with free intraperitoneal fluid.[62] The early results from this study have been encouraging and further confirmation is now awaited.

CT scanning

The place of CT scanning in the early assessment of the acute abdomen is difficult to evaluate. Its role in the investigation of severity of acute diverticulitis has already been discussed, and it can also be used to identify miscellaneous intra-abdominal collections resulting from other conditions. However, with the exception of acute pancreatitis, where contrast-enhanced CT has an important role in demonstrating the presence of pancreatic necrosis (see Chapter 7), CT scanning has little role to play in the early management of the acute non-traumatic abdomen.

Peritoneal investigations

Ultimately the surgeon assessing the acute abdomen wishes to determine exactly what is going on within the peritoneal cavity. Needle paracentesis has been successfully used for many years to detect conditions such as intestinal perforation, infarction and peritonitis, by demonstrating foul-smelling fluid in aspirated fluid.[84] More recently surgeons have attempted to quantify these results in a more meaningful fashion using both peritoneal lavage[85] and fine catheter aspiration cytology.[86]

Peritoneal lavage

In this technique a standard peritoneal lavage is carried out using the 'open' technique and the effluent evaluated for white cell concentration, amylase, bacteria and bile. A review of the literature[85] demonstrated impressive results, with a mean accuracy of 93%, 1.6% false positive rate and 1% false negative rate.

Fine catheter peritoneal cytology

This was first introduced by the late Richard Stewart from Wellington, New Zealand,[86] and is more simple than lavage and appears equally accurate. It involves the insertion of a venous cannula into the peritoneal cavity under local anaesthesia through which a fine umbilical catheter is inserted. Peritoneal fluid is aspirated back, placed on a slide, stained and examined under a light microscope for percentage of polymorphonuclear cells. A percentage greater than 50% suggests a significant underlying inflammatory process, but obviously cannot identify the exact cause. This procedure can be carried out at the bedside or even in the Accident and Emergency department and has been shown to significantly improve surgical decision-making, whether it is used in all patents with acute abdominal pain,[87] or just those with suspected acute appendicitis,[88] when the sensitivity and specificity have been reported as 91% and 94% respectively.[89]

Laparoscopy

The first reported use of laparoscopy to evaluate acute abdominal pain was in 1978 when Sugarbaker and colleagues performed laparoscopy before laparotomy in a group of patients in whom the decision to operate was uncertain.[90] They showed that following laparoscopy 18 patients were spared an unnecessary laparotomy, whereas six of 27 patients going straight to laparotomy did not require surgery. Following on from this other surgeons became interested in laparoscopy, a technique which had previously been left to the gynaecologists for the best part of half a century since its early use by gastroenterologists to investigate liver disorders, intra-abdominal masses and malignancies between its introduction in 1902 and the following three decades.

Many studies have now demonstrated that laparoscopy significantly improves surgical decision-making in patients with acute abdominal pain,[91] particularly when the need for operation is uncertain.[37] If one specifically looks at suspected appendicitis, then the argument for laparoscopy increases. In a study from St Mary's Hospital London,[92] of 90 patients with suspected appendicitis, 50 were thought definitely to require appendicectomy and in 40 the decision was uncertain, but the surgeon had elected to 'look and see' rather than 'wait and see'. The error rate in the 50 patients going straight to appendicectomy was 22%, but only 8% in the uncertain group who all underwent laparoscopy first, those with a normal appendix undergoing no further surgery. In a hypothetical situation without laparoscopy, the overall unnecessary appendicectomy rate in the whole series would have been 25/90 with the error rate in women of 19/49 (39%) being more than twice that in men (6/41, 15%). Thus there is a very strong argument in support of the view that all women with suspected appendicitis should undergo laparoscopy before appendicectomy. As mentioned earlier more than 13% of all women admitted to a surgical ward with acute abdominal pain have a gynaecological cause,[14] which may only come to light at laparoscopy.

With the recognised complication rate associated with the removal of a normal appendix lying somewhere between 17% and 21%, depending on whether other conditions have been found,[93] continuing to accept an unnecessary appendicectomy rate of around 20% or higher[94] is no longer defensible. There is of course the question as to what to do if at laparoscopy a normal appendix is seen but no other condition can be identified which could account for the patient's symptoms. Some surgeons might argue that in this case the appendix should be removed, either by formal open appendicectomy or by using the laparoscopic approach, because a normal looking appendix can be found to have histological evidence of mucosal inflammation.[95] However, there have been other studies which have shown that even histologically normal appendices can subsequently be shown to contain inflammatory changes if more advanced analyses are used.[96] A pragmatic approach would be to remove the appendix when it looks inflamed at laparoscopy, but do nothing further if it looks normal. The decision may differ in each patient and the final course of action has to be left to the operating surgeon. The author has always taken this pragmatic view and has never knowingly had reason for regret. This area remains controversial and is discussed further in Chapter 6.

Summary   The art of good management of patients with acute abdominal pain lies in an accurate history, careful examination and logical decision-making, taking into account results from appropriate investigations. Regular re-assessment of patients is an essential part of this process and emergency surgeons who do not make use of the investigative options discussed in this chapter are in danger of falling short of the standards of care which patients with acute abdominal pain have a right to expect.

References

1. Senate of the Royal Surgical Colleges of Great Britain and Ireland. Consultant Practice and Surgical Training in the UK. London, October 1994.
2. Hobbs R. Rising emergency admissions. Br Med J 1995; 310: 207–8.
3. Ellis BW, Rivett RC, Dudley HAF. Extending the use of clinical audit data: a resource planning model. Br Med J 1990; 301: 159–62.
4. Darby CR, Berry AR, Mortensen N. Management variability in surgery for colorectal emergencies. Br J Surg 1992; 79: 206–10.
5. Consultant Surgeons of the Lothian and Borders Health Boards. Lothian and Borders large bowel cancer project: immediate outcome after surgery. Br J Surg 1995; 82: 888–90.
6. Campling EA, Devlin HB, Hoile RW, Lunne JN. Report of the National Confidential Enquiry into Peri-operative Deaths 1990. National enquiry into peri-operative deaths, London, 1992.
7. Irvin TT. Abdominal pain: a surgical audit of 1190 emergency admissions. Br J Surg 1989; 76: 1121–5.

8. Gray DWR, Collin J. Non-specific abdominal pain as a cause of acute admission to hospital. Br J Surg 1987; 74: 239–42.

9. Paterson-Brown S. The acute abdomen: the role of laparoscopy. In: Williamson RCN, Thompson JN (eds) Baillières clinical gastro-enterology: gastrointestinal emergencies, Part I, London: Baillière Tindall, 1991; pp. 691–703.

10. Gallegos NC, Hobsley M. Abdominal wall pain: an alternative diagnosis. Br J Surg 1990; 77: 1167–70.

11. Hall PN, Lee APB. Rectus nerve entrapment causing abdominal pain. Br J Surg 1988; 75: 917.

12. Gray DWR, Seabrook G, Dixon JM, Collin J. Is abdominal wall tenderness a useful sign in the diagnosis of non-specific abdominal pain? Ann R Coll Surg Engl 1988; 70: 233–4.

13. De Dombal FT, Matharu SS, Staniland JR et al. Presentation of cancer to hospital as 'acute abdominal pain'. Br J Surg 1980; 67: 413–16.

14. Paterson-Brown S, Eckersley JRT, Dudley HAF. The gynaecological profile of acute general surgery. J R Coll Surg Edinb 1988; 33: 13–15.

15. Pearce JM. Pelvic inflammatory disease. Br Med J 1990; 300: 1090–1.

16. Wood JJ, Bolton JP, Cannon SR, Allan A, O'Connor BH, Darougar S. Biliary-type pain as a manifestation of genital tract infection: the Curtis–Fitz–Hugh syndrome. Br J Surg 1982; 69: 251–3.

17. Shanahan D, Lord PH, Grogono J, Wastell C. Clinical acute cholecystitis and the Curtis–Fitz–Hugh syndrome. Ann R Coll Surg Engl 1988; 70: 45–7.

18. Gatt D, Heafield T, Jantet G. Curtis–Fitz–Hugh syndrome: the new mimicking disease? Ann R Coll Surg Engl 1986; 68: 271–4.

19. de Dombal FT, Leaper DJ, Staniland JR, McCann AP, Horrocks JC. Computer-aided diagnosis of acute abdominal pain. Br Med J 1972; 2: 9–13.

20. Gunn AA. The diagnosis of acute abdominal pain with computer analysis. J R Coll Surg Edinb 1976; 21: 170–2.

21. Adams ID, Chan M, Clifford PC, Cooke WM et al. Computer aided diagnosis of acute abdominal pain: a multicentre study. Br Med J 1986; 293: 800–4.

22. Clifford PC, Chan M, Hewett DJ. The acute abdomen: management with microcomputer aid. Ann R Coll Surg Engl 1986; 68: 182–4.

23. Scarlett P, Cooke WM, Clarke D, Bates C, Chan M. Computer aided diagnosis of acute abdominal pain at Middlesbrough General Hospital. Ann R Coll Surg Engl 1986; 68: 179–81.

24. Sutton GC. Computer-aided diagnosis: a review. Br J Surg 1989; 76: 82–5.

25. Batstone GF. Educational aspects of medical audit. Br Med J 1990; 301: 326–8.

26. Gruer R, Gunn AA, Gordon DS, Ruckley CV. Hospital practice: audit of surgical audit. Lancet 1986; ii: 23–5.

27. Marteau TM, Wynne G, Kaye W, Evans TR. Resuscitation: experience without feedback increases confidence but not skill. Br Med J 1990; 300: 849–50.

28. Lawrence PC, Clifford PC, Taylor IF. Acute abdominal pain: computer aided diagnosis by non-medically qualified staff. Ann R Coll Surg Engl 1987; 69: 233–4.

29. Paterson-Brown S, Vipond MN, Simms K, Gatzen C, Thompson JN, Dudley HAF. Clinical decision-making and laparoscopy versus computer prediction in the management of the acute abdomen. Br J Surg 1989; 76: 1011–13.

30. de Dombal FT. Picking the best tests in acute abdominal pain. J R Coll Phys Lond 1979; 13(4): 203–8.

31. Bennett DH, Tambeur LJMT, Campbell WB. Use of coughing test to diagnose peritonitis. Br Med J 1994; 308: 1336–7.

32. Dixon JM, Elton RA, Rainey JB, McLeod DAD. Rectal examination in patients with pain in the right lower quadrant of the abdomen. Br Med J 1991; 302: 386–8.

33. Howie CR, Gunn AA. Temperature: a poor diagnostic indicator in abdominal pain. J R Coll Surg Edinb 1984; 29(4): 249–51.

34. Attard AR, Corlett MJ, Kidner NJ, Leslie AP, Fraser IA. Safety of early pain relief for acute abdominal pain. Br Med J 1992; 305: 554–6.

35. Keszler H. A cruel practice experienced. Br Med J 1994; 308: 1577.

36. Clavien PA, Burgan S, Moossa AR. Serum enzymes and other laboratory tests in acute pancreatitis. Br J Surg 1989; 76: 1234–43.

37. Paterson-Brown S, Eckersley JRT, Sim AJW, Dudley HAF. Laparoscopy as an adjunct to

decision-making in the acute abdomen. Br J Surg 1986; 73: 1022–4.

38. Bradbury AW, Brittenden J, McBride K, Ruckley CV. Mesenteric ischaemia: a multi-disciplinary approach. Br J Surg 1995; 82: 1446–59.

39. Thomson HJ, Jones PF. Active observation in acute abdominal pain. Am J Surg 1986; 152: 522–5.

40. Thompson MM, Underwood MJ, Dookeran KA, Lloyd DM, Bell PRF. Role of sequential leucocyte counts and C-reactive protein measurements in acute appendicitis. Br J Surg 1992; 79: 822–4.

41. Davies AH, Bernau F, Salisbury A, Souter RG. C-reactive protein in right iliac fossa pain. J R Coll Surg Edinb 1991; 36: 242–4.

42. Middleton SB, Whitbread T, Morgans BT, Mason PF. Combination of skin temperature and a single white cell count does not improve diagnostic accuracy in acute appendicitis. Br J Surg 1996; 83: 499.

43. Dunlop MG, King PM, Gunn AA. Acute abdominal pain: the value of liver function tests in suspected cholelithiasis. J R Coll Surg Edinb 1989; 34: 124–7.

44. Stower MJ, Hardcastle JD. Is it acute chole-cystitis? Ann R Coll Surg Engl 1986; 68: 234.

45. Miller RE, Nelson SW. The roentgenologic demonstration of tiny amounts of free intra-peritoneal gas: experimental and clinical studies. Am J Roentgenol 1971; 112(3): 574–85.

46. Lee PWR. The plain X-ray in the acute abdomen: a surgeon's evaluation. Br J Surg 1976; 63: 763–6.

47. Stower MJ, Amar SS, Mikulin T, Kean DM, Hardcastle JD. Evaluation of the plain abdominal X-ray in the acute abdomen. J R Soc Med 1985; 78: 630–3.

48. de Lacey GJ, Wignall BK, Bradbrooke S, Reidy J, Hussain S, Cramer B. Rationalising abdominal radiography in the Accident and Emergency Department. Clin Radiol 1980; 31: 453–5.

49. Eissenberg RL, Heineken P, Hedgcock MW, Federle M, Goldberg HI. Evaluation of plain abdominal radiographs in the diagnosis of abdominal pain. Ann Intern Med 1982; 97: 257–61.

50. Campbell JPM, Gunn AA. Plain abdominal radiographs and acute abdominal pain. Br J Surg 1988; 75: 554–6.

51. Field S, Guy PJ, Upsdell SM, Scourfield AE. The erect abdominal radiograph in the acute abdomen: should its routine use be abandoned? Br Med J 1985; 290: 1934–6.

52. Simpson A, Sandeman D, Nixon SJ, Goulbourne IA, Grieve DC, Macintyre IMC. The value of an erect abdominal radiography in the diagnosis of intestinal obstruction. Clin Radiol 1985; 36: 41–2.

53. Matheson NA, Dudley HAF. Contrast radiography: an aid to postoperative management. Lancet 1963; i: 914–17.

54. Zer M, Kaznelson D, Feigenberg Z, Dintsman M. The value of gastrografin in the differential diagnosis of paralytic ileus versus mechanical intestinal obstruction: a critical review and report of two cases. Dis Colon Rectum 1977; 20(7): 573–9.

55. Ott DJ, Gelfand DW. Gastrointestinal contrast agents: indications, uses and risks. JAMA 1983; 249(17): 2380–4.

56. Wellwood JM, Wilson AN, Hopkinson BR. Gastrografin as an aid to the diagnosis of perforated peptic ulcer. Br J Surg 1971; 58: 245–9.

57. Fraser GM, Fraser ID. Gastrografin in perforated duodenal ulcer and acute pancreatitis. Clin Radiol 1974; 25: 397–402.

58. Donovan AJ, Vinson TL, Maulsby GO, Gewin JR. Selective treatment of duodenal ulcer with perforation. Ann Surg 1979; 189: 627–36.

59. Crofts TJ, Park KGM, Steele RJC, Chung SSC, Li AKC. A randomized trial of non-operative treatment for perforated peptic ulcer. N Engl J Med 1989; 320: 970–3.

60. Stewardson RH, Bombeck CT, Nyhus LM. Critical operative management of small bowel obstruction. Ann Surg 1978; 187: 189–93.

61. Pain JA, Collier D St J, Hanka R. Small bowel obstruction: computer-assisted prediction of strangulation at presentation. Br J Surg 1987; 74: 981–3.

62. Ogata M, Imai S, Hosotani R, Aoyama H, Hayaashi M, Ishikawa T. Abdominal ultra-sonography for the diagnosis of strangulation in small bowel obstruction. Br J Surg 1994; 81: 421–4.

63. Dunn JT, Halls JM, Berne TV. Roentgeno-graphic contrast studies in acute small-bowel obstruction. Arch Surg 1984; 119: 1305–8.

64. Riveron FA, Obeid FN, Horst HM, Sorensen VJ, Bivins BA. The role of contrast radiography in presumed bowel obstruction. Surgery 1989; 106: 496–501.

65. Joyce WP, Delaney PV, Gorey TF, Fitzpatrick JM. The value of water-soluble contrast radiology in the management of acute small bowel obstruction. Ann R Coll Surg Engl 1992; 74: 422–5.

66. Caroline DF, Herlinger H, Laufer I, Kressel HY, Levine MS. Small-bowel enema in the diagnosis of adhesive obstructions. Am J Roentgenol 1984; 142: 1133–9.

67. Murphy JB. Ileus. JAMA 1896; 26: 15–22.

68. Dudley HAF, Paterson-Brown S. Pseudo-obstruction. Br Med J 1986; 292: 1157–8.

69. Stewart J, Finan PJ, Courtney DF, Brennan TG. Does a water soluble contrast enema assist in the management of acute large bowel obstruction: a prospective study of 117 cases. Br J Surg 1984; 71: 799–801.

70. Koruth NM, Koruth A, Matheson NA. The place of contrast enema in the management of large bowel obstruction. J R Coll Surg Edinb 1985; 30(4): 258–60.

71. Munro A, Youngson GG. Colonoscopy in the diagnosis and treatment of colonic pseudo-obstruction. J R Coll Surg Edinb 1983; 28(6): 391–3.

72. Shrier D, Skucas J, Weiss S. Diverticulitis: an evaluation by computer tomography and contrast enema. Am Coll of Gastroenterol 1991; 86: 1466–71.

73. McKee RF, Deignan RW, Krukowski ZH. Radiological investigation in acute diverticulitis. Br J Surg 1993; 80: 560–5.

74. Laing FC, Federie MP, Jeffrey RB, Brown TW. Ultrasonic evaluation of patients with acute right upper quadrant pain. Radiology 1981; 140: 449–55.

75. Samuels BL, Freitas JE, Bree RL, Schwab RE, Heller ST. A comparison of radionuclide hepatobiliary imaging and real-time ultrasound for the detection of acute cholecystitis. Radiology 1983; 47: 207–10.

76. Schofield PF, Hulton NR, Baildam AD. Is it acute cholecystitis? Ann R Coll Surg Engl 1986; 68: 14–16.

77. Addison NV, Finan PJ. Urgent and early cholecystectomy for acute gallbladder disease. Br J Surg 1988; 75: 141–3.

78. Puylaert JBCM, Rutgers PH, Lalisang RI et al. A prospective study of ultrasonography in the diagnosis of appendicitis. N Engl J Med 1987; 317: 666–9.

79. Schwerk WB, Ruschoff BWJ, Rothmund M. Acute and perforated appendicitis: current experience with ultrasound-aided diagnosis. World J Surg 1990; 14: 271–6.

80. McGrath FP, Keeling F. The role of early sonography in the management of the acute abdomen. Clin Radiol 1991; 44: 172–4.

81. Parys BT, Barr H, Chantarasak ND, Eyes BE, Wu AVO. Use of ultrasound scan as a bedside diagnostic aid. Br J Surg 1987; 74: 611–12.

82. Davies AH, Mastorakou I, Cobb R, Rogers C, Lindsell D, Mortensen NJ. Ultrasonography in the acute abdomen. Br J Surg 1991; 78: 1178–80.

83. Williams RJLI, Windsor ACJ, Rosin RD, Mann DV, Crofton M. Ultrasound scanning of the acute abdomen by surgeons in training. Ann R Coll Surg Engl 1994; 76: 228–33.

84. Baker WNW, Mackie DB, Newcombe JF. Diagnostic paracentesis in the acute abdomen. Br Med J 1967; 3: 146–9.

85. Hoffmann J. Peritoneal lavage in the diagnosis of the acute abdomen of non-traumatic origin. Acta Chir Scand 1987; 153: 561–5.

86. Stewart RJ, Gupta RK, Purdie GL, Isbister WH. Fine catheter aspiration cytology of peritoneal cavity improves decision-making about difficult cases of acute abdominal pain. Lancet 1986; ii: 1414–15.

87. Baigrie RJ, Saidan Z, Scott-Coombes D et al. Role of fine catheter peritoneal cytology and laparoscopy in the management of acute abdominal pain. Br J Surg 1991; 78: 167–70.

88. Baigrie RJ, Scott-Coombes D, Saidan Z, Vipond MN, Paterson-Brown S, Thompson JN. The selective use of fine catheter peritoneal cytology and laparoscopy reduces the unnecessary appendicectomy rate. Br J Clin Pract 1992; 46: 173–6.

89. Caldwell MTP, Watson RGK. Peritoneal aspiration cytology as a diagnostic aid in acute appendicitis. Br J Surg 1994; 81: 276–8.

90. Sugarbaker PH, Bloom BS, Sanders JH, Wilson RE. Pre-operative laparoscopy in diagnosis of acute abdominal pain. Lancet 1975; i: 442–5.

91. Paterson-Brown S. Emergency laparoscopic surgery. Br J Surg 1993; 80: 279–83.

92. Paterson-Brown S, Thompson JN, Eckersley JRT, Ponting GA, Dudley HAF. Which patient with suspected appendicitis should undergo laparoscopy? Br Med J 1988; 296: 1363–4.

93. Chang FC, Hogle HH, Welling DR. The fate of the negative appendix. Am J Surg 1973; 126: 752–4.

94. Baigrie RJ, Dehn TCB, Fowler SM, Dunn DC. Analysis of 8651 appendicectomies in England and Wales during 1992. Br J Surg 1995; 82: 933.

95. Lau WY, Fan ST, Yiu TF, Chu KW, Suen HC, Wong KK. The clinical significance of routine histopathological study of the resected appendix and safety of appendiceal inversion. Surg Gynecol Obstet 1986; 162: 256–8.

96. Wang Y, Reen DJ, Puri P. Is a histologically normal appendix following emergency appendicectomy always normal? Lancet 1996; 347: 1076–9.

2 Perioperative management

Nicholas J. Everitt
William E. G. Thomas

Introduction

The aphorism states that surgery is simple; all that is required is that the appropriate operation is performed on the right patient at the ideal time. This wisdom can not be discredited, but it is also true that a successful procedure does not guarantee a successful outcome. Although patients may recover despite our interventions, optimal peri-operative care will do much to ensure a complete convalescence.

The aim of this chapter is to outline an approach to the various problems encountered in the management of critically ill or emergency surgical patients. The discussion is divided into four sections. The first three describe aspects of pre-, intra- and postoperative management, respectively. In the final section, the management of conditions which frequently influence more than one of these phases is discussed. When drug doses are quoted they refer to adult requirements.

Preoperative investigation

The history

Preoperative investigation begins with elucidation of the history. A full history is the ideal but may not be possible to obtain from the critically ill, or in an emergency. Under such circumstances certain key features should be obtained whenever possible. The history of the presenting complaint is paramount; if the patient cannot give adequate account, the observations of witnesses should be sought. The timing of symptoms, and of delay in referral, may indicate the need and extent of preoperative resuscitation. After trauma, a description of the mechanism of the event may indicate the likely pattern of injury. A clue to any chronic medical problems, which might influence management, may be deduced not only from the past medical history but also the patient's usual medication. Any history of allergy should be sought, with detail as to the nature of the reaction wherever possible. Many 'allergies', particularly to antibiotics, will be found to be minor intolerances which in this situation need not preclude potentially life-saving drugs. The social history may not be of immediate relevance, but it can indicate the patient's usual level of performance. The management of a normally fit patient may differ from that of the chronically bed-ridden. It is important to stress that no matter how valuable the history may prove, its elucidation should not interfere with immediate resuscitation of the critically ill patient.

The examination

Physical examination is a logical continuation of the history; the aim is to determine the nature of the presenting complaint and to identify other conditions which may influence subsequent management. It should be thorough, but again may be limited by the circumstances of the patient's presentation. The Advanced Trauma Life Support (ATLS)[1] system of primary survey of the **A**irway, **B**reathing and **C**irculation (ABC), can be advocated in all circumstances as a guide to initial resuscitation. When the surgeon is satisfied that adequate resuscitation is underway, further examination may proceed. After trauma, it cannot be assumed that any part of the body is uninjured, and a thorough examination is essential. However, treatment of life-threatening injuries must take priority and complete examination may have to be postponed. Whatever the circumstances of the initial presentation, a deterioration in the patient's condition demands immediate repetition of the primary survey. The timing of all observations should be recorded.

Laboratory tests

Laboratory tests should be requested for specific indications, and not merely as routine. They may not be required for young fit patients who are to undergo minor surgical procedures. However, the majority of patients who require emergency surgery do not fall into this group. Indications for the more frequently required investigations are given in Table 2.1, but are not intended to replace protocols at the reader's hospital.

The surgeon should consider the need for blood products. A cross-match ensures that the requested number of units of blood are immediately available. Each unit will be ABO and Rhesus typed, and will have been tested against the patient's serum to ensure compatibility. Cross-matching is indicated when significant blood loss is likely, or when the patient is anaemic. A 'Group and Save' determines the patient's ABO and Rhesus type, and screens their blood for red cell antibodies. Blood can then be cross-matched within 15 min. 'Group and Save' is indicated when major blood loss is possible, but unlikely to occur. If clotting factors or platelets are likely to be required, their availability should be discussed with the haematologist beforehand. The use of blood products and their alternatives is described below.

Table 2.1 *Suggested scheme for preoperative laboratory tests*

Full blood count	Any major surgical procedure Pathology likely to be associated with anaemia Symptoms or signs of anaemia, or major blood loss
Urea and electrolytes	Any major surgical procedure History of hypertension, diabetes, hepatic or renal disease Diuretics, cardiac drugs, corticosteroids, chronic NSAID History of obstruction, vomiting, or diarrhoea Proteinuria
Sickle test or haemoglobin electrophoresis	Afro-Caribbean, Mediterranean, or Arabian patient Family history of haemoglobinopathy
Random blood glucose	Known diabetes mellitus, or glycosuria Emergency surgery for abscess
Clotting studies	Personal, or family history of abnormal bleeding tendency Anticoagulant therapy Jaundice or symptoms or signs of liver failure Major haemorrhage, or significant blood transfusion
Arterial blood gases	Dyspnoea at rest, or cyanosis Intended thoracotomy
Chest radiography	Acute respiratory symptoms Possible pulmonary metastases Chronic cardiorespiratory disease when a radiograph from the last 6 months is not available Recent immigrants from areas where TB is endemic Major chest trauma, or intended thoracotomy
Electrocardiogram	Hypertension History or signs of cardiorespiratory disease Patient aged >50 for major surgery Any patient aged >70

Provided that cardiac output and oxygen exchange are normal, oxygen delivery is unlikely to be impaired until the haemoglobin concentration is less than $8 \, g \, dl^{-1}$. In the haemodynamically stable patient, preoperative transfusion is best avoided within 24 h of surgery because the administered blood will not be an effective carrier of oxygen at the time of operation. When the patient is actively bleeding, preoperative transfusion should not delay prompt surgical arrest of haemorrhage.

Certain surgical procedures require intraoperative radiological studies; for example, fluoroscopic screening, cholangiography or angiography. The surgeon should ensure that equipment and technical staff will be available *before* the patient is transferred to the operating theatre.

Assessment of patient fitness

Patient fitness will have an impact on postoperative morbidity and mortality, and specific illness can influence postoperative outcome. Surgery performed within six months of myocardial infarction risks a further infarct (40% within three months and 15% within six), with a mortality of 50%. However, fitness is usually multifactorial, and is determined by the immediate pathology and chronic factors of ill health. A variety of scoring systems have been developed. The TRISS (Trauma Related Injury Severity Score)[2] and APACHE (Acute Physiology and Chronic Health Evaluation)[3] associate the effect of injury or disease to overall prognosis. The ASA (American Society of Anaesthetists) Score[4] relates patient fitness to outcome after anaesthesia, but does not take account of age (Table 2.2). It should be remembered that all scoring systems are validated against patient *populations*; they predict, but do not determine, patient outcome. Therefore, patient fitness is a relative concept. Before an elective procedure is performed, it is usually possible to take time to improve the patient's physical condition. In an emergency, treatment of the primary pathology may take precedence. When urgent surgery is

Table 2.2 *American Society of Anaesthetists (ASA) grading[4]*

Class	Definition	Mortality (%)
I	Normally healthy individual	0.1
II	Mild systemic disease	0.2
III	Severe, but not incapacitating, systemic disease	1.8
IV	Incapacitating systemic disease constantly threatening life	7.8
V	Moribund patient not expected to survive 24 hours irrespective of intervention	9.4
E	Suffix for emergency surgery	

anticipated, early assessment by an anaesthetist will often help to optimise preoperative resuscitation.

Outcome from surgery is adversely influenced by poor nutritional status. In the absence of sophisticated tests of body composition, clinical assessment of nutritional status remains a sensitive indicator of potential risk. Plasma albumin concentration is frequently, and erroneously, regarded as a marker of nutritional status.[5] Plasma protein concentration is influenced not only by the total body pool of the protein, but more importantly by the plasma volume. Unless kwashiorkor is present, a low plasma concentration is most likely to represent redistribution of albumin and water across abnormally permeable cell membranes. Thus, although hypo-albuminaemia is a marker of increased surgical risk, it usually represents sepsis rather than nutritional status. Sepsis is a broad term which implies cytokine activation; it may be caused by Gram-negative infection, but also by extensive tissue necrosis, acute pancreatitis or multiple fractures. The majority of patients with multiple organ failure (MOF) will behave as though septic, although in many cases clear evidence of infection is difficult to demonstrate.[6] It does not follow that hypo-albuminaemia and malnutrition may not co-exist; but normal plasma albumin levels are unlikely to return while any sepsis remains. Nutritional support is no substitute for appropriate surgical intervention.

Management of shock

Shock exists when the circulation is unable to maintain tissue perfusion and oxygenation. Shock represents a mismatch between cardiac output and the capacity of the circulation. Whenever shock occurs, administration of supplemental oxygen is required.

Hypovolaemic shock is a consequence of fluid loss; in the surgical patient this is most commonly due to haemorrhage or extensive burns. Other causes include profuse diarrhoea and vomiting, particularly in the infant. The management comprises fluid replacement with prompt arrest of haemorrhage. In *septic shock* cytokine activation is associated with systemic vasodilatation and suppression of the myocardium. It is characterised by a hyperdynamic circulation and fever, although in the later stages it may be indistinguishable from hypovolaemic shock. The underlying cause of sepsis must be treated in addition to maintenance of the circulation. *Neurogenic shock* is a result of the loss of sympathetic tone which may be associated with spinal injury. The diastolic blood pressure is low, and there may be relative or absolute bradycardia because of damage to the cervical sympathetic nerves. Fluid replacement is required, possibly with use of pressor agents. It must be remembered that, in victims of trauma, shock may also be due to acute haemorrhage. *Anaphylactic/anaphylactoid* shock represents an overwhelming immune response to a foreign substance, and is uncommon in surgical practice. However great caution should be exercised when prescribing for patients with a previous history of anaphylaxis or atopy. Massive release of histamines and kinins is associated with increase in the volume and permeability of the circulation, and with myocardial suppression. Airway spasm and oedema are common. Adrenaline 1 mg, hydrocortisone 100 mg and chlorpheniramine 20 mg should be given promptly and nebulised bronchodilators may be indicated. Fluid replacement is essential, and crystalloids only should be infused; anaphylaxis may even be promoted by plasma expanders.

Cardiogenic shock occurs when there is acute pump failure; it can occur in the surgical patient as a consequence of cardiac trauma, or cardiac surgery. It may be a consequence of impaired venous return, secondary to cardiac tamponade or tension pneumothorax, in which case immediate pericardiocentesis or thoracocentesis are indicated, respectively. Perioperative myocardial infarction and dysrhythmia, as well as fluid overload due to overzealous replacement or renal failure may also cause cardiac failure. Cardiogenic shock is characterised by a failing cardiac output in the presence of a normal, or elevated central venous pressure. Fluid replacement is contraindicated.

Fluid resuscitation

Signs of return of organ perfusion are the hallmark of successful fluid resuscitation. Improved capillary return, slowing of tachycardia, and normalisation of blood and pulse pressure indicate successful management. In severe shock mental function may be impaired, and an improved level of consciousness is again a favourable sign. Bladder catheterisation allows measurement of urine output; a satisfactory diuresis suggests adequate fluid replacement. Measurement of central venous pressure (CVP) may aid resuscitation and act as an indicator of the volume of fluid required for resuscitation. Restitution of circulating volume should be accompanied by an increase in CVP to a normal level. However, central venous catheterisation is not without complications. The risk of injury to structures in the root of the neck, particularly the pleura, is increased when the central veins are underfilled. Pressure measurement must be interpreted with caution; the trend is more informative than the absolute value. Central venous pressure is influenced by the location of the catheter tip and by changes in the patient's position. When CVP is measured, it is assumed that it reflects left ventricular end-diastolic pressure (LVEDP), and hence left ventricular filling. The hypothesis may be invalid if there is variation in central venous tone, right heart function, or the tone of the pulmonary circulation. Vasopressor drugs may also alter CVP, but such agents should not be used as a substitute for adequate fluid replacement. When intercurrent disease, such as sepsis, renders CVP measurement unreliable, assessment of pulmonary capillary wedge pressure (PCWP) by means of Swan Ganz catheterisation enables LVEDP to be estimated without the influence of systemic venous and right heart factors. However, in the presence of abnormal left ventricular compliance, or mitral stenosis, PCWP is an unreliable guide to LVEDP. The Swan Ganz catheter also contains a thermistor and can be used to measure core temperature. Cardiac output can be calculated by a thermal dilution method after injection of a bolus of fluid of known temperature (4°C). Systemic vascular resistance (SVR) is calculated by dividing the difference between mean arterial and central venous pressure by the cardiac output.

Preoperative fluid and electrolyte replacement

Many patients, admitted as emergencies, will have considerable fluid and electrolyte deficits. Significant amounts may be sequestered within an inflamed peritoneal cavity or obstructed bowel lumen. In the presence of sepsis, expansion of the interstitial space may be associated with a relative intravascular hypovolaemia. Patients who are victims of trauma or who are burned will usually require rapid fluid replacement. A low threshold for fluid replacement is crucial; in the previously healthy adult, up to 1500 ml of fluid may be lost before physical signs are obvious. Significant acute fluid loss (greater than 15% of circulating volume) will be recognised by classical signs of hypovolaemic shock such as delayed capillary return and tachycardia. However, systolic hypotension may not be manifest until greater than 30% of circulating volume is lost. Profuse haemorrhage is usually an indication for immediate surgical intervention, but when bleeding is excluded the majority of surgical patients will benefit from a period of determined fluid resuscitation. The choice of fluid depends on the pathology involved. Gastrointestinal fluid losses are best replaced with crystalloid fluids. When there is relative hypovolaemia secondary to sepsis, colloid replacement with plasma or a synthetic substitute can be considered. If there is concomitant anaemia, blood is preferable. In acute haemorrhage, whole blood is preferable to packed cells, but the former is not always available. Therefore clotting factors and platelets will be required if haemorrhage is massive.

Electrolyte losses due to acute gastrointestinal disease may be considerable. Diarrhoea and loss of colonic mucus may cause hypokalaemia. Rapid replacement of potassium should be undertaken with caution, as cardiac arrhythmias may follow. Electrocardiographic monitoring and frequent serum potassium measurements must be made. It should be recognised that prompt restoration of serum potassium does not necessarily imply that intracellular homeostasis is restored. Hyponatraemia may be due to profuse vomiting and sodium replacement is required. However, low serum sodium may also be a consequence of sepsis. In this instance sodium replacement is not indicated, and correction of hyponatraemia should not delay appropriate surgical intervention.

Pre-operative treatment

Optimisation of pulmonary function

Most critically ill patients will benefit from supplementary oxygen. Pulmonary function may be improved further before surgery by physiotherapy, in an attempt to clear retained secretions. Wheezing patients should be tested for airway reversibility, and nebulised bronchodilators administered as appropriate. Similarly, patients who are already prescribed bronchodilators should receive them before induction of anaesthesia. If the patient has pulmonary oedema, appropriate diuresis and cardiac support should be initiated.

Optimisation of cardiac function

Adequate cardiac filling and myocardial oxygenation are the goals; any dysrhythmia will impair both. Many cardiac rhythm anomalies can be precipitated by disturbances of electrolyte or acid–base balance, or by hypoxia, and may resolve when the metabolic cause is rectified. Atrial fibrillation can be controlled by digitalisation, after hypokalaemia has been excluded. In an emergency, preoperative cardioversion is indicated for paroxysmal atrial fibrillation. Other arrhythmias should be corrected by appropriate drug therapy whenever possible. Detailed management is outside the remit of this chapter and cardiological advice should be sought.

Some patients will need preoperative pacing. A permanent pacemaker may be required by a patient with symptomatic heart block, presenting with a history of either syncope or evidence of cardiac failure. Other patients may be asymptomatic, but will have patterns of block that require insertion of a temporary pacemaker. These include third degree block, Möbitz II second degree block, and first degree block with bifascicular bundle branch block. Caution must be exercised when the patient with a pacemaker undergoes surgery; there may be a risk that diathermy will interfere with the function of the device. The risk is influenced by the pattern of pacing, and the type of diathermy. The matter is discussed under Patient Safety.

Optimisation of renal function

To optimise renal function, hypovolaemia should be corrected before surgery whenever possible. When the patient presents with stigmata of renal impairment, obstructive uropathy must be considered. Decompression of the urinary tract, by catheter or nephrostomy, may result in prompt resolution of biochemical abnormalities. Caution must be exercised because a large diuresis may follow relief of obstruction. Urinary tract drainage is of particular importance when there is concomitant urinary tract infection, or a solitary obstructed kidney. When the patient with established renal failure requires surgery, consideration should be given to the need for preoperative dialysis. It should be remembered that the patient must be anticoagulated to undergo haemodialysis, and this may have significant implications for surgery. The management of oliguria is described later.

Tube thoracostomy

Insertion of a tube thoracostomy, performed by open cut-down, is essential management of pneumothorax, or significant haemothorax. It should be considered for all victims of chest trauma who are to undergo anaesthesia with positive pressure ventilation, in whom an unrecognised tension pneumothorax may prove rapidly fatal. The nature of injury, or presence of multiple rib fractures should alert the clinician. A chronic pleural effusion will impair ventilatory function, but rapid drainage may lead to significant shunting and may be detrimental immediately before anaesthesia.

Nasogastric intubation

The principal indication for preoperative nasogastric intubation is to prevent tracheobronchial aspiration of nasogastric contents. Gastric emptying is likely to be impaired in the presence of gastrointestinal obstruction and after major trauma. When gastric outlet obstruction is suspected, preoperative gastric lavage via a wide bore tube may be required. Gross dilatation of the stomach may also be associated with hypoventilation, secondary to diaphragmatic splinting, and in these patients nasogastric intubation may well improve gas exchange. Measurement of nasogastric aspirate can be an invaluable guide to fluid and electrolyte replacement when gastrointestinal motility is impaired.

After trauma in which a fracture of the cribriform plate of the skull is suspected, blind nasogastric intubation should not be performed, because the tube may enter the vault. In this situation the nasogastric tube can be safely passed orally.

Bowel preparation

When colonic resection is anticipated, the presence of faecal loading may predispose to contamination of the peritoneal cavity and wound and preclude the possibility of a primary anastomosis. However, in the majority of surgical emergencies which involve the colon, preoperative bowel preparation may be impossible, inadvisable, or contraindicated. When there is peritonitis it is inappropriate to delay surgery until the bowel is cleared, indeed cathartics may exacerbate faecal peritonitis if the colon is perforated. Catharsis is also contra-indicated in the presence of colonic obstruction. However, in certain circumstances, for example refractory colitis, it may still be possible to prepare the colon before surgery. Provided that the patient can tolerate oral fluids, sodium picosulphate (Picolax®) or polyethylene glycol (KleenPrep®) are suitable choices. It should be remembered that cathartics cause substantial fluid and electrolyte loss, and a concomitant intravenous infusion may be required to prevent dehydration. If the colon is obstructed, on-table colonic lavage may permit a primary anastomosis without the need for a covering stoma. The additional time which it requires must be balanced against the patient's fitness and the surgeon's expertise.

Siting of a stoma

Formation of an ileostomy or colostomy is usually a simple procedure, yet a poorly sited stoma will prove a constant source of frustration to the patient and will, on occasion, require revision. Whenever possible, potential stoma sites should be marked before the patient is taken to theatre. Ideally, the patient should be examined seated and standing. The anterior superior iliac spine, skin flexures, and skin creases caused by previous scars should be avoided because the seal between bag and skin will be compromised. Consideration must also be paid to the patient's style of dress and the stoma should not be directly under the waistband. Lastly, the stoma should be sited in a position which the patient can see and reach with ease.

Bladder catheterisation

There are a number of situations in which preoperative bladder catheterisation should be considered. Catheterisation enables hourly measurement of urine output, and hence confirmation of fluid replacement. A urethral catheter will decompress the bladder and reduce the risk of vesical injury during lower midline incisions. Bladder decompression also improves access within the pelvis. The presence of a catheter within the urethra may facilitate its identification in perineal surgery. Many patients will be bed-bound for several days after surgery and catheterisation of the urethra allows bladder drainage during a period when retention of urine might otherwise occur, especially in males. Moreover, catheterisation will guard against contamination of open perineal wounds by urine. However, urethral catheterisation is not without risk. The catheter should pass with ease and dilation of the urethra, or the use of a rigid introducer should only be performed by those with urological experience. When the bladder is palpable, the suprapubic route is preferable to forceful or traumatic attempts at urethral catheterisation. In the trauma victim a high index of suspicion for urethral injury should be maintained, especially in those with pelvic fractures. The presence of blood at the urethral meatus or within the scrotum, perineal extravasation of urine, or a high prostate on rectal examination, are contraindications to blind urethral catheterisation.

Prophylaxis

Prevention of deep venous thrombosis

Patients who undergo surgical procedures are at risk of deep venous thrombosis (DVT), and hence pulmonary embolism. A hypercoagulable state is a component of the metabolic response to stress which is promoted by induction of anaesthesia and the subsequent operation. The metabolic response to stress is activated in many who require emergency surgery, even before they reach hospital. Trauma, underlying malignancy and sepsis, and dehydration all render intravenous thrombosis more likely. Prevention of deep venous thrombosis therefore begins on admission with adequate fluid replacement. Graded compression stockings may be used provided that their fit is good, there is no history of peripheral vascular disease, and foot pulses are present. When immobility is anticipated subcutaneous heparin (5000 units sc bd) should be given as soon as the patient has been assessed, and certainly before transfer to the operating theatre. Heparin acts by inactivation of thrombin and factor X_a, via enhancement of the action of antithrombin III. Newer low-molecular-weight heparins, for example enoxaparin (20–40 mg sc od), inactivate factor X_a only. They need only be administered once daily. It was expected that the risk of perioperative bleeding would be less with low-molecular-weight heparin, but current evidence does not support this hypothesis. In a large meta-analysis low-molecular-weight heparin was associated with a lower incidence of DVT,[7] but pulmonary embolism was more common than with conventional heparin. Patient positioning is paramount (see below) and use of pneumatic compression boots should be considered. A suggested protocol for thromboembolic prophylaxis[8] is summarised in Table 2.3.

Antibiotic prophylaxis

Antibiotic prophylaxis refers to the use of antibiotics to prevent the complications of transient bacteraemia. It is implicit in the definition that the antibiotic should be given before the surgical procedure is started; usually a single dose is all that is required. The antibiotic(s) chosen should cover the spectrum of pathogens expected during any bacteraemic episode. They should be given in a dose and presentation, and at a time, to ensure that bactericidal concentrations are achieved in the circulation at the time at which bacterial contamination is anticipated. If the antibiotic is given intravenously at induction of anaesthesia then plasma levels are likely to be optimal when required. Other routes may be used, for example rectal metronidazole before emergency appendicectomy. However, in this latter instance plasma levels are acceptable between two and six hours after administration, and hence surgery must be performed within this period. The antibiotics chosen for prophylaxis should be bactericidal, and should differ from those used for therapeutic courses. By following this policy the incidence of antibiotic resistance can be minimised.

The risk of infection is dependent on the nature of the procedure. During a *clean* procedure mucosal surfaces are not breached, and there is no local infection or soiling. In a *clean-contaminated* procedure mucosal surfaces are exposed, but the procedure is otherwise clean. A *contaminated* procedure is one in which there is established local infection, or soiling of the tissues. It is estimated that 75% of all

Table 2.3 *Prophylaxis against deep venous thrombosis[8]*

High risk		Past history of DVT, PE, or CVA*	Heparin SC and TED stockings
	or	Major pelvic or abdominal surgery	
	or	Surgery for malignancy	
Moderate risk		Patient >40 years	Heparin SC and/or TED stockings
	and	Surgery >30 min	
	or	Oral contraceptive use	
	or	Inflammatory bowel or cardiopulmonary disease	
Low risk		Patient <40 years	Early mobilisation
	and	No additional risk factors	
	or	Patient >40 years	
	and	Surgery <30 min	
	and	No additional risk factors	

Risk factors include obesity, varicose veins, pregnancy, immobility, hypercoagulable states, and recent surgery.
Active haemorrhage, or coagulopathy, may be considered relative contraindications to subcutaneous heparin.

*Consider pneumatic compression (Flotron®) boots whilst under anaesthesia.

procedures are clean,[9] but this proportion is substantially reduced when emergency surgery is considered. Other factors which influence the risk of sepsis are abdominal surgery in any form, a procedure of greater than two hours' duration, and surgical technique. The critically ill are particularly at risk and the incidence of sepsis has been shown to be increased when there are three or more diagnoses on the discharge sheet. Antibiotic prophylaxis is therefore indicated when surgical manipulation is likely to cause specific infective complications. Four categories can be identified: (1), in clean-contaminated or contaminated cases, when wound infection is likely, (2) in the toxic patient, when surgical manipulation might precipitate a septicaemic episode; for example percutaneous drainage of an obstructed biliary tree; (3) when transient bacteraemia may result in endocarditis, particularly of valves damaged by rheumatic fever; and (4) when bacteraemia may cause infection of a prosthesis, for example prosthetic cardiac valves, vascular grafts and orthopaedic prostheses. Most hospitals will have their own guidelines for antibiotic prophylaxis.

It should be borne in mind that antibiotic prophylaxis is no substitute for surgical debridement, drainage and lavage. Prophylaxis should not be expected to prevent intra-abdominal sepsis, nor to influence the likelihood of anastomotic failure. When the operative procedure reveals gross contamination, or when the patient is immunocompromised, it may be appropriate to institute a therapeutic course of postoperative antibiotics.

Prevention of stress ulceration

The critically ill are at risk of gastric and duodenal stress ulceration; the hazard is increased when enteral intake is denied. Intravenous ranitidine 50 mg tds may reduce the risk. It has been suggested that gastric acid suppression promotes colonisation of the stomach by coliform bacteria, and that aspiration of gastric organisms contributes to hospital-acquired pneumonia. Sucralfate 1 g qds protects the gastric mucosa without reducing gastric acidity and can be administered via a nasogastric tube. Early enteral feeding may reduce the incidence of stress ulceration further.

Consent

Whenever possible written informed consent must be obtained from the patient. Consent should be obtained by the operator, who is best suited to explain the proposed procedure and any likely departures from it; for example the need to bring out a stoma or amputate. Patients who refuse blood products should be asked to sign a specific consent form. If the patient is of sound mind, but cannot write, verbal consent can be sought. It is prudent for verbal consent to be witnessed in writing by another member of medical staff. However, patient consent is not always possible, because of acute or chronic incapacity. Under such circumstances the consent of a relative or guardian must suffice. In an emergency, expedience may not allow written consent from a second party to be obtained; telephoned verbal consent may need to be obtained and clearly documented. When the patient is aged less than 16 years, the written consent of a parent or legal guardian is advised. However, the surgeon may legally accept the consent of a minor if he is convinced that the child is sufficiently mature to understand the consequences. If the surgeon believes that the wishes of a parent, or guardian, are against the interests of the child it is advisable to have the patient made a ward of court. The mentally impaired may give their own consent if it is believed that they can comprehend the implications. When this is not the case the surgeon should, if possible, liaise with the managing psychiatric team. In any circumstance, as a last resort, the surgeon may proceed without consent of any form, when immediate intervention is in the patient's best interest.

Preoperative marking

The surgeon must consider marking the side and site of the operation. Side must always be marked before the patient is transferred to theatre. The mark should be placed away from the proposed incision to avoid tattooing of the skin. On occasion, the site or the incision itself must be marked. In such circumstances non-tattooing ink must be used.

Anticipation of postoperative requirements

It will often be evident, before surgery, that postoperative management will require either high dependency, or intensive care. Some liver and cardiac procedures will require cardiopulmonary bypass. Availability of resources should be ascertained in advance. If such facilities are unavailable, preoperative transfer to another hospital should be considered, provided that the patient's condition can be stabilised to allow this.

Intraoperative management

Patient safety

Whatever the procedure, the safety of the patient within the operating theatre must be maintained. The surgeon should confirm that the patient who arrives in the anaesthetic room is indeed the one expected. The consent form, and side and site of the operation, should be checked. Transfer of the patient between trolley and table should be undertaken with care to prevent injury to both patient and attendants. Correct lifting techniques must be used, and it is usual for the anaesthetist to coordinate all manoeuvres so that the airway and neck are protected at all times. The positioning of the patient on the operating table is the responsibility of the surgeon. He should ensure that the patient's position is adequate for the intended procedure, but also that it does not risk injury. Joints should be moved slowly, particularly when the normal range is restricted by arthrosis. Sudden and excessive movements risk articular and nerve plexus injury. Bolsters and strapping are used to prevent unwanted change in position, but adhesive tape should be used with caution in patients with a known allergy, or delicate skin. Pressure areas should be protected with padding and trauma to the calves, which might otherwise precipitate deep venous thrombosis, should be avoided. If diathermy is to be used, contact between the patient and any metal surface must be prevented. All metallic jewellery should be removed or, if this is impossible, completely covered by insulating tape. The choice of skin disinfectant is the prerogative of the surgeon. If an alcoholic solution is used, the skin should be thoroughly dried to avoid ignition of the solution by an electrical current. Specific care is required in the region of skin flexures where the solution may pool. Diathermy current may interfere with cardiac pacemaker performance; bipolar diathermy is less hazardous than unipolar but may not be appropriate for the procedure to be performed. When unipolar diathermy is used, the plate should be placed as far from the pacemaker generator as possible.

Short bursts of current only should be used, during which the anaesthetist should monitor the elecrocardiogram (ECG) for arrhythmia. If diathermy is used close to the generator there is a risk of current conduction down the electrode wires and thus of myocardial burning.

The immobile patient is at risk of hypothermia. Cooling is prevented by maintenance of the theatre temperature at an appropriate level (adults 24–28°C, infants 32–34°C). In addition a warming blanket and insulating covers may be of value. Fluids, for infusion and irrigation, should be warmed to body temperature before use.

Operative procedure

The details of the operative procedure will vary according to the underlying pathology; nonetheless general surgical principles apply. Tissue perfusion must be maintained, and necrotic tissue must be excised and sepsis drained. Although generous debridement may be required, tissues must always be handled gently and with respect. In the critically ill, delayed wound closure may be preferable to primary suture. As an alternative, wounds may be left to close by secondary intention. If they are large, delayed skin grafting can be considered. Similarly, when the gastrointestinal tract is damaged, or resected, diversion via an appropriate stoma may be preferable to primary anastomosis. A 'second look' procedure may be beneficial when wounds or body cavities are grossly contaminated, when tissue viability is dubious, and if sepsis or MOF develop.

Drains

Use of surgical drains is very much dictated by the procedure performed, however some general principles apply. Drains may reduce formation of serous collections, but should not be expected to prevent haematomas. Coagulating blood will block all but the largest of tubes, and drainage is no substitute for meticulous haemostasis. There is no evidence that abdominal drains reduce the incidence of anastomotic failure, nor is it likely that a drain will prevent peritonitis when an anastomosis leaks. Peritoneal soiling will be influenced by the degree to which adjacent tissues 'wall off' the defect, and clinical signs will indicate the need to intervene. There is some evidence that a neighbouring drain may actually initiate anastomotic leakage by erosion. Anastomotic healing is dependent on adequate blood supply, and is principally influenced by surgical technique. If there is concern that an anastomosis may leak it should either be defunctioned, or avoided by an alternative procedure. Drains may be used to manage sepsis, but will not be able to cope with solid necrotic tissue. Adequate debridement and lavage are essential, and may need to be repeated when there is pancreatic necrosis or gross faecal soiling. Under such circumstances some surgeons would advocate a laparostomy or abdominal zip.

Drains come in many forms. Tube drains are ideal when low viscosity fluids must be evacuated. When a tube is used, suction can be applied, and closed drainage systems may reduce the incidence of retrograde infection. Use of a suction drain (Redivac®) can reduce dead space, but is not without complications. The drain may be compromised if neighbouring tissues are drawn into the tube, and these tissues may become necrotic. Sump drains allow continuous suction to be applied with minimal risk of blockage by surrounding structures. Sometimes all that is required is that a path for drainage remains patent. The simplest example is the seton used to drain a high fistula in ano. A corrugated drain may be used when a large cavity is encountered; but if trauma from contact with the drain is feared, soft latex tubing (Penrose drain) may be used.

The adage tells us that it is time to remove a drain when it has stopped draining but, although this remains true most of the time, exceptions exist. Some serous collections, particularly after lymphadenectomy, will persist indefinitely whilst drained. Once the drainage volume has significantly reduced, the drain can be removed and any seroma drained by needle aspiration. Progressive shortening of a tube or corrugated drain may allow a large cavity to obliterate before the drain wound closes. Under other circumstances it may be necessary to allow a track of granulation tissue to form before a drain can be removed. If so the drain must remain for a specific period of time, irrespective of the volume of effluent. In general, a drain should cause as little tissue reaction as possible, but when a track is required the material from which it is made should provoke adhesion of the structures around it. A biliary T-tube track allows controlled drainage of bile from the site at which the tube enters the bile duct, and may be a conduit by which the duct lumen can be explored.

Use of blood products

Assessment of blood loss

Peroperative blood loss may be assessed by various means, but all are likely to underestimate the deficit. Swabs may be collected and weighed, or washed and the effluent subjected to colorimetric assessment of haemoglobin content. During lengthy procedures intraoperative measurement of circulating haemoglobin concentration may be appropriate, but the true haemoglobin level will not be apparent until the changes in intravascular volume associated with the metabolic response to surgery are complete.

Replacement of acute blood loss

In the previously healthy adult, acute blood loss of less than 1500 ml may be corrected by rapid infusion of crystalloid solutions alone. Continued loss and prior anaemia are indications for blood transfusion. During haemorrhage all components of blood are lost; they can be replaced by transfusion of whole blood, yet whole blood is rarely available. Blood for transfusion is usually available as packed red cells; each unit has a volume of approximately 450 ml and should be expected to raise the circulating haemoglobin concentration by $1 \, \text{g} \, \text{dl}^{-1}$ in a stable patient. Ideally, transfused blood should be fully cross-matched, yet in an emergency there may be insufficient time for this procedure. If the patient's ABO and Rhesus subtypes are known, grouped blood can be requested. If immediate transfusion is required, O Rhesus negative blood may have to suffice.

Autologous blood transfusion

Autologous transfusion of blood harvested before surgery is unlikely to be possible in patients who require emergency surgery. However, it may be possible to salvage blood lost during the procedure and re-infuse it. A cell-saver is a machine which allows shed blood to be collected; it requires expertise in use. The cells are washed and re-suspended before infusion. The Solcotrans® system is more simple; it is attached to the surgical sucker and lost blood is collected in a special container which has previously been primed with heparin. When the container is full it is given to the anaesthetist who can reinfuse its contents through a filter. Blood can be collected from the thoracic or abdominal cavities. When the surgical field is contaminated, or infected, autologous transfusion is contraindicated. Similarly, the technique should not be used when malignancy is suspected.

Correction of clotting abnormalities

Fresh frozen plasma contains most clotting factors, but is deplete in fibrinogen and factor VIII. It is indicated for replacement of clotting factors, reversal of warfarinisation, and treatment of disseminated intravascular coagulopathy (DIC). Cryoprecipitate contains both factor VIII and fibrinogen; fibrinogen may be used to treat DIC. Specific factor deficiencies can be corrected with factor concentrates. Platelets are provided as concentrates, and are indicated to correct both quantitative and qualitative platelet deficiencies, and again DIC. When coagulopathy exists in the presence of major haemorrhage it is preferable to arrest bleeding surgically, and then administer clotting factors and platelets.

Complications of the use of blood products

Blood products may act as vehicles of infection. Donor screening reduces the risk of infection by many organisms, but the hazard persists if donation occurs before antigenaemia develops. The risks are greater when products are prepared from pooled donation. Screening for hepatitis B and C, human immunodeficiency virus, and *Treponema pallidum* is routinely performed in the UK. In endemic areas malaria may be transmitted by blood products. Bacterial infection may occur during transfusion if strict asepsis is not practised.

Massive blood transfusion (transfusion of greater than the patient's blood volume) may be associated with a variety of problems.[10] Fluid overload may occur whenever large volumes are administered, and a blood warmer should be used to prevent hypothermia. Coagulopathy may develop because of clotting factor and platelet deficiency. Fresh frozen plasma (four units) and platelets (six units) should be given. Stored blood usually contains citrate; large transfusions may be associated with hypocalcaemia and the risk is greater in the presence of liver disease and during liver surgery. Hyperkalaemia may also occur, and may be an indicator of underlying hypocalcaemia. Acidosis is a further risk, but administration of bicarbonate is rarely required, unless the patient is acidotic before transfusion.

The immunological properties of blood give rise to a variety of potential transfusion reactions; over 90% are due to clerical errors in labelling or administration of blood products. Immediate haemolytic transfusion reactions (IHTR) are initiated during transfusion. Mild IHTR may be manifest by fever only and may not be recognised. Moderate reactions cause anxiety, dyspnoea, rigors and palpitations; jaundice develops within hours. The transfusion must be stopped and hydrocortisone 100 mg and chlorpheniramine 10 mg should be administered. Major IHTR is accompanied by development of chest and abdominal pain, tachycardia, hypotension and oliguria. Haemoglobinuria may be obvious, and free haemoglobin is present in the blood. The management is as for a moderate reaction, but in addition urine output must be maintained by vigorous crystalloid infusion, together with a loop diuretic or mannitol.

Delayed haemolytic transfusion reactions occur one to three weeks after transfusion. They are characterised by development of jaundice, fever and generalised aches, and progressive anaemia. They are usually a response to Rhesus antigens and can be confirmed by a positive direct antiglobulin test; specific treatment is often not required. Whenever a transfusion reaction is suspected the advice of a haematologist should be sought. Non-haemolytic reactions occur when pyrogens are released by granulocytes. The usual signs are flushing and pyrexia, but respiratory distress may follow. Treatment with paracetamol may be all that is required, but it may be difficult to exclude IHTR. Blood transfusion may induce immune tolerance. This may be of benefit in renal transplantation when graft survival is improved, but there is evidence to suggest that the outcome after surgery for colorectal cancer is impaired by peroperative transfusion. Graft-versus-host disease may occur rarely in the immunocompromised.

Alternatives to blood for volume replacement

When blood is unavailable, or its use is unacceptable to the patient, plasma expanders can be considered as an alternative. Modified gelatin products (Haemaccel®) have a half-life of 5 h, but may not be acceptable for patients in whom beef products are forbidden. Hydroxyethyl starch derivatives (Hespan®) have a half-life of 24 hours and are acceptable in the majority of patients. The use of albumin as a plasma expander cannot be justified as it is expensive, and in the majority of circumstances is no more effective than cheaper synthetic alternatives. Nor should albumin be used as a nutritional solution for replacement of amino acids. Albumin is indicated to restore colloid oncotic pressure when the plasma albumin concentration is less than $15 \, \text{g} \, \text{dl}^{-1}$. It may also be of use in the treatment of the nephrotic syndrome, and after drainage of massive ascites. Albumin solutions have a high sodium content (greater than $160 \, \text{mmol} \, \text{l}^{-1}$).

Postoperative management

Control of pain

Pain is an unpleasant sensation and this is reason enough for its prevention, but postoperative discomfort may prove deleterious in other ways. Pain, particularly from chest and upper abdominal wounds, may impair ventilation and hence predispose to atelectasis, hypoxia and chest infection. When pain limits the ability to mobilise, pressure sores and deep venous thrombosis will be more common. Unless the anaesthetist provides analgesia in addition to anaesthesia during the operation, the metabolic and physiological responses to noxious stimuli will be heightened. Adequate intraoperative analgesia may reduce the depth of anaesthesia required, and hence recovery from anaesthesia may be enhanced. Thus regional anaesthesia, in addition to standard general anaesthesia, may be advantageous. Postoperative analgesic requirements are greater when the patient is anxious before the procedure, and when the patient is in pain on recovery from anaesthesia. Preoperative counselling has been shown to reduce postoperative analgesic requirements. Infiltration of local anaesthetic, by the surgeon, before completion of the procedure may also reduce the quantity of postoperative analgesia required.

Opiate analgesia

Oral opiates are usually ineffective in the immediate postoperative period because gastric emptying is delayed. Therefore, opiate analgesia has traditionally been administered by intermittent intramuscular injection. However, the technique is often ineffective. Pressures on nursing staff may mean that, rather than receiving analgesia on regular review, the patient has to request a further dose after pain has returned. Moreover, there is substantial interpatient variability in the timing and magnitude of peak plasma opiate concentration when the intramuscular route is used. Intramuscular drug injection is unreliable in patients who are hypotensive, or who exhibit peripheral vasoconstriction. Entry of the drug into the bloodstream may be delayed, and thus analgesia impaired. Further doses are then given to achieve pain relief but, when peripheral circulation is restored, drug sequestered in the muscle may suddenly prove toxic. Intravenous bolus administration of an opiate offers rapid analgesia, but the dose must be slowly titrated against the patient's response. Therefore, bolus intravenous analgesia usually requires the presence of medically qualified staff.

Continuous intravenous opiate infusions provide uninterrupted analgesia, but may be associated with significant respiratory depression. On the ward, where intramuscular analgesia cannot be administered on time, regular measurement of ventilation rate is also likely to be difficult. Patient-controlled analgesia (PCA) offers a satisfactory alternative; an infusion pump delivers metered drug boluses when the patient presses a switch. Inadvertent overdose is prevented by a programmed 'lock-out' period during which it is impossible for the patient to administer another dose. More sophisticated PCA pumps deliver a continuous low-dose background infusion of analgesia in addition to a bolus on demand. In this manner the patient receives pain relief even when asleep. PCA is not universally effective; the elderly or confused may not comprehend the technique, whereas the weak or disabled may not be able to press their switch.

The dose of opiate required may be reduced by use of co-analgesics, or peroperative regional anaesthetic techniques. Non-steroidal drugs such as diclofenac are particularly effective for relief of musculoskeletal pain and can be administered as a suppository before reversal of anaesthesia.

Regional analgesia

Bupivicaine is commonly used for regional analgesia. Peripheral nerve blockade typically provides analgesia for between 8 and 12 h; addition of adrenaline to the solution may delay absorption and prolong the duration of pain relief. Spinal analgesia, in which the drug is injected into the subarachnoid space, may last for up to 4 h. Top-up doses may be administered via a subarachnoid catheter, but the consequences of infection render this technique unattractive. Spinal analgesia is best used to control pain below the umbilicus, and is excellent for patients in whom respiratory disease is a relative contraindication to general anaesthesia. Analgesia distal to the level of subarachnoid puncture is produced, and dense motor blockage is expected. Thoracic subarachnoid analgesia may be associated with hypotension because of sympathetic blockade, and extension to the high cervical cord may cause apnoea. In epidural blockade the drug is delivered into the extradural space; a band of analgesia is produced around the level of the catheter and motor blockade is less common. Addition of a lipid-soluble opiate, such as fentanyl, to the infusion may increase the density of the region of anaesthesia. A bolus dose may be effective for 4 h; insertion of an indwelling catheter is safer than in spinal blockade and hence top-up doses or a continuous infusion can be given. The physiological effects are similar to subarachnoid blockade; but because the extradural space is larger than the subarachnoid, greater doses of analgesic are required. Systemic drug absorption may cause myocardial suppression. Both spinal and extradural blockade are contraindicated in the presence of coagulopathy and infection, and their effects on circulatory reflexes render them unattractive in the presence of hypotension or cardiac disease.

Inhalational analgesia

Inhalation of a 50% oxygen/50% nitrous oxide mixture (Entonox®) can provide good analgesia, particularly during painful postoperative procedures such as dressing changes. The patent holds a mask, or mouthpiece, which has a demand valve; if drowsiness occurs the patient will drop the mask and hence toxicity is avoided. The mixture is contraindicated when pneumothorax or gastrointestinal obstruction cannot be excluded. Diffusion of nitrous oxide may increase pressure in the pleural cavity or bowel lumen with disastrous consequences.

Postoperative fluid and electrolyte balance

Postoperative fluid balance should be uncomplicated for the majority of patients. Provided that fluid resuscitation in the preoperative period is adequate, and intraoperative losses are not excessive, daily post-operative requirements should be predictable and consistent. Such patients require fluid to replace insensible loss and maintain an adequate diuresis. Insensible losses will be greater in the presence of fever. Normal daily electrolyte requirements are sodium 1 mmol kg^{-1} day^{-1} and potassium 1 mmol kg^{-1} day^{-1}. Care must be taken with the elderly, and patients with cardiac, hepatic or renal failure who are poorly tolerant of fluid and sodium loads. However, in some patients significant fluid volumes may be sequestered because of ileus. Others may lose large quantities of fluid and electrolytes via other routes. Volumes of vomitus and diarrhoea should be taken into account, as must nasogastric aspirates and losses via drains and fistulae. Typical electrolyte contents of various gastrointestinal fluids are given in Table 2.4. Pancreatic fluid typically contains a significant quantity of bicarbonate; and a high output pancreatic fistula may be associated with a metabolic acidosis.

Table 2.4 *Electrolyte composition of various body fluids (mmol l^{-1})*

	Sodium	Potassium	Chloride	Bicarbonate
Plasma	135–145	3.5–5.5	95–105	24–32
Urine	70–160	40–120	–	–
Gastric	50	15	140	0–15
Bile	140	5	100	40
Pancreatic	130	5	55	110
Jejunal	140	0	130	a
Ileal	140	10	70	a
Colonic	30–140	30–70	–	20–80

[a]Bicarbonate content varies with the presence of bile and pancreatic juice.

Clinical assessment is the mainstay of fluid and electrolyte balance. The adequately hydrated patient should not be thirsty; the tongue moist and skin turgor normal. However, patients who mouth-breathe because of nasogastric intubation, or those who receive oxygen by mask may have a dry mouth. The jugular venous pulse should not be elevated and there should be no evidence of peripheral or pulmonary oedema. A daily fluid balance chart is essential for all patients who receive intravenous fluids. It should include all losses. For the adult, a urine output of 40–50 ml h^{-1} is ideal. In the early post-operative period when the body is maximally preserving fluids a urine output of 20 ml h^{-1} is acceptable. Attention should be paid to the pulse and blood pressure; tachycardia or hypotension may reflect profound fluid deficit. Measurement of daily weight may aid assessment of fluid requirements; rapid weight change is likely to indicate loss or retention of fluid rather than alteration in lean body mass. As a rough guide, each kilogram change represents one litre of fluid. Measurement of plasma urea, creatinine and electrolytes is essential when patients are prescribed intravenous fluids. Elevation of urea and creatinine indicate significant renal impairment. Therefore, normal plasma values alone cannot be regarded as evidence of adequate fluid replacement. The interpretation of changes in plasma electrolytes is discussed below.

Management of electrolyte disorders

The bulk of body potassium is intracellular; changes in plasma potassium reflect changes in whole body potassium. Hypokalaemia is treated by gradual potassium replacement, whereas hyperkalaemia requires potassium restriction in the first instance. In contrast, the majority of body sodium is extracellular; changes in serum sodium most frequently represent alteration in extracellular volume. Hyponatraemia is most commonly due to water excess, and therefore fluid restriction is indicated. Sodium supplementation is not indicated, because the total body sodium is normal and extra solute will cause further water retention and a paradoxical reduction in serum sodium concentration. In surgical patients dilutional hyponatraemia may be a consequence of sepsis. Serum sodium will return to normal when the underlying pathology resolves. Nevertheless, when gastrointestinal fluid losses are marked, true sodium depletion may cause hyponatraemia, and sodium replacement is indicated. Measurement of urinary sodium may aid management of hyponatraemia. Provided that renal tubular function is normal, a low urinary sodium indicates true sodium deficiency whereas a normal, or elevated urinary sodium indicates water excess. Plasma osmolality should also be measured when the possibility of water imbalance is considered.

Postoperative blood transfusion

Postoperative blood transfusion is indicated for hypotension in the presence of anaemia, or when the patient has other symptoms of anaemia. However, transfusion is seldom required if the haemoglobin concentration is stable and greater than 10 g dl^{-1}.

Management of postoperative oliguria

Poor urine output is an important sign which represents deteriorating renal function, frequently as a consequence of hypovolaemia. It demands prompt patient assessment. The majority of patients at risk of postoperative oliguria should have a urinary catheter inserted before surgery, not least to enable intraoperative assessment of urine output. If there is any doubt that a non-catheterised patient may be oliguric, a catheter must be inserted. An algorithm for management of oliguria (less than 20 ml h^{-1} for 2 or more hours) is given in Fig. 2.1. When fluid replacement is warranted, the choice of infusion will depend on the nature of the loss. Blood is required for haemorrhage; crystalloid to replace nasogastric aspirate. It must not be assumed that free urinary drainage is assured; the position of a catheter must be checked, as well as the integrity of the drainage system, before potentially aggressive therapy is instituted.

Postoperative laboratory investigations

Just as with preoperative investigation, 'routine' tests should be avoided. A rationale for postoperative investigation is given in Table 2.5. It is usually unnecessary to perform blood tests on patients who undergo uncomplicated minor and intermediate procedures.

Respiratory support

The aim of respiratory support is to maintain tissue oxygenation. Adequate tissue oxygenation depends upon **A**irway, **B**reathing, and **C**irculation. An adequate safe airway is vital. Ventilation must be maintained and sufficient oxygen administered to ensure saturation, and hypovolaemia and anaemia should be corrected. The management of hypovolaemia has already been discussed, and haemoglobin concentration is assessed by the full blood count. Oxygen saturation reflects the partial pressure of oxygen in arterial blood ($Pa\mathrm{O}_2$). Oxygen tension may be assessed directly by arterial blood sampling. When repeated samples are required, an arterial catheter should be inserted. Such a catheter also allows continuous monitoring of blood pressure, and blood samples may be collected for other haematological and biochemical investigations. Pulse oximetry offers a non-invasive alternative for assessment of arterial oxygen saturation; but may be inaccurate in the presence of peripheral vasoconstriction or jaundice. The presence of carboxyhaemoglobin and methaemoglobin also render pulse oximetry unreliable.

Figure 2.1
Algorithm for the management of oliguria.

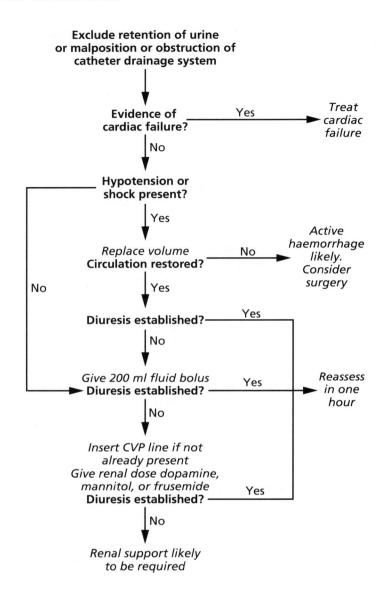

Exclude retention of urine or malposition or obstruction of catheter drainage system

Evidence of cardiac failure? — Yes → *Treat cardiac failure*

No

Hypotension or shock present?

Yes

Replace volume Circulation restored? — No → *Active haemorrhage likely. Consider surgery*

Yes

Diuresis established? — Yes

No

Give 200 ml fluid bolus Diuresis established? — Yes → *Reassess in one hour*

No

Insert CVP line if not already present Give renal dose dopamine, mannitol, or frusemide Diuresis established? — Yes

No

Renal support likely to be required

Respiratory failure

Respiratory failure is characterised by hypoxia. Two patterns exist; in Type I (hypoxaemic) failure, PaO_2 is reduced but the arterial pressure of carbon dioxide ($PaCO_2$) is normal or reduced because of hyperventilation. In Type II (ventilatory) failure, gas exchange is impaired, PaO_2 is reduced and $PaCO_2$ elevated. Hypoxaemic respiratory failure occurs in the presence of a ventilation–perfusion mismatch; examples include pulmonary embolism, cyanotic heart disease and adult respiratory distress syndrome (ARDS). Ventilatory failure implies a defect

Table 2.5 *Suggested scheme for postoperative laboratory tests*

Urea and electrolytes	Check on the first postoperative day in patients who have an intravenous infusion which will not be taken down that day. Check on alternate days thereafter until return to free oral fluids is achieved. Check daily for patients who have abnormal results, or large fluid losses.
Full blood count	Check on the first postoperative day only if the patient was anaemic before surgery, or peroperative losses were significant. Check on the second postoperative day for all patients who have undergone major surgery. Once the haemoglobin is stable, no further measurement is necessary. Check on alternate days when heparin prescribed (risk of thrombocytopenia). Monitor platelets after splenectomy until the count has stabilised.
Blood glucose	Patients who receive insulin are at risk of both hypo- and hyperglycaemia, and require regular measurement of blood glucose. Patients who receive IVN are at risk of hyperglycaemia. In the first instance blood glucose should be measured. If the blood sugar is stable, urinalysis can then be substituted. Hypoglycaemia is a risk after major liver resection, and in fulminant hepatic failure.
Coagulation studies	Measure after major transfusion, when intraoperative haemostasis proved difficult, or on development of signs of bleeding. Measure regularly during therapeutic anticoagulation.

in the control, or mechanics of breathing. Central control of ventilation may be impaired by head injury or drugs such as opiates. High cervical spine injuries (above C4) may paralyse respiratory muscles and trauma which disrupts the integrity of the thoracic wall will also impair ventilation. Adequate chest movement is prevented by pain, and by diaphragmatic splinting due to intestinal obstruction or intraperitoneal fluid. Chest wall deformity, encircling chest dressings and cicatrising thoracic burns also impair ventilation. Effective lung volume is reduced by pneumothorax, atelectasis, consolidation or contusion. Gas exchange is further hampered by pulmonary oedema.

Airway management

Loss of the airway will rapidly prove fatal. Nonetheless, in the trauma victim, care must be taken to protect the cervical spine during airway manoeuvres until unstable injuries have been excluded. A patent airway may be restored by simply clearing the mouth and pharynx of debris or secretions, and performing a jaw lift or thrust. Insertion of an oropharyngeal airway will maintain the upper air passage, but may precipitate vomiting in the conscious patient; a nasopharyngeal airway may be better tolerated. When ventilation is required, or the patient is at risk of aspiration of gastric contents a definitive airway is indicated. Usually a cuffed endotracheal tube will be used, but acute obstruction of the upper airway may dictate a cricothyroidotomy.

The indications for tracheostomy are several. Prolonged endotracheal intubation may be associated with permanent damage to the glottis; a tracheostomy is usually required after the tube has been in place for 10 days. A tracheostomy allows easy passage of catheters for bronchial toilet in the patient who breathes spontaneously, but has copious secretions. A minitracheostomy can be easily inserted on the general ward and may be a satisfactory alternative for short-term use. Permanent tracheostomy is inevitable when radical resection of the larynx or pharynx is performed, and temporary tracheostomy may be required after head and neck trauma, and radiotherapy to the neck.

Lower airway secretions may be cleared by physiotherapy, possibly with postural drainage. Use of nebulisers may aid mucolysis, and bronchoscopy may be required to remove mucus plugs.

Oxygen delivery

Supplemental oxygen may be administered by a variety of means, but should always be humidified. Inspired oxygen concentration (FiO_2) depends on the oxygen flow and the patient's pattern of ventilation. At an oxygen flow of $4\,l\,min^{-1}$, nasal cannulae and simple masks may provide a FiO_2 of 30–40%. High-flow masks provide a FiO_2 which is constant and independent of the pattern of ventilation. Depending on the mask type and oxygen flow, FiO_2 of 28–60% may be achieved. A low FiO_2 is used for patients reliant on hypoxic drive to maintain ventilation, whereas a high FiO_2 may be required by the patient with a pulmonary shunt (ventilation/perfusion mismatch). Continuous positive airway pressure (CPAP) masks provide a tight seal around the face and may facilitate recruitment of collapsed alveoli and disperse pulmonary oedema. Similar effects can be achieved by use of positive end expiratory pressure (PEEP) during mechanical ventilation, or by increasing the duration of the inspiratory phase (reverse I:E ratio).[11] CPAP and PEEP may cause intrathoracic barotrauma and may reduce cardiac output by impairment of venous return. In addition both may increase CVP. Increased airway pressure may also increase pulmonary vascular resistance. Continuous use of a CPAP mask can cause pressure necrosis, particularly over the nasal bridge.

Indications for ventilation

Ventilation is indicated in the presence of respiratory failure that cannot be corrected by more conservative methods. It is also indicated when raised intracranial pressure is present, or likely; ventilation allows Pa_{CO_2}, and thus intracerebral vasodilitation, to be reduced. Patients who undergo major surgical procedures, particularly those who are malnourished, are at risk of postoperative fatigue and for them a period of ventilation may be advisable. Some emergency surgical patients require multiple surgical procedures within a short period of time, for example second-look laparotomy or change of abdominal packs. Postoperative ventilation is usually indicated in such circumstances. Ventilation is also indicated for the patient who cannot protect his airway, as a consequence of local trauma, or because of reduced level of consciousness.

Adult respiratory distress syndrome (ARDS)

ARDS is a clinical syndrome characterised by hypoxaemia, pulmonary shunting and reduced pulmonary compliance. It may be precipitated by a variety of disorders which include direct and inhalational chest injuries, sepsis including pancreatitis, aspiration of gastric contents, hypovolaemia and massive transfusion. It is thought that the common factor is activation of cytokines and free radicals. ARDS may develop as part of the MOF syndrome. The earliest sign may be hypoxaemia alone, and a high index of clinical suspicion is required. Swan Ganz catheterisation may reveal shunting, and if the patient is mechanically ventilated the decrease in pulmonary compliance may be evident. The classical radiological changes of pulmonary infiltrates occur relatively late. Treatment is predominantly supportive; oxygenation and circulating volume must be maintained, without fluid overload. CPAP may be beneficial, but mechanical ventilation with PEEP is usually necessary. Nutritional support is usually required and although high dose steroids have been recommended by some, their use is controversial.[12] Inhaled nitric oxide reduces pulmonary artery pressure, and hence improves blood flow in ventilated lung segments without causing systemic vasodilatation. The role of nitric oxide in ARDS remains to be confirmed by a randomised trial. The precipitating cause should be rectified; sepsis should be drained or debrided, and early fixation of long bone fractures may be beneficial.

Cardiovascular support

Postoperative cardiac failure may be a progression of pre-existing cardiac impairment, or an indication of perioperative myocardial infarction or arrhythmia. The principles of optimisation of preload and myocardial oxygenation, with prevention of arrhythmia, apply as well in the postoperative period as in the period before surgery. In addition, reduction of afterload may do much to support the failing heart. Cardiac filling must be maintained, but not at the expense of volume overload. Many of the drugs required for cardiovascular support have varying actions which depend on dose, and most can precipitate cardiac dysrhythmia. When they are used, a continuous ECG and invasive monitoring by means of arterial, CVP, or Swan Ganz catheters are essential. Postoperative circulatory failure may be a consequence of tension pneumothorax or cardiac tamponade. Both are most likely to be seen after trauma or cardiothoracic surgery, but may complicate central venous catheterisation. Immediate thoracocentesis or pericardiocentesis will be necessary. Tension pneumothorax may be attributable to barotrauma from positive pressure ventilation, particularly when CPAP or PEEP are used.

Cardiac output is determined by stroke volume and heart rate. Stroke volume is increased by use of β-adrenergic agonists such as dopamine $5–10 \ \mu g \ kg^{-1} \ min^{-1}$ or dobutamine $2–15 \ \mu g \ kg^{-1} \ min^{-1}$. Both are positive inotropes, but also increase heart rate and myocardial oxygen consumption. Phosphodiesterase inhibitors, for example enoximone $10 \ \mu g \ kg^{-1} \ min^{-1}$, are positive inotropes but do not increase heart rate or myocardial oxygen consumption. They also reduce SVR and should not be used in the presence of hypotension. When bradycardia is a problem, atropine $600 \ \mu g$ may be of benefit. Adrenaline infused at a low dose ($1–2 \ \mu g \ min^{-1}$) has a predominant β-agonist effect and may be used as a second-line inotrope.

When preload or afterload are excessively high, infusion of a vasodilator may be indicated. Isosorbide dinitrate reduces preload by dilatation of the peripheral capacitance veins. The drug rarely causes systemic hypotension unless other antihypertensive agents are prescribed. Glyceryl trinitrate acts predominantly on the venous circulation, and improves myocardial blood flow. It reduces afterload by moderate dilatation of arterioles and hypotension may occur during infusion. Sodium nitroprusside is a potent dilator of both arteries and veins. It can cause profound hypotension and this may be exploited in the management of dissecting aortic aneurysm, and to protect suture lines after cardiac surgery. Its short half-life means that changes in infusion rate are rapidly reflected in the physiological response. In heart failure the dose is titrated against the change in cardiac output. When used as an antihypertensive, nitroprusside infusion is adjusted according to the change in systolic pressure. Nitroprusside infusion may cause methaemoglobinaemia and thus invalidate pulse oximetry.

When SVR is low, for example in sepsis, a vasopressor may be required. Noradrenaline $2–4 \ \mu g \ min^{-1}$ may be used, but it is essential to ensure that volume replacement is satisfactory.

Myocardial contractility is impaired, and irritability increased, in the presence of malnutrition and nutritional support may have an unquantifiable benefit in the management of postoperative cardiac problems.

Mechanical assist devices

Cardiac output, and myocardial oxygenation may be improved by intra-aortic balloon counterpulsation. The technique is principally used as an adjunct to cardiac surgery, and is not appropriate for end-stage cardiac failure. A balloon is inserted into the thoracic aorta via the femoral artery. Its inflation and deflation is synchronised with the ECG. Inflation during diastole increases left ventricular end-diastolic pressure and increases coronary artery flow. Peripheral blood flow is also improved as the balloon displaces blood from the distal aorta. Deflation during systole allows blood to circulate, and the sudden increase in aortic volume reduces myocardial work.

Renal support

Postoperative renal failure is most commonly due to hypovolaemia, possibly exacerbated by jaundice or sepsis, and the importance of maintenance of renal perfusion cannot be overemphasised. Jaundice and sources of sepsis will require drainage or debridement. In many cases acute tubular necrosis will be transient and resolution can be expected after six weeks if interim support is provided.

Acute renal failure is established when there is persistent oliguria in the presence of a normal CVP, and a failure to concentrate the urine to an osmolality greater than that of plasma (290–300 mosmol l^{-1}). In the early stages, plasma urea and creatinine may not be substantially elevated. Fluid intake should be restricted to the previous hour's urine output plus 20 ml to allow for insensitive loss. Volume overload is the principal cause of morbidity in acute renal failure; the patient must be carefully examined for signs of fluid retention, and should be weighed daily if possible. Plasma potassium and arterial hydrogen ion concentration must be closely monitored, and the advice of a nephrologist obtained. In the early stages of acute tubular necrosis renal function may be stimulated by a low-dose ('renal dose') dopamine infusion 2–5 μg kg^{-1} min^{-1}. Alternatively a potent diuretic such as frusemide 250 mg, or bumetanide 1 mg, may be used. Infusion of 100 ml 20% mannitol may also restore a diuresis. If these measures prove ineffective it is likely that artificial renal support will be required.

Artificial renal support

Indications for artificial renal support include removal of excess fluid, hyperkalaemia, acidosis and rapidly climbing plasma creatinine (>500 μmol l^{-1}). It is not uncommon in the critically ill for the volume of drug infusions to exceed the hourly permissible volume; this is particularly true when intravenous nutrition is required. Artificial renal support may be required to 'make space'. Haemodialysis or haemofiltration may be used, but peritoneal dialysis is unlikely to be appropriate after emergency surgery, particularly following laparotomy. During haemodialysis countercurrent diffusion removes large fluid volumes in a relatively short period of time. The flux may cause hypotension which is poorly tolerated by the critically ill. In haemofiltration the patient's blood is pumped through a filter, and the filtrate is discarded. Fluid is removed continuously, and at a slower rate, than during haemodialysis, and hence haemofiltration causes less cardiovascular disturbance.

Admission to high dependency or intensive care units (HDU/ICU)

Although many postoperative patients can be managed on the general ward, limitations in staffing levels or experience may dictate admission to an HDU or ICU. The HDU is supervised by the managing surgical team, whereas the ICU usually has dedicated anaesthetic cover. Many of the facilities offered by an HDU and ICU are similar, but ventilation is usually only available on an ICU. When there is a risk of airway obstruction, for example after facial trauma or burns, the ICU is the ideal environment. Patients on ICU receive continuous one-to-one nursing care, whereas one nurse to two patients is more likely on HDU. Continuous monitoring of vital signs occurs in both units. Either unit is suitable for patients whose clinical condition is, or may become, unstable in the perioperative period. Haemodialysis or haemofiltration, or intensive cardiovascular support are best conducted on a HDU or ICU. Although the majority of patients will be admitted to an HDU or ICU in the postoperative period, preoperative admission should be considered for critically ill patients. A period of intensive monitoring may allow optimal resuscitation before surgery. In general, close cooperation between surgeons, anaesthetists and the nursing staff on both the HDU and the ICU will permit the most appropriate management to be instituted for each patient.

Management of the surgical patient with specific problems

The diabetic patient

The diabetic patient poses a twofold problem. Not only are there the specific metabolic consequences of diabetes mellitus, but the systemic complications of diabetes may also influence the outcome after surgical illness. Diabetic patients are frequently arteriopaths, and are at greater risk of ischaemic heart and cerebrovascular disease. Many have chronic renal failure. Diabetes mellitus predisposes to sepsis and small vessel disease may hamper wound healing. In particular, survival of myocutaneous grafts may be impaired. Microangiopathy may be associated with autonomic neuropathy. Gastric emptying may be slowed and, if hypertension is present, it may be labile. Sepsis itself may cause glucose intolerance, and therefore diabetic ketoacidosis may be a sign of underlying surgical disease.

The major perioperative metabolic risk is *hypoglycaemia*, which will occur if diabetic medication is continued in the absence of available glucose. Under anaesthesia, many of the symptoms and signs of hypoglycaemia may be masked. Therefore it is preferable to allow the patient's blood glucose to remain slightly high. Nonetheless, uncontrolled hyperglycaemia will result in coma and must be prevented. Diabetic patients should be placed first on the operating list whenever possible and their preparation should be discussed with the anaesthetist who will supervise the patient. Possible management strategies are outlined in Table 2.6. If possible, patients on long-acting insulins should be stabilised preoperatively with short-acting soluble insulin (Actrapid®) administered by either the intravenous or subcutaneous route. The alternative is an inravenous insulin–potassium–glucose infusion (Alberti regimen).[13] When insulin alone is used a sliding scale, in which the dose is related to the degree of hyperglycaemia, is recommended. Blood glucose should be regularly monitored and should not be allowed to fall below 7 mmol l^{-1}. Administration of insulin will cause potassium to shift from the intravascular to the intracellular space, and hence hypokalaemia may occur. In the Alberti regimen, 16 units soluble insulin and 10 mmol potassium chloride in 500 ml 10% glucose are infused at 100 ml h^{-1}. The infusion is started 1 h before surgery, and blood glucose checked after 2 h. If greater than 10 mmol l^{-1}, the dose of insulin should be increased by 4 units, and the blood glucose rechecked.

Table 2.6 *Perioperative management of the diabetic patient*

Diet controlled	• No specific action required. • If hyperglycaemia occurs consider either a sliding scale insulin, or glucose–potassium–insulin infusion.
Oral hypoglycaemics	• Omit oral hypoglycaemic on day of surgery. Long-acting oral hypoglycaemics (e.g. chlorpropamide) should be stopped the day before surgery. • Monitor blood glucose in postoperative period. If hyperglycaemia occurs consider either a sliding scale insulin, or glucose–potassium–insulin, infusion. • Resume oral hypoglycaemic on full return to enteral diet
Insulin dependent	• Omit morning dose of insulin. • If prompt return to enteral intake anticipated on recovery from anaesthesia consider a glucose–potassium–insulin infusion. • If return to enteral intake is likely to be delayed, start a sliding scale insulin infusion.

Surgical stress and sepsis are associated with peripheral insulin resistance and mild hyperglycaemia. As the patient's condition improves after surgery a reduced insulin requirement should be anticipated, otherwise hypoglycaemia may occur. Similarly, a sudden increase in insulin requirement, in a previously stable patient, may be the first sign of an evolving septic complication.

The jaundiced patient

Jaundice is a marker of increased risk for the perioperative patient and may represent either parenchymal liver disease or obstruction of the biliary tree; an underlying malignancy should always be considered. Impaired hepatic function may be associated with altered drug and hormone metabolism, and with a coagulopathy. Jaundiced patients frequently demonstrate secondary hyperaldosteronism, and are poorly tolerant of sodium loads. Furthermore, there is an increased risk of postoperative renal failure and an impaired tolerance of hypovolaemia. Obstructive jaundice is often associated with endotoxaemia[14] and intraoperative manipulation of the biliary tree may precipitate septicaemia.

It is essential to maintain adequate hydration and an intravenous infusion should be considered for any jaundiced patient who is starved for investigations or surgery. Sodium overload should be avoided in the presence of hepatic failure or ascites by prescribing 5% dextrose only, with potassium as required. Preoperative infusion of low-dose dopamine may protect the kidneys. Coagulation studies should be performed and vitamin K 10 mg given by intravenous injection; fresh frozen plasma may be required to correct any established coagulopathy. If time allows, preoperative biliary drainage should be considered.[15] Internal endoscopic drainage has a lower morbidity than external percutaneous drainage.[16] Acute hepatic failure may be precipitated in patients with chronic liver disease by the sudden protein load which follows massive gastrointestinal haemorrhage and therefore oral lactulose should be given to reduce the risk of encephalopathy. Moreover, lactulose binds endotoxin and may protect renal function in jaundiced patients.[17]

The anticoagulated patient

Surgery performed in the anticoagulated patient risks haemorrhage; yet in some, for example those with prosthetic heart valves, the risk of reversal of anticoagulation for a significant period may exceed that of bleeding. The management of the anticoagulated patient will vary with the clinical context. Some guidelines are give below.

Elective surgery

If the patient is heparinised, the infusion should be stopped four hours before surgery, and the Kaolin Cephalin Clotting Time (KCCT) checked after two hours to ensure that it is normal. If the patient is warfarinised, the drug should be stopped and the International Normalised Ratio (INR) allowed to return to normal before surgery. For warfarinised patients in whom complete cessation of anti-coagulation is undesirable, therapeutic heparinisation should be started and the KCCT monitored until the INR is normal. The patient is then managed as described above. Provided that bleeding is not a problem anticoagulation may be started promptly in the postoperative period. Warfarin should not be reversed with vitamin K otherwise re-warfarinisation in the postoperative period may be delayed for a considerable time.

Emergency surgery or major haemorrhage
In an emergency there may not be sufficient time to implement the methods described above, and again the relative risks of continued anticoagulation against haemorrhage must be assessed. All anti-coagulation should be stopped and, in the case of bleeding, coagulation and platelets should be checked and DIC excluded. Fresh frozen plasma and platelets should be ordered, and consideration given to administration of vitamin K 10 mg. The effects of heparin may be counteracted by administration of protamine (0.5–1.0 mg/1000 units heparin), and fibrinolysis may be inhibited by tranexamic acid (500–1000 mg tds).

Disseminated intravascular coagulopathy
Disseminated intravascular coagulopathy is characterised by con-sumption of clotting factors and platelets due to synchronous generation of thrombin and fibrinolysis.[18] Fibrin degradation prod-ucts (FDP) impair thrombin activity and fibrinolysis. Precipitants of DIC include trauma and fat embolism, sepsis, and transfusion of ABO incompatible blood. In the acute form, fibrinolysis dominates and haemorrhage occurs as coagulation factors are consumed. Acute DIC is manifest by oozing bleeding not only from surgical wounds, but also from intravenous cannulation sites. Widespread spontaneous petechiae and bruising may also appear. In chronic DIC, deposition of fibrin within small vessels leads to renal failure and ARDS. DIC may precede, or be a consequence of, MOF.

In DIC, coagulation times (KCCT, prothrombin time) are prolonged while the platelet count falls precipitously. Fibrinogen levels are low, and the level of FDP is abnormally elevated. The underlying cause must be treated promptly and circulating volume maintained. Blood is given to treat anaemia, and fresh frozen plasma, cryoprecipitate, factor concentrates and platelets may be required when there is active haemorrhage or invasive procedures are necessary. Vitamin K should also be given because stores may be depleted during DIC. When intravascular fibrin deposition predominates, anticoagulation with heparin must be considered but is evidently hazardous. The advice of a haematologist is essential in the management of DIC.

The patient on steroids

Chronic steroid use is associated with poor wound healing. Thinning of the skin may predispose to extensive tissue loss from trivial trauma. Care must be taken when the patient is positioned on the operating table, and when adhesive tapes and orthopaedic casts are applied. High dose steroids may be associated with glucose intolerance, or frank diabetes. Steroids may mask acute abdominal signs, and a high suspicion of peritonitis must be maintained. A daily dose of prednisolone 10 mg or greater will be associated with complete suppression of the pituitary–adrenal axis. In the critically ill, corticosteroid requirements may be greater than usual, and the physiological stress of anaesthesia and surgery increase requirements further. Thus corticosteroid supplementation is necessary and hydrocortisone 100 mg should be given intravenously on induction of anaesthesia, and continued six hourly until the patient's condition is stabilised. The dose may then be steadily reduced as required. Acute corticosteroid insufficiency may precipitate an Addisonian crisis. The signs of hypotension and tachycardia can mimic circulatory collapse due to haemorrhage but electrolyte measurement may reveal hyponatraemia and hyperkalaemia. Rapid administration of intravenous hydrocortisone 100 mg, and infusion of saline should restore the circulation.

Nutritional support in the perioperative period

Although this subject is extensively discussed elsewhere in this volume, it is appropriate to discuss certain aspects of perioperative nutritional support in this section. There is little evidence to suggest that preoperative nutritional support is of benefit for the majority of patients.[19] Malnourished patients who require surgery fall into two groups. The first comprises malnourished patients who, although at increased risk of complication, have pathology for which definitive treatment cannot be delayed while nutritional repletion occurs. Repletion of lean body mass is a relatively slow process, and may be impossible until underlying pathology is treated. The second group consists of malnourished patients in whom surgery is required, but can be delayed for several *months* while nutritional repletion is achieved. An example might be the patient with multiple fistulae due to Crohn's disease. The majority of patients who are critically ill and require emergency surgery will fall into the first group.

Awareness of the need for early postoperative nutritional support is essential. It will be required when the patient is malnourished, or is unable to maintain nutritional status, and should be provided in *anticipation* of delay in normal dietary intake.[20] The surgeon should consider placement of a gastrostomy or jejunostomy tube during surgery. The enteral route should be used for nutritional support provided that gastrointestinal motility is not impaired and that there is adequate mucosa available for absorption. If these conditions cannot be assured, intravenous nutrition (IVN) is indicated. There is no evidence to suggest that, when the enteral route is available, IVN is more efficacous. Intragastric feeding is appropriate provided that the stomach empties normally. Gastric emptying may be assessed by instillation of a test feed of 5 ml kg^{-1}; failure to aspirate the feed after 1 h indicates that infusion may continue.[21] However, intragastric feeding in the presence of inadequate emptying predisposes to aspiration. Small bowel motility may be normal even when gastric emptying is delayed and in these cases jejunostomy feeding with nasogastric drainage may be appropriate. Enteral feeding is not contraindicated in the ventilated patient, nor by the absence of bowel sounds. However, abdominal distension and obstructive sounds usually indicate the need for IVN. Enteral nutrition is, in general, more simple, safe and cheaper than IVN. Moreover, there is a growing body of evidence to suggest that the route of feeding may influence outcome. The enteral route may be associated with preservation of the gut-mucosal barrier, and possible prevention of MOF in the critically ill. It is apparent that certain nutrients may have specific therapeutic properties in addition to their nutritional role.[22]

References

1. Advanced Trauma Life Support Student Manual. Chicago: American College of Surgeons, 1993.
2. Boyd CR, Tolson MA, Copes WS. Evaluating trauma care: the TRISS method. Trauma 1987; 27: 370–8.
3. Knauss WA, Draper EA, Wagner DP, Zimmerman JE. APACHE II: A severity of disease classification system. Crit Care Med 1985; 13: 818–29.
4. Vacanti CJ, van Houten RJ, Hill RC. A statistical analysis of the relationship of physical status to postoperative mortality in 68 388 cases. Anesth Analges 1970; 49: 564.
5. O'Keefe SJD, Dicker J. Is plasma albumin concentration the assessment of nutritional status of hospital patients? Eur J Clin Nutr 1988; 42: 41–5.
6. Goris RJ, Beokhorst PA, Nuytinck KS. Multiple organ failure: generalized auto-destructive inflammation. Arch Surg 1985; 120: 1109–15.
7. Nurohamed MT, Rosendaal FR, Buller HR *et al*. Low-molecular-weight heparin versus standard heparin in general and orthopaedic surgery – a meta analysis. Lancet 1992; 340: 152–6.
8. Preventing and treating deep vein thrombosis. Drug Ther Bull 1992; 30: 9–12.
9. Paluzzi RC. Antimicrobial prophylaxis for surgery. Med Clin North Am 1993; 77: 427–41.
10. Brozović B, Brozović M. Manual of clinical blood transfusion. Edinburgh: Churchill Livingstone, 1986.
11. Shapiro BA, Peruzzi WT. Changing practices in ventilator management: a review of the literature and suggested clinical correlations. Surgery 1995; 117; 121–33.
12. Kollef MH, Schuster DP. The acute respiratory distress syndrome. N Engl J Med 1995; 332: 27–37.
13. Johnston DG, Alberti KGMM. Diabetic emergencies: practical aspects of the management of diabetic ketoacidosis and diabetes during surgery. Clin Endocrinol Metab 1980; 9: 437.
14. Fogarty BJ, Parks RW, Rowlands BJ, Diamond T. Renal dysfunction in obstructive jaundice. Br J Surg 1995; 82: 877–84.
15. Trede M, Schwall G. The complications of pancreatectomy. Ann Surg 1988; 207: 39–47.

16 Speer AG, Russel RCG, Hatfield ARW *et al.* Randomised trial of endoscopic versus percutaneous stent insertion in malignant obstructive jaundice. Lancet 1987; ii: 57–62.

17. Pain JA, Cahill CJ, Gilbert JM, Johnson CD, Trapnell JE, Bailey ME. Prevention of postoperative renal dysfunction in patients with obstructive jaundice: a multicentre study of bile salts and lactulose. Br. J. Surg. 1991; 78: 467–9.

18. Baglin T. Disseminated intravascular coagulation: diagnosis and treatment. Br Med J 1996; 312: 683–7.

19. The Veterans Affairs Total Parenteral Nutrition Cooperative Study Group. Perioperative total parenteral nutrition in surgical patients. N Engl J Med 1991; 325: 525–32.

20. ASPEN Board of Directors. Guidelines for the use of total parenteral nutrition in the hospitalised adult patient. J Parenter Enteral Nutr 1986; 10: 441–5.

21. Columb MO, Shah MV, Sproat LJ *et al.* Assessment of gastric dysfunction. Current techniques for the measurement of gastric emptying. Br J Intens Care 1992; 2: 75–80.

22. Deitch EA. Multiple organ failure. Pathophysiology and potential future therapy. Ann Surg 1992; 216: 117–34.

3 Surgical nutrition

Steven D. Heys
William G. Simpson
Oleg Eremin

Introduction   The adverse effect of 'malnutrition' on the morbidity and mortality of patients was first recognised by Hippocrates many centuries ago. However, 'malnutrition' is difficult to define and to assess accurately, therefore, 'weight loss', which is readily measurable, is more commonly used in determining nutritional assessment. In more recent times, the importance of weight loss in patients undergoing surgery was emphasised by Studley in 1936.[1] He stated that 'weight loss was a basic indicator of surgical risk' and demonstrated that in patients who were undergoing elective peptic ulcer surgery, a weight loss of 20% or more was associated with an eightfold increase in postoperative mortality, when compared with patients who had lost less than 20% of their body weight. The prevalence of malnutrition among patients in hospital has been reported to be up to 40%. Furthermore, in patients undergoing gastrointestinal surgery, the prevalence of 'mild' and 'moderate' malnutrition has been reported to be approximately 50% and 30%, respectively. The clinical importance of malnutrition has been demonstrated by Detsky *et al.*[2] who found that in patients undergoing gastrointestinal surgery, there was a sixfold increase in the risk of significant complications in patients who were identified as being 'severely' malnourished prior to surgery.

In the presence of malnutrition, surgical wounds and anastomoses are less likely to heal, resulting in an increased risk of wound complications and anastomotic dehiscence. Malnutrition also results in alteration of skeletal muscle metabolism and impairment of skeletal muscle function, reduced cardiac mass and contractility, impaired respiratory muscle function, gut smooth muscle atrophy and dysfunction of the immune system. This chapter will discuss (1) normal nutrient requirements and nutrient absorption from the gut, (2) the metabolic response to trauma and sepsis, (3) the identification of malnourished patients, (4) the indications for, and use of, enteral and parenteral nutrition, and (5) the use of specific nutrients to modulate metabolism and immune responses in patients who have been traumatised and in those with sepsis and cancer.

Nutritional requirements

Proteins and amino acids

Ingestion of protein is required for the maintenance of normal health and cellular function. Proteins have many functions, such as being required as essential components of cellular structure and for the synthesis of a variety of secretory proteins produced by many organs. In an average (70 kg) man, there is approximately 11 kg of protein, with 43% of this being found in skeletal muscle, 16% in blood, 15% in the skin, and less than 2% in the liver.[3] The average daily intake of protein is approximately 80 g per day, with a recommended daily intake of 0.8 g kg^{-1} body weight, with nitrogen comprising approximately 16% of its weight.

The synthesis of these various proteins requires their precursor amino acids. Although more than 300 amino acids exist, only approximately 20 of these are found in animal proteins and all are of the L-optical configuration. Conventionally, amino acids have been classified as being either 'essential' or 'non-essential'. The essential amino acids cannot be synthesised endogenously and are required in the diet, whereas the non-essential amino acids can be synthesised by the human body. Both groups of amino acids, however, are necessary for maintenance of nitrogen balance and normal tissue growth and metabolism. Dietary intake and endogenous synthesis of amino acids in the body maintains the relevant pool of amino acids, replacing those that have been lost as a result of excretion in the urine, from the skin and gastrointestinal tract, utilisation as precursors for non-protein synthetic pathways, irreversible modification and irreducible oxidation (Fig. 3.1).

It has become recognised that under certain circumstances (e.g. sepsis, trauma, growth) the endogenous synthesis of some of the amino acids, which normally are considered to be 'non-essential', is inadequate for the body's nitrogen fluxes. Therefore, unless these amino acids are present in the diet abnormal tissue protein metabolism may occur. These amino acids, therefore, are described as being 'conditionally essential'. It seems likely that only three amino acids (L-alanine, L-glutamate and L-aspartate), which are produced by a simple transamination reaction, are actually non-essential.

Energy requirements

Energy transduction is accomplished by the breakdown of carbohydrate, fat and proteins. The energy available from various common nutrients is: fat, 9.3 kcal g^{-1}; glucose, 4.1 kcal g^{-1}; protein, 4.1 kcal g^{-1}, and alcohol, 7.1 kcal g^{-1}. In some less well developed countries up to 80% of the daily calorie intake may come from carbohydrate, whereas in the Western world, the calorie intake from carbohydrates may be as low as 40%. The principal carbohydrates in the diet are polysaccharides (starch and dietary fibre), dextrins and free sugars (monosaccharides, disaccharides, oligosaccharides and sugar alcohols).

Figure 3.1
Diagrammatic representation of the interorgan fluxes of amino acids between the liver, gut and skeletal muscle.

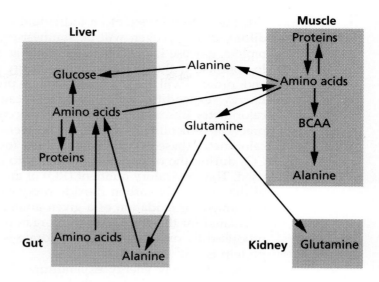

Dietary fat includes triglyceride, containing long-chain fatty acids (C_{16}–C_{18} long-chain triglycerides), and medium-chain fatty acids (C_6–C_{12} medium-chain triglycerides) and cholesterol.

Energy is required for many processes including protein synthesis (tissue and secretory proteins), membrane transport, heat production, secretion and detoxification, and for the function of other organs including muscle. Various tissues in the body will oxidise nutrients (fat, ketone bodies, glucose and amino acids) through the Krebs (tricarboxylic acid) cycle to produce readily transducible forms of energy supply, such as adenosine triphosphate (ATP) (Fig. 3.2).

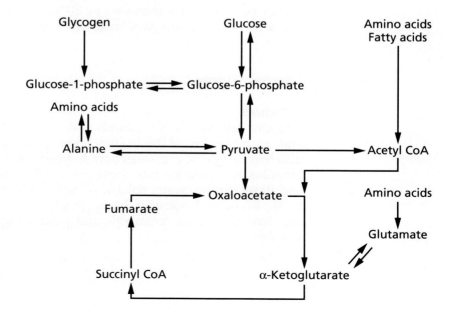

Figure 3.2 *Energy production pathways from the common nutrients.*

If the energy intake of an individual is greater than energy expenditure, then glycogen will be synthesised; when glycogen stores are replete, glucose is metabolised to fatty acids and fat synthesis occurs. In contrast, if there is a negative energy balance, then fat, glycogen and protein will be broken down to provide the required energy. Energy expenditure of individuals can be calculated by direct calorimetry (measuring the heat produced by the body), but this has practical difficulties and may take several hours. Therefore, indirect calorimetry (based on the requirement for oxygen and production of CO_2 during the oxidation of nutrients to produce heat) is more often used. The respiratory quotient (RQ) of an energy substrate is the ratio of the volume of carbon dioxide produced to the volume of oxygen consumed for oxidation of a given amount of a nutrient. This can be calculated for the whole body, an organ or individual tissues. The RQ produced by oxidation of carbohydrate is 1, that of fat is 0.70 and of protein is 0.8.[4]

The total daily energy expenditure (TEE) is made up of different components. The basal metabolic rate (BMR) is defined as the energy expenditure of a person at rest, living in a thermoneutral environment, at least 12 hours after the last meal. This is influenced by the individual's age, sex, body size, nutritional state, hormonal status, geographical or genetic factors and body composition. Physical activity is an important consideration in energy expenditure and may account for 20–40% of the TEE. In addition, food ingestion also will result in an increase in energy expenditure. This has been called the specific dynamic action of food, postprandial thermogenesis or diet-induced thermogenesis, and accounts for approximately 10% of the TEE. Under normal circumstances, approximately 25–30 kcal kg^{-1} body weight are required every day. In hypermetabolic conditions this can be increased substantially. For example, following elective abdominal surgery the energy requirement is increased by 20%, in severe sepsis by up to 50% and with severe burns may increase by up to 100%.

Micronutrients

Vitamins
Vitamins are organic compounds that are essential for normal growth and maintenance of body functions, playing key roles in many different metabolic processes both in health and in disease. In general, vitamins are classified into those that are fat soluble (A, D, E and K), and those that are water soluble (C and the B vitamins (folic acid, B_{12}, B_1, B_2, B_3, pantothenic acid, biotin and B_6)). The sources, requirements and functions of the fat-soluble and water-soluble vitamins are listed in Tables 3.1 and 3.2.

Table 3.1 *Fat-soluble vitamins: sources, functions and requirements*

Vitamin	Daily requirements	Sources in diet	Functions
A (retinol)	250–700 μg	Carotene, fish, dairy produce	Stabilises epithelial cell membranes, stimulates epithelialisation, fibroblast differentiation and collagen secretion; necessary for rod vision. Stored in the liver (3–12 month supply), released as retinol and bound to retinol binding protein in the circulation.
D	0–10 μg	Synthesis by skin, vegetables, dairy produce	Role in regulation of calcium and phosphate metabolism, stimulates reabsorption of calcium and phosphate from gut and kidney. Body stores can last for several months, deficiencies result in rickets and osteomalacia.
E	10–15 mg	Vegetables	α-tocopherol is the main form of vitamin E, found mainly in fat and located predominantly in the cell membrane. Important in free radical scavenging and prevention of peroxidation of lipids in cell membranes by various oxidants. Stimulates phagocytosis and other aspects of immune function. Deficiency in adults results in peripheral nerve damage, haemolysis, anaemia and platelet aggregation.
K	1 μg kg^{-1}	Vegetables, liver	Required for hepatic synthesis of clotting factors II, VII, IX, X, by acting as a coenzyme for γ-glutamyl carboxylase. Minimal storage in the body (lung and liver), but is also manufactured by intestinal bacteria.

Adapted from: The Principles and Scientific Basis of Surgical Practice, Oxford University Press, in press.

Trace elements

Trace elements are inorganic elements that are also important in the regulation of many metabolic processes.[5] The requirements for health and the functions of the trace elements are detailed in Table 3.3.

It should be remembered that micronutrients, if given at high doses, can be toxic to tissues and organs. In particular, toxicity can be a problem with excess vitamins A and D, iron, selenium, zinc and copper. Care must be taken, therefore, when these micronutrients are provided for a prolonged period to patients.

Table 3.2 *Water-soluble vitamins: sources, requirements and function*

Vitamin	Daily requirements	Sources in diet	Functions
Thiamine	0.4 mg/1000 kcal	Plants, bacteria, pork	Metabolised to a coenzyme (thiamine pyrophosphate) involved in carbohydrate metabolism and synthesis of ATP and NAD. Also plays a role in nerve conduction. Deficiency results in Wernicke's encephalopathy. In severe cases, high output cardiac failure can occur.
Riboflavin (B_2)	1.3 mg	Plants, meat, bacteria	Precursor of coenzymes (flavin mononucleotide, flavin adenine dinucleotide), involved in oxidative metabolism. Deficiency results in angular stomatitis, cheilosis.
Pyridoxine (B_6)	2.0 mg	Vegetables, meat	Precursor for pyridoxal phosphate which is a coenzyme for amino acid deamination and transamination. Deficiency occurs after 3 weeks of a deficient diet, resulting in cheilosis and angular stomatitis, anaemia, neuropathy, skin rashes.
Cobalamine (B_{12})	5 μg	Animal tissues, fish	Important component of coenzymes involved in protein, fat and nucleic acid metabolism. Stored in the liver (adequate supplies for 3 years). Deficiency results in pernicious anaemia and neurological symptoms (affecting the posterior columns).
Ascorbic acid	40 mg	Fruit, vegetables	Important in hydroxylation reactions (e.g. prolene to hydroxyprolene), electron transport; is an antioxidant. It is also important in wound healing, immune function and the maintenance of vascular integrity and for iron absorption. Deficiency results in scurvy.
Folic acid	200 μg	Green vegetables, fruit, meat	Converted into active forms (dihydrofolate and tetrahydrofolate). Required for synthesis of purines and pyrimidines, amino acid metabolism and red blood cell maturation.
Niacin	6.6 mg/1000 kcal	Meat, cereals, vegetables	Is a precursor for the coenzymes NAD, NADP, which are required for a variety of oxidation/ reduction reactions involved in carbohydrate and protein metabolism and respiration.
Biotin	10–200 μg	Meat, vegetables	Is a cofactor for enzymes involved in decarboxylation of fat and carbohydrates. Also required for the initiation of fatty acid synthesis

Adapted from: The Principles and Scientific Basis of Surgical Practice, Oxford University Press (in press).

Table 3.3 *Trace elements: requirements and functions*

Trace element	Daily requirements	Functions
Iron	10–18 mg	Body contains up to 5 g, 65% in haem, 30% in the reticulo-endothelial system as ferritin, 10% in myoglobin. It is absorbed from the small intestine predominantly as the Fe^{2+} form, transported in circulation by transferrin and stored in the tissues bound to ferritin or haemosiderin. It is a key component of enzymes and proteins involved in energy transfer and oxygen transport (e.g. haemoglobin, myoglobin, cytochromes, flavoproteins) and is an antioxidant. Deficiency results in hypochromic microcytic anaemia.
Copper	2–3 mg	Body contains 150 mg, 90% in liver, bone and muscle. Cofactor in many enzymes, (e.g. cytochrome *c* oxidase and superoxide dismutase), involved in electron transfer, free radical scavaging and collagen synthesis. Transported bound to albumin and incorporated into caeruloplasmin in the liver. Caeruloplasmin also oxidises the ferrous to the ferric ion to allow its transport by ferritin. Vitamin C impairs its bioactivity and zinc and phytates impair its absorption from the gut. Deficiency may result in hypochromic anaemia and defects in collagen synthesis.
Zinc	15 mg	Body contains 1.5–3 g of zinc, predominantly in bones, teeth and soft tissues. Bound to albumin and globulins in circulation. Cofactor in more than 100 enzymes which are involved in protein and nucleic acid synthesis – DNA, RNA polymerase and metallo-enzymes. Required for tissue healing and immune function. It may also be an antioxidant. Chronic deficiency results in acrodermatitis enteropathica (skin rashes, diarrhoea, hair loss).
Manganese	2.5–5.0 mg	Body contains 10–20 mg, mainly in mitochondria. Cofactor in many enzymes (arginase, pyruvate carboxylase, DNA, RNA polymerases, and enzymes required for polysaccharide synthesis). Potentiates iron deficiency by competing for binding sites in intestinal absorption. Deficiency results in skin changes, skeletal abnormalities and anaemia.
Selenium	50–200 µg	Absorbed from the duodenum and transported in the circulation bound to low- and very low-density lipoproteins. It is used to synthesise selenoamino acids which are required for the synthesis of the antioxidant enzyme glutathione peroxidase which protects cell membranes against peroxidation, and is also necessary for prostaglandin metabolism. Deficiency is rare but may result in muscle pain and cardiomyopathy.
Iodine	0.15 mg	Body contains 10–20 mg, mainly in the thyroid gland. Required for the synthesis of thryoid hormones and deficiency results in goitre and hypothyroidism.
Chromium	50–200 µg	Absorbed from the small intestine and bound to transferrin. Main function is to potentiate the action of insulin.
Molybdenum	0.2–5 mg	This is a cofactor in xanthine oxidase, sulphate oxidase, aldehyde oxidase.

Adapted from: The Principles and Scientific Basis of Surgical Practice, Oxford University Press (in press).

Table 3.4 *Absorption of nutrients by the gastrointestinal tract*

Absorption of	Upper small intestine	Mid small intestine	Lower small intestine	Colon
Sugars (glucose, galactose etc.)	++	+++	++	–
Amino acids	++	+++	++	–
Water-soluble vitamins	+++	++	–	–
Pyrimidines	+	+	?	?
Fatty acid absorption and conversion into triglycerides	+++	++	+	–
Bile salts	+	+	+++	
Vitamin B_{12}	–	+	+++	–
Na^+	+++	++	+++	+++
K^+	+	+	+	sec
Ca^{2+}	+++	++	+	?
Fe^{2+}	+++	++	+	?
Cl^-	+++	++	+	+
SO_4^{2-}	++	+	–	?

Amount of absorption is graded from + to +++; sec, secreted when intraluminal K^+ is less than 25 mm; ? not known.

Reproduced from: Ganong WF. Review of medical physiology, Norwalk, CT: Appleton & Lange, 1995 (with permission).

Absorption of nutrients by the gastrointestinal tract

Absorption of nutrients occurs in the gastrointestinal tract following breakdown of ingested food into a variety of smaller molecules. These are discussed in more detail below and summarised in Table 3.4.

Amino acids

Protein in the gastrointestinal tract is derived from several sources: the ingestion of food, shedding of intestinal epithelial cells into the gut lumen, and secretion of proteins into the gut. These various proteins are initially broken down by enzymes present within the lumen of the gastrointestinal tract. In the stomach, proteins are enzymatically digested by gastric pepsins, and then by the pancreatic peptidases (trypsin, chymotrypsin, elastase, carboxypeptidases), and aminopeptidases of the brush border of the intestinal lumen. In addition, the brush border of the intestinal lumen also has dipeptidases to hydrolyse dipeptides.

As a result of the actions of these enzymes, there is a release of free amino acids and small peptides, two to six amino acid residues in length. These are then absorbed across the brush border of the intestinal epithelium by carrier-mediated processes (active transport mechanism in which amino acids are usually co-transported with sodium). There are four main sodium-dependent transport systems, in the intestinal epithelial cells which transport certain groups of amino acids: (1) neutral amino acids, (2) dibasic amino acids and L-cystine, (3) glycine, L-proline and L-hydroxyproline and (4) acidic amino acids.[6] There is a separate transport mechanism for the absorption of di- and tripeptides, which are then quickly broken down by intracellular peptidase enzymes to produce free amino acids. These amino acids then diffuse into the extracellular fluid by passive diffusion and facilitated diffusion. Their absorption is most rapid in the duodenum and proximal jejunum, but is slower in the ileum. In addition, there is a significant absorption of amino acids (derived from intestinal secretions and desquamated intestinal epithelial cells) occurring in the colon, with the colonic microflora digesting these proteins. Approximately 50% of the digested protein comes from ingested food substances, 25% from digestive juice proteins and 25% from desquamated intestinal mucosal cells.

Absorption of fats
Dietary fat is liquidised within the stomach as a result of its temperature, and emulsified by agitation. Lipases (from tongue, stomach and pancreas, aided by pancreatic colipase, digest the triglycerides to di-, then monoglyceride (thus releasing fatty acids). Cholesterol esterase (also from the pancreas) hydrolyses cholesterol esters. The products of digestion of fat, mainly monoglycerides, combine with bile acids, cholesterol (from bile) and phospholipids, to form water-soluble micelles. They are then transported to the intestinal brush border and absorbed. Triglycerides are then re-formed from long-chain fatty acids (shorter chains of 12 or less passing in the free form into the portal circulation). This triglyceride and cholesterol (some re-esterified), forms chylomicrons which enter lacteals and drain into the thoracic duct. Normally, over 98% of dietary fat is absorbed; the small amount in the stool is derived predominantly from desquamated epithelial cells and intestinal microorganisms.

Absorption of vitamins
The fat-soluble vitamins are also dependent on their solubilisation in micelles for absorption from the intestine. It is thought that these vitamins may be hydrolysed prior to absorption. However, if there is impairment of fat absorption then uptake of these vitamins from the gut is also reduced. The absorption of water-soluble vitamins is rapid, with most of the vitamins being absorbed in the upper small intestine. Vitamin B_{12}, however, is absorbed in the distal ileum, after binding to intrinsic factor which is produced by the stomach.

Absorption of carbohydrates
The main carbohydrates in the diet are starches (polysaccharides), lactose and sucrose (disaccharides) and glucose and fructose (monosaccharides). A number of enzymes are involved in carbohydrate

breakdown – amylases (from saliva and pancreas), α-limit dextrinases (from the succus entericus intestinal of the mucosa in the gut lumen), sucrase, lactase, maltase (in the brush border of the intestinal epithelial cells). The resultant hexose and pentose monosaccharides are rapidly absorbed by the small intestine in conjunction with sodium ions, via active transport processes. A small amount of starch and non-starch polysaccharides enter the colon and are metabolised by the colonic microorganisms which ferment them. This results in the production of short-chain fatty acids (e.g. acetate, propionate and butyrate) and various gases (e.g. CO_2, H_2, CH_4).

The metabolic response to trauma and sepsis

Following trauma, a complex series of changes in tissue metabolism occurs. It is noteworthy that John Hunter recognised that changes in the body occurred in tissues distant to the site of trauma over 200 years ago. Subsequently, Claude Bernard demonstrated that the circulating blood glucose concentration was increased following injury. A major advance in the understanding of these changes took place more than 50 years ago when David Cuthbertson described the loss of nitrogen from skeletal muscle that occurred following traumatic injury (in patients who had sustained long bone fractures).[7] In addition, there was an associated loss of potassium, phosphorus, sulphur and zinc in the urine. He concluded that the response to injury could be considered as occurring in two phases: (1) the 'ebb' phase, which is a short-lived response associated with hypovolaemic shock, increased sympathetic nervous system activity and a reduced metabolic rate, and, (2) the 'flow' phase, which is associated with a loss of body nitrogen and resultant negative nitrogen balance (Fig. 3.3).

These changes result in an increased resting energy expenditure (REE), increased heat production, pyrexia, increased muscle catabolism and wasting and loss of body nitrogen, increased glucose production, glucose intolerance, increased breakdown of fat and reduced fat synthesis. The role of hormones and cytokines, which are important mediators of these changes, are being understood and elucidated. These are discussed in more detail below.

Mediation of the responses to trauma

The central nervous system and the neuroendocrine axis play key roles in mediating the metabolic changes that occur following trauma. Initial experiments carried out in animal models demonstrated that unless the central nervous system was intact (at least to the level of the midbrain) the hormonal responses that occur following trauma could not be triggered. The sympathetic–adrenal axis is responsible for initiating these responses. Afferent nerve impulses also stimulate the hypothalamus to secrete hypothalamic releasing factors which, in turn, stimulate the pituitary gland to release prolactin, vasopressin, growth hormone and adrenocorticotrophic hormone.

Figure 3.3
Diagrammatic representation of the ebb and flow phases in the metabolic response to injury.

(Reproduced with permission from Broom J. Sepsis and trauma. In: Garrow J, James WPT (eds) Human nutrition and dietetics. Edinburgh: Churchill Livingstone, 1993.)

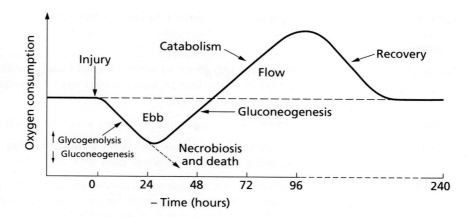

The changes in hormone levels in plasma following trauma are outlined in Table 3.5. The so-called stress hormones (adrenaline, cortisol and glucagon) play a key role in these responses and the changes they elicit are shown in Table 3.6. Studies in human volunteers have shown that many of the metabolic changes that occur following trauma are induced by intravenous infusions of cortisol, adrenaline and glucagon.

Energy expenditure

Following trauma, increases in the resting energy expenditure (REE), which is defined as the summation of the basal energy expenditure and the energy required to maintain normal body functions, have been found to occur. In patients undergoing hip arthroplasty, for example, there may be a modest increase in REE (up to 5–10%), but in patients with severe trauma this is usually more pronounced. An increase of up to 30% may be seen in patients with peritonitis, and up to 100% increase in patients with severe burns. The maximal rise in REE has been shown to correlate with the maximal increase in protein breakdown, which occurs approximately 1 week after the traumatic event. The reasons for this increased REE have not been fully clarified but it may be due to one or more of the following: (1) increased oxygen utilisation by tissues which have been traumatised; (2) increased energy expenditure by other organs such as the heart; (3) so called 'futile cycling' which involves the breakdown and synthesis of glucose and triglycerides, but without any apparent gain in stored glucose or fat, and the dissipation of energy as heat. Under normal physiological conditions, 'futile cycling' is termed substrate cycling and is part of normal metabolic control.

Protein metabolism

The increased loss of nitrogen following trauma arises as a result of protein breakdown occurring at a rate in excess of synthesis. Some studies of whole body protein metabolism have suggested that after elective surgical operations, whole body protein synthesis is decreased

Table 3.5 *Changes in hormone levels in plasma following trauma*

Hormone	Changes
Catcholamines	Increases in concentrations of adrenaline and noradrenaline rapidly within a few minutes of injury due to increased activity of sympathetic nervous system. Levels returns to normal within 24 h.
Glucagon	Rises within a few hours; maximal levels at 12–48 h post-trauma.
Insulin	Initially plasma levels are low following trauma, but rise to above normal levels reaching a maximum several days after the injury.
Cortisol	Rapid increase in cortisol (due to stimulation by ACTH), returning to normal 24–48 h later; may remain elevated for up to several days. Has 'permissive' effects with other hormones such as catecholamines.
Growth hormone	Levels increased following trauma, usually return to normal levels within 24 h.
Thyroid hormones	Following trauma, systemic thyroxine level is normal but tri-iodothyronine is low and reverse tri-iodothyronine is high.
Renin, aldosterone	Aldosterone levels increased after trauma, returning to normal within 12 h. Its secretion is stimulated by renin which in turn is produced in response to reduced renal perfusion.
Testosterone	Plasma levels fall after trauma and may remain low for up to 7 days.
Vasopressin	Plasma levels rise following trauma and may remain elevated for several days.
Prolactin	Secretion increased following trauma but function in trauma is unknown.

but there is no change in protein breakdown.[8] By contrast, in more severe trauma there is an increase in whole body protein synthesis but this is associated with an even greater rise in breakdown. The changes in protein metabolism in individual tissues, mainly skeletal muscle (the major store of protein) and liver, have been studied in some detail (Fig. 3.4).

Skeletal muscle contains 80% of the body's free amino acid pool, of which 60% is glutamine.[9] Following trauma, there is a generalised increase in breakdown of skeletal muscle protein, raising the intra-cellular concentration of free amino acids. This increase is particularly with amino acids of the aromatic and branched chain series which may be used as a fuel source within the myocyte. At the same time, the efflux of amino acids into the circulation is increased, particularly of the non-essential amino acids alanine and glutamine (which comprise 70% of the total amino acids released).[10] These latter amino acids are formed from other amino acids as a result of transamination and deamination reactions. The increased release of amino acids are used for (1) synthesis of proteins necessary for structural repair in the traumatised area, (2) hepatic production of proteins with immuno-

Table 3.6 *Factors responsible for the metabolic changes occurring following trauma*

Metabolic alterations	Factor responsible
Decreased ketone body production	Increased systemic insulin and adrenaline
Increased lipolysis	Increased systemic catecholamines, cortisol, glucagon, growth hormone, and insulin suppression
Increased hepatic glycogenolysis	Enhanced sympathetic activity, circulating catecholamines, and increased glucagon
Increased gluconeogenesis	Increased circulating catecholamines and corticosteroids
Inhibition of insulin release	Enhanced sympathetic activity and circulating catecholamines
Decreased peripheral utilisation of glucose	Insulin resistance, and increased systemic corticosteroids
Release of amino acids from muscle	Increased systemic corticosteroids, adrenaline, glucagon (other unknown factors)

logical or tissue repair functions, (3) hepatic production of glucose from alanine, (4) alternative energy substrates for the gut (e.g. L-glutamine).

The intracellular concentration of L-glutamine in skeletal muscle falls by approximately 50% after trauma with its release in to the circulation. A key role for L-glutamine is its utilisation by the gut and other rapidly proliferating tissues (for example lymphocytes) as a fuel.[11] In addition, it is converted into L-alanine and L-citrulline in the gut. It has also been suggested that this reduction in intracellular L-glutamine may be responsible for the decrease in skeletal muscle protein synthesis occurring after trauma.[12] In addition, some studies have demonstrated that there is a negative correlation between skeletal muscle intracellular L-glutamine levels and mortality following trauma. In the liver, there is an increased synthesis of both structural and acute phase proteins (for example C-reactive protein).

Fat metabolism

After trauma, there is an increase in the turnover of fatty acids and glycerol. Lipolysis of triglycerides (sometimes referred to as triacylglycerols) is increased with the production of free fatty acids and glycerol. Some is oxidised in the adipocyte, the remainder being released with a resultant rise in circulating concentrations, fatty acids in the circulation being carried by albumin. The glycerol can be used by the liver for gluconeogenesis and the fatty acids can also be used as a fuel source (e.g. one molecule of palmitic acid giving rise

Figure 3.4
Relationship between nitrogen losses and degree of injury stress.

(Reproduced with permission from Broom J. Sepsis and trauma. In: Garrow J, James WPT (eds) Human nutrition and dietetics. Edinburgh: Churchill Livingstone, 1993.)

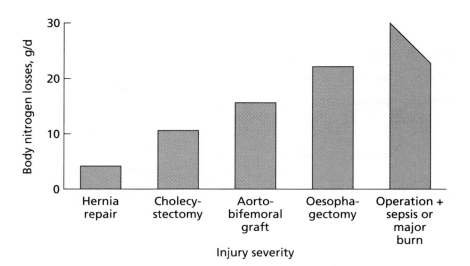

to 129 molecules of ATP), although mammals cannot synthesise glucose from fatty acids. However, this response may be complicated by other factors. For example, hypovolaemic shock will induce a lactic acidosis which results in an increased re-esterification of triglycerides, with a rise in plasma levels.[13] There is an increase in the rate of oxidation of fatty acids (and ketogenesis).[14] Ketone body production is dependent on the patient's intravenous fluid support. If carbohydrate is not available, ketogenesis is increased and ketone bodies are used as fuels by the peripheral tissues in preference to glucose. However, if patients are receiving intravenous infusions of dextrose then this response is ablated.

Carbohydrate metabolism

Glucose is the main fuel used for many different tissues. It is obtained by absorption from the gastrointestinal tract, endogenous production from glycogen (glycogenolysis) or from other precursors such as amino acids (gluconeogenesis). Glucose can be utilised for energy transduction aerobically (each molecule producing 38 molecules of ATP and six each of carbon dioxide and water) or anaerobically (producing two molecules of both ATP and lactate) or converted into glycogen or fat. The anaerobic pathway is considerably less efficient, but allows for very rapid energy transduction during short periods of relative hypoxia.

Following trauma, there is an increase in the hepatic glycogen breakdown (caused by increased sympathetic activity).[15] These stores are substantially depleted within 24 h (although not usually completely depleted unless there is continuing catecholamine drive, for example in severe burns or sepsis).[16] There is also an associated reduction in the peripheral utilisation of glucose. This results in an increase in plasma glucose concentration and an increase in insulin release.

The rate of production of glucose is inversely linked to plasma glucose concentration. In some patients who have been traumatised, however, the liver produces glucose at an increased rate under the influence of hormones and cytokines such as glucagon and interleukin 1 (IL1). Production of glucose is, therefore, increased despite an increased blood glucose concentration. Similarly, endogenous production by the liver is not suppressed to the same extent by exogenous glucose administration.[17] The breakdown of glycogen in the liver is only one pathway for glucose production and is limited in duration. Other pathways for the production of glucose are (1) conversion of lactate (in the Cori cycle), (2) synthesis from pyruvate, and (3) produced from amino acids (e.g. L-alanine and L-glutamine).[18]

Resistance to insulin occurs in patients who have been injured. The circulating concentrations of glucose and insulin are both elevated following injury, but there is a more marked rise in insulin concentrations. The circulating insulin level usually reaches a maximum several days after the injury, before returning towards normal basal levels. In addition, there is a decrease in peripheral glucose utilisation by the tissues and it has been suggested that glucose oxidation may be less efficient in patients who have been injured. It has been suggested that these changes are a mechanism to maintain the availability of glucose.

Figure 3.5
Differences between the metabolic response to trauma, starvation and sepsis.

(Reproduced with permission from Broom J. Sepsis and trauma. In: Garrow J, James WPT (eds) Human nutrition and dietetics. Edinburgh: Churchill Livingstone, 1993.)

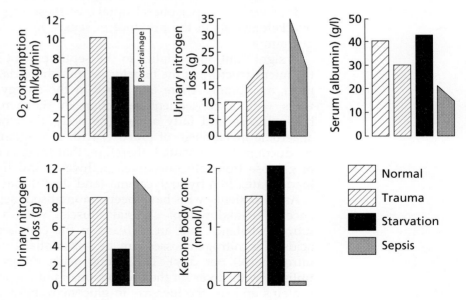

Sepsis

The metabolic response to sepsis is also characterised by alterations in protein, carbohydrate and fat metabolism. However, the changes occurring in patients with sepsis have defined differences, when compared with those occurring in response to trauma (Fig. 3.5).[19]

In patients who are septic, there is an increased production of glucose by the liver (e.g. both gluconeogenesis and glycogenolysis) resulting in an elevated plasma glucose concentration. There is an increased rate of glucose uptake and oxidation by the peripheral tissues. The septic patient, however, may also become 'insulin resistant'. In this state, despite elevated levels of insulin, the production of glucose by the liver is not suppressed nor is the peripheral uptake of glucose enhanced.

There continues to be a debate as to the changes that occur in the metabolism of free fatty acids. Some studies have observed that the circulating levels of free fatty acids increase in patients with sepsis, whereas other authors have found decreases.[20] The reasons for these differences may possibly be explained by the differing times during the septic episode at which concentrations were measured. There is, however, an increase in breakdown of fat stores in adipose tissue by lipolysis. This occurs as a result of an increased activity of hormone-sensitive lipase, whose activity is stimulated by catecholamines. In addition, there is hypertriglyceridaemia, with an increased production of very low density lipoprotein triglyceride by the liver. There is also a decrease in the peripheral uptake of these triglycerides and defective ketogenesis in the presence of sepsis, in contrast to the situation in trauma.

A significant abnormality in the septic patient is the disruption of the microstructure of the hepatocyte mitochondria, in particular, of the inner membrane. There is a block in the energy transduction pathways with a consequent reduction in the aerobic metabolism of both glucose and fatty acids. The body, therefore, depends on the anaerobic metabolism of glucose, with a resultant increase in lactate production. It is essential, therefore, that there is an adequate supply of glucose from gluconeogenic pathways, and if this is impaired or inadequate, then hypoglycaemia (and death) may ensue.

As in patients who have been traumatised, septic patients experience a breakdown of skeletal muscle, with a resultant negative nitrogen balance and an increase in the circulating levels of amino acids. The nitrogen losses can be substantial (more than 15–20 g of nitrogen (N) per day). The amino acids released from muscle are utilised by the liver for the production of both acute phase and visceral proteins and for the increase in gluconeogenesis that is required.

Assessment of nutritional status

A reliable and reproducible assessment of nutritional status has proved difficult to identify and, as yet, there is no definitive test. However, assessment may be considered to have two components. First, there is the determination of body composition (the content of protein, fat, carbohydrate, vitamins, water, etc.) and secondly, an evaluation of organ and cellular function (skeletal and respiratory muscle function, immune responses, synthesis of certain proteins). These components of nutritional status will each be discussed in more detail below.

Assessment of body composition

Anthropometric indices

Height and weight

Height and weight are some of the most commonly used indices of nutritional status. A body weight value for a particular patient can be compared with a series of standard values in order to assess the degree of leanness or adiposity. The tables most commonly used are those of the Metropolitan Life Assurance Company.[21] These tables refer to 'frame size' but do not give any information as to the criteria for selection of 'frame size'. Some would suggest, therefore, that these tables should not be used for assessing nutritional status in the clinical situation. The Quatelet Index, defined as weight/height,[2] has been used with increasing frequency and has been suggested to be the best anthropometric indicator of total body fat in adults.

Loss of body weight has been used as an indicator of nutritional status. This loss of body weight is usually determined by subtracting the patient's current weight from either their recall weight when they were 'well', or, if this cannot be determined, from their 'ideal' weight which is obtained from published tables. Although patients' recall of weight can be inaccurate, the loss of more than 10% of body weight, or more than 4.5 kg of their recall weight, is associated with a significant increase in postoperative mortality in patients undergoing surgery. Furthermore, the shorter the period of time over which weight is lost, the more significant this is in predicting an increased risk of postoperative complications. Some authors have utilised a combination of both these absolute weights and rate of weight loss in an attempt to improve accuracy in identifying patients who are malnourished. For example, Pettigrew[22] has suggested that malnutrition is defined as a body mass index of less than the 10th percentile with a weight loss of 5% or more.

Subcutaneous fat thickness

Techniques have been developed to measure total body fat, such as body densitometry, isotope dilution techniques, inert gas uptake, isotopic determinations of total body water and potassium, and soft tissue imaging. These techniques have various difficulties which have limited their use in clinical situations. However, the most commonly used index of total body fat is skinfold thickness. Approximately 50% of the total body fat is in the subcutaneous layer, although it varies in thickness depending on age, sex and which particular fat pad is measured. Therefore, although the triceps skin-fold thickness is the one most commonly measured, assessment of skin folds at multiple sites has become increasingly common, and has a good correlation with total body fat content. Regression equations for the estimation of total body fat from these measurements have been developed.[23] It has been shown that this is an accurate way of measuring total body fat. However, measurements of skin-fold thicknesses are particularly susceptible to intra- and interobserver variability and may be particularly difficult in patients who are very obese or are oedematous. Therefore, when such measurements are being used it is important that the observer is trained correctly, and that sequential measurements are carried out by the same individual.

Mid-arm circumference of mid-arm muscle area

The mid-upper arm circumference (MUAC) and mid-arm muscle area have been used as an index of protein/energy malnutrition and as an index of skeletal muscle mass in ill patients:[24]

$$\text{Arm muscle area} = (\text{MUAC} - \pi)^2 / 4\pi$$

This equation assumes that both the arm and arm muscles are circular and that the bone area can be neglected. However, the arm and arm muscle are fusiform and measurements of circumference and skin-fold thickness, therefore, must be taken at the same level. In addition, it has been demonstrated that assessments of lean body mass using these measurements may overestimate this by up to 25%. However, other studies have failed to demonstrate a correlation between total body nitrogen content and muscle circumferences. Furthermore, there is an interobserver variation of up to 33% in arm muscle area calculated.

Chemical analyses

More complicated techniques for assessing the body's different compartments (e.g. fat, fat-free mass, total body nitrogen and total body mineral contents) have also become available although these often require specialised equipment and may not be readily applicable to clinical practice, especially in critically ill patients. Relatively simple techniques, such as bioelectrical impedance, are easily used in clinical practice. Other techniques, such as dual-energy X-ray absorptiometry, total body water, total body potassium and *in vivo* neutron activation analysis currently have limited application to clinical practice but are valuable research tools.

Bioelectrical impedance

This entails the passage of an alternating electrical current between electrodes attached to the hand and foot. The current passes through the water and electrolyte compartment of lean tissues and the drop in voltage between the two electrodes is measured.[25] This change in voltage gives an estimation of total body resistance, which depends principally on the total body water and electrolyte content, i.e. lean body mass. The passage of current through the intracellular fluid compartment is impeded by the non-conductive cell membrane. This gives rise to a 'phase-shift' and a decrease in current at low (<1 kHz) frequencies. At higher frequencies (>50 kHz), current will be less impeded. Although bioelectrical impedance is an accurate measure of body composition in stable subjects, it becomes less reliable in patients with oedema and electrolyte shifts, and its value in critically ill patients is unclear.[26]

Biochemical indices

Serum proteins

Albumin is the major protein in serum. The total body content of albumin is approximately 350 g. It is produced by the liver at the rate of approximately 1.5 g per day. The relationship between serum protein concentration and protein/energy malnutrition was first recognized over 150 years ago.[27] Subsequently, serum albumin concentration has been used in population studies as an indicator of visceral protein depletion and studies have shown that low serum albumin levels are associated with an increased risk of complications in patients undergoing surgery.[28]

A low serum albumin has been demonstrated to correlate with a low dietary protein intake.[29] In experimental starvation, however, serum albumin levels may not fall for several weeks,[30] because although synthesis decreases, only 30% of the total exchangeable albumin is in the intravascular space with the remainder being in the extravascular compartment. In addition, albumin has a relatively long half-life of approximately 21 days. It has been suggested that the extravascular compartment replenishes the intravascular pool, which then only falls when this can no longer occur. In fact, it has been estimated that the flux of albumin between the intravascular and extravascular compartments is about ten times the rate of albumin synthesis.[31] Serum albumin is also lowered in malignancy, trauma and sepsis, despite an adequate intake, and hence it should not be used as an assessment of nutritional state.

Alternatives to using albumin as a marker of nutritional status by measuring other serum protein concentrations have been evaluated. These are transferrin (half-life ($t_{1/2}$), 7 days), retinol binding protein ($t_{1/2}$, 1–2 h) and pre-albumin ($t_{1/2}$, 2 days). The changes in their serum concentrations should, therefore, more accurately reflect acute changes in nutritional state than does albumin. The serum levels of these proteins are, however, also altered in stress, sepsis and cancer, and this must be considered when interpreting data containing such information. Thus, it may be that the levels of these serum proteins are an index of illness severity rather than nutritional status. Proteins other than those already discussed have been used as indices of nutritional status. One example is C-reactive protein (CRP) whose levels change by a factor of thousands following injury. Although the magnitude of the rise in CRP following surgery is affected by nutritional status,[32] its serum levels are thought to be a better indicator of an inflammatory response rather than nutritional status, hence it is useful in interpreting the levels of other proteins.

Creatinine

Skeletal muscle contains both creatine and creatinine. The 24 h urinary excretion of creatinine has also been used as a marker for body muscle mass, because it is derived from muscle creatine. The 'creatinine height index' (CHI) – the ratio of 24 h urinary creatinine to that expected from a normal subject of the same height and sex – has been used in assessments of nutritional status.[33] A ratio of 60–80% indicates moderate depletion of skeletal muscle, and if less than 60%, indicates severe depletion. However, although some studies have demonstrated that CHI does predict which patients experience complications, others have failed to show this relationship, possibly because of the potential errors involved in urine collections. Accurate 24 h urine collections are difficult to obtain and there is a coefficient of variation of 36% in creatinine excretion in samples collected for five days. In addition, ingestion of meat can lead to an increase in urinary creatinine output because of the creatine phosphate content and, therefore, a creatinine-free diet is essential for this type of measurement.

Nitrogen balance

Most of the nitrogen lost from the body is excreted in urine and mainly as urea (approximately 80% of the total urinary nitrogen). Urea alone may be measured as an approximate indicator of losses, or total urinary nitrogen may be measured, although this latter technique is less widely available. In addition, there are also losses of nitrogen from the skin and in stool of approximately 2–4 g per day. One equation used for balance studies is:

$$\text{Nitrogen balance} = (\text{Dietary protein} \times 0.16)$$
$$- (\text{Urea nitrogen (urine)}$$
$$+ 2\,\text{g stool} + 2\,\text{g skin})$$

where urine urea nitrogen (g) = urine urea (mmol) × 28

Although nitrogen balance has not been shown to be a prognostic indicator, it is still an important way of assessing a patient's nutritional requirements and of assessing the response to the provision of nutritional support.

Tests of physiological function

Immune competence

Malnutrition predisposes to abnormalities of immune function. There is a reduction in the total circulating lymphocyte count, impaired lymphocyte responsiveness to mitogens *in vitro*, deficiencies in IgG and complement component C_3, reduction in the production of key cytokines, decreased skin reactivity to mumps, candida and tuberculin antigens and a reduction in the lymphoid cells in the spleen, lymph glands and thymus.[34] A correlation between depressed immune function and postoperative morbidity and mortality in cancer patients has been demonstrated, and a depression of total circulating lymphocyte count is also associated with a poorer prognosis in patients undergoing surgery.[35]

However, these alterations in immune function are non-specific and although they may be prognostic indicators, a variety of factors other than mulnutrition can also modulate the immune response. For example, trauma, surgery, anaesthetic and sedative drugs, pain and psychological stress (all important in the surgical patient) may inhibit various aspects of the immune response.[36] Therefore, tests of immune function are not specific indicators of nutritional status.

Muscle function

Skeletal muscle

Various aspects of skeletal muscle structure and function are deranged in the presence of malnutrition. Skeletal muscle fibres become atrophic (with loss of the fast twitch fibres preferentially) together with degeneration of the Z bands.[37] In addition, there are alterations in pH and electrolyte composition. More importantly, these changes are reflected by alterations in muscle function.

Klidjian *et al.*[38] demonstrated that in patients who were undergoing elective gastrointestinal surgery, measurements of hand grip strength (which are cheap and easy to perform) predicted accurately those patients who subsequently develop postoperative complications (with a sensitivity >90%). However, grip strength may be influenced by other factors such as the patient's motivation and cooperation. Furthermore, such tests may be difficult to apply to patients who are critically ill.

Stimulation of the ulnar nerve at the wrist, with a variable electrical stimulus, results in contraction of the adductor pollicis muscle. The changes in the force frequency curve obtained from this muscle and the measurement of its contraction force and maximal relaxation rate have been shown to reflect nutritional intake.[39] However, it is not clear whether such measurements will identify patients at risk of developing complications.

Respiratory muscle

The function of the respiratory muscles is also impaired by malnutrition and this can be detected by deteriorations in various indices of standard respiratory function tests, in particular vital capacity.[40] Measurements of inspiratory muscle strength have the advantage that they can be performed even in patients who are intubated and who are affected by other intercurrent illnesses.

Prognostic nutritional indices

Combinations of variables used to assess nutritional status have been used in an attempt to predict those patients with an increased risk of postoperative morbidity and mortality. Mullen *et al.*[41] documented such a series of nutritional variables which identified those patients who underwent elective surgery and were at risk from developing postoperative complications. These were: (1) serum albumin less than 30 g l[-1], (2) a serum transferrin concentration less than 220 mg dl[-1], and (3) failure of the immune system to react to skin antigens. A prognostic nutritional index (PNI) was developed using these variables and the same group then applied this to patients undergoing surgery. It was found that if the PNI was greater than 40%, postoperative sepsis was predicted with a sensitivity of 89%. However, less than 50% of those patients who were categorized as high risk using this system actually developed complications.[42] Further studies have suggested that the information provided by the PNI is comparable to that provided by weight loss alone or by serum proteins alone. Therefore, prognostic nutritional indices have had limited application in the general clinical setting.

Subjective global assessment

Subjective global assessment (SGA) evaluates nutritional status by taking into consideration a range of factors. These are: (1) the extent and rate of weight change and alterations in dietary intake, (2) gastrointestinal symptoms, (3) functional capacity, (4) underlying disease, (5) findings on physical examination (muscle wasting, loss of subcutaneous fat, ascites, ankle and sacral oedema), (6) the underlying illness, and the metabolic demands it makes on the patient.

Using this technique, the clinician gives a subjective weighting to each of these factors, but there is the ability to accommodate for interactions between the various factors. For example, weight change may be a less reliable indicator in the presence of oedema. Using the SGA assessment method, patients are categorised as being well nourished, moderately malnourished, or severely malnourished.[43]

Studies of substantial numbers of individuals have demonstrated that patients who fall into the severely malnourished category have complication rates of at least five times that of those in the moderately malnourished group, and approximately ten times that of patients in the well nourished group. Furthermore, others have shown that the time spent in hospital, occurrence of infections and antibiotic usage are also correlated with the nutritional state assessed using this method.[44] The reproducibility of SGA has been demonstrated (agreement on degree of malnutrition in over 80% of cases). However, the role of SGA in evaluating nutritional status in critically ill patients requires further clarification.

How should nutritional status be assessed in clinical practice?

The various techniques for assessing nutritional status have been outlined above. Although they can predict the risks of complications in some (but not all) patients, there is, at present, no reliable technique for assessing nutritional status. Useful indicators for the bedside assessment of nutritional status in clinical practice have been suggested.[45] These include: (1) an estimation of protein and energy balance, (2) assessment of body composition, and most importantly, (3) an evaluation of physiological function. These are described in more detail below.

Protein and energy balance
This can be either an analysis by a dietician or by the clinician assessing the frequency and size of meals eaten by the patient. This information is compared with the patient's rate of loss of body weight.

Assessment of body composition
Loss of body fat can be determined by observing the physical appearance of the patient (loss of body contours) and feeling the patient's skinfolds between the clinician's finger and thumb. In particular, if the dermis can be felt on pinching the biceps and triceps skinfolds, then considerable weight loss has occurred.

The stores of protein in the body can be assessed by examining various muscle groups. Those to be examined are the temporalis, deltoid, suprascapular, infrascapular, biceps and triceps and the interossei of the hands. When the tendons of the muscles are prominent and the bony protuberances of the scapula are obvious, greater than 30% of the total body protein stores have been lost.

Assessment of physiological function
Assessments of function are made by observing the patient's activities. Grip strength can be determined by asking the patient to squeeze the clinician's index and middle fingers for at least 10 s and respiratory function by asking the patient to blow hard on a strip of paper held approximately 10 cm from the patient's lips. The measurement of metabolic expenditure requires specialised equipment, but additional metabolic stresses on the patient can also be determined from clinical examination. Extra metabolic stresses will be occurring if

trauma or surgery has occurred recently, if there is evidence of significant sepsis (elevated temperature and/or white blood cell counts, tachycardia, tachypnoea, positive blood cultures), active inflammatory bowel disease. In addition, patients should be asked about their ability to heal wounds (scratches etc.), changes in exercise tolerance and their 'tiredness'.

Nutritional support in surgical practice

Once a decision has been made that the patient's oral intake of nutrients is insufficient to meet their requirements, nutritional supplementation is required. The route of administration of nutritional support may be through either the gastrointestinal tract (enteral) or the intravenous (parenteral) route. Both of these routes of nutrient delivery have advantages and disadvantages which will be discussed in more detail below. However, in general, the enteral route is the preferred method of nutrient delivery whenever possible.

Enteral nutritional support

If a patient will not or cannot eat enough to meet his/her requirements, but has an intact and functioning gastrointestinal tract, then enteral feeding is the route of choice. However, enteral feeding is contraindicated in patients with intestinal obstruction, paralytic ileus, vomiting or diarrhoea, high output intestinal fistulae or in the presence of major intra-abdominal sepsis. The response of the body to the absorption of nutrients from the intestinal lumen is quite different from that produced by presentation of nutrients via the systemic circulation. For example, glucose that has been absorbed enterally will tend to be stored as hepatic glycogen, whereas glucose entering via the systemic circulation is metabolised to produce lactate. The intestine controls the rate of absorption of the products of digestion. Normally, there are marked fluctuations in the rate of presentation of nutrients to the intestine but, with the assistance of the liver, delivery of substrates into the systemic circulation is maintained at an approximately constant rate. The gut performs a process of 'detoxification' of food, by processing products, in the main via the portal tract. The intestine also performs a significant excretory role in addition to its absorptive functions. A number of substances are secreted in the various fluids of digestion which would otherwise accumulate within the body. An example of failure of such a mechanism is the accumulation of copper in Wilson's disease, where there is failure of copper excretion by the biliary system.

Experimental studies in animals have shown that in the absence of the provision of nutrients into the intestinal lumen changes occur in the intestinal mucosa. There is a loss of height of the villus, a reduction in cellular proliferation and the mucosa becomes atrophic.[46,47] In addition, stimulation of the intestinal tract by nutrients is important for the release of the many gut-related hormones, including those responsible for gut motility and stimulation of production of secretions, which are necessary for normal maintenance of the mucosa. The activities of the enzymes found in association with the mucosa are also reduced and the permeability of the mucosa to macromolecules is increased.[48] The gut also acts as a barrier to bacteria, both physically and by the release of chemical and immunological substances. There is evidence from experimental studies to suggest that atrophy of the intestinal mucosa is associated with loss of intercellular adhesion and the opening of intercellular channels. This is believed to predispose to an increased translocation of bacteria and endotoxin from the gut lumen into the portal venous and lymphatic systems.[49] Loss of gut integrity, therefore, is believed to account for a substantial proportion of septicaemic events in severely ill patients.

Routes of access for enteral nutritional support

Nasoenteric tubes

Nasogastric feeding via fine bore tubes (with an internal diameter of 1–2 mm, and made either of polyvinylchloride (PVC) or polyurethane) may be used in patients who require nutritional support for a short period of time. Large bore tubes (e.g. Anderson or Ryle's tubes) should not be used as they are very uncomfortable and their use may result in trauma to the nose and oropharynx, oesophageal reflux and stricture formation. However, in patients receiving enteral nutritional support with nasoenteric tubes, gastric emptying should be adequate to ensure that there is not an accumulation of the feed within the stomach and that it passes on to the rest of the gastrointestinal tract.

There has been considerable debate as to whether the positioning of the feeding tube beyond the pylorus into the duodenum or jejunum (using guide wires and placed under fluoroscopic or endoscopic control) will result in a reduction in the risks of regurgitation of gastric contents and pulmonary aspiration. In patients with nasogastric tubes, up to 30% will experience aspiration of gastric contents. This is most likely to occur in those patients with impaired gastric motility. In the latter patients the fine bore tube can be manipulated through the pylorus into the duodenum, reducing the risk of gastric aspiration. Other complications associated with the use of nasoenteric tubes include pulmonary atelectasis, oesophageal necrosis and stricture formation, tracheo-oesophageal fistulae, sinusitis and post-cricoid ulceration. Dual lumen tubes are now available which allow feeding into the duodenum whilst aspirating from the stomach, thus reducing the risk of aspiration.

Gastrostomy techniques

Gastrostomy has been performed for more than 100 years in clinical practice. A gastrostomy tube is placed into the stomach either at the time of laparotomy, or more recently by using percutaneous endoscopic or percutaneous fluoroscopic techniques.

Percutaneous endoscopic gastrostomy Percutaneous endoscopic gastrostomy allows the insertion of a feeding tube directly into the stomach without the patient requiring a laparotomy. It was initially described by Gauderer *et al.*[50] approximately 15 years ago, but many variations of the original technique are used in clinical practice. An upper gastrointestinal endoscopy is performed and the stomach is distended with air so that the anterior gastric wall is pushed up against the anterior abdominal wall. The endoscope is then turned within the stomach so that the anterior stomach wall is illuminated and the endoscope light can be seen shining through the anterior abdominal wall. The skin of the abdominal wall is then prepared with antiseptic solution and an incision in the skin (under local anaesthesia) is made directly over the point of light that can be seen through the abdominal wall. An intravenous cannula can then be pushed through this incision, traversing the abdominal and stomach walls straight into the lumen of the stomach. The needle is withdrawn from the cannula and a fine suture passed through the cannula, into the stomach. This suture can then be grasped by forceps that have been inserted through the gastroscope. The gastroscope, forceps and suture are removed from the stomach and oesophagus. The next step is to attach the suture to the gastrostomy tube. The gastrostomy tube is then pulled into the stomach by traction on the suture until the tube abuts against the intravenous cannula which is still positioned in the stomach. Both the cannula and external portion of the gastrostomy tube are then withdrawn through the abdominal wall and the tube can then be sutured to the abdominal wall. Patients are given prophylactic broad-spectrum antibiotic cover for this procedure.

An alternative technique is to pass a flexible wire through the cannula into the stomach. It can then be grasped by the forceps and pulled out through the patient's mouth. A special gastrostomy tube can then be threaded over the wire into the stomach until it abuts against the cannula. The abdominal operator can then pull both the cannula and tube out through the abdominal wall and secure the tube in the correct position.

Percutaneous fluoroscopic gastrostomy This is performed using a Seldinger technique that requires an initial air-insufflation of the stomach through a nasogastric tube. The anterior abdominal and stomach walls are punctured using an intravenous cannula. A stiff guide wire is then passed through the intravenous cannula into the stomach. The resulting tract can then be dilated to sufficient diameter to allow the insertion and placement of a Foley or special gastrojejunostomy catheter.[51,52] This method of insertion has advantages over the endoscopic technique in that only one operator is required and abdominal wound infections are less common. However, it does require radiological imaging equipment and, therefore, is more difficult to do at the patient's bedside, especially in an intensive care unit.

Complications of gastrostomy   The establishment and usage of a gastrostomy does have certain disadvantages and a recognised morbidity. For example, it is an invasive procedure and may be associated with infection of the skin at the puncture site, necrotising fasciitis or deeper sited sepsis, damage to adjacent intra-abdominal viscera, leakage of gastric contents into the peritoneal cavity (resulting in peritonitis), haemorrhage from the stomach and persistent gastrocutaneous fistula following removal of the feeding tube. The overall mortality rate for a gastrostomy is approximately 1–2%, with major and minor complications occurring in up to 15% of patients. Mechanical complications associated with the tube itself include tube blockage, fracture and displacement. Also, complications such as 'dumping' and diarrhoea are more common when the tip of the tube lies in the duodenum or jejunum.[53]

Jejunostomy

A feeding jejunostomy is usually carried out at the time of laparotomy if it is envisaged that a patient will need nutritional support for a long period. A fine bore tube, e.g. a small diameter urinary catheter, can be used in this procedure.

This is performed by making a stab incision in a suitable place on the abdominal wall – usually laterally. A fine bore tube, or a small diameter Foley catheter, is then placed through this stab incision into the peritoneal cavity. A purse-string suture is placed into the anti-mesenteric border of the jejunum and the catheter is inserted into the jejunal lumen through a small incision in the jejunal wall. The purse-string suture is tied and the jejunum then brought into apposition with the anterior abdominal wall and sutured in place, thus ensuring that there is no leakage of jejunal contents into the peritoneal cavity. There are several advantages of a feeding jejunostomy, when compared with a gastrostomy; (1) there is less stomal leakage with a jejunostomy, (2) gastric and pancreatic secretions are reduced because the stomach is by-passed, (3) there is less nausea, vomiting or bloating, (4) the risk of pulmonary aspiration is reduced.[54]

Nutrient solutions available for enteral nutrition

A range of nutrient solutions is currently available for use in enteral nutritional support and examples can be found in specialised texts. However, there are four main categories of enteral diet and these will be discussed in more detail.

Polymeric diets

These are also termed 'nutritionally complete' diets and are provided to patients whose gastrointestinal function is good. They contain whole protein as the source of nitrogen, and energy is provided as complex carbohydrates (glucose polymers) and fat. They also contain vitamins, trace elements and electrolytes in the standard amounts.

Elemental diets

These diets are required if the patient is unable to produce an adequate amount of digestive enzymes or has a reduced area for absorption, e.g. severe pancreatic insufficiency or short bowel syndrome. Elemental diets contain the nitrogen source as either free amino acids or oligopeptides. The energy source is provided as glucose polymers and as fat (long- and medium-chain triglycerides).

Special formulations

The specially formulated diets have been developed for patients with particular diseases. Examples of such diets include (1) those which have increased concentrations of branched chain amino acids (L-leucine, L-isoleucine and L-valine) and are low in aromatic amino acids (L-phenylalanine, L-tyrosine, L-tryptophan) for use in patients with hepatic encephalopathy, (2) those with a higher fat but lower glucose energy content for use in patients who are artificially ventilated, (3) diets containing key nutrients which modulate the immune response (see later sections).

Modular diets

These are not commonly used but allow the provision of a diet rich in a particular nutrient for use in an individual patient. For example, the diet may be enriched in protein if the patient is hypoproteinaemic, or sodium, if hyponatraemic, etc. These modular diets can be used to supplement other enteral regimens or oral intake if required.

Delivery of enteral nutrition

Enteral nutrition is provided to the patient by whichever route has been selected. Previously, it was accepted that when starting an enteral nutrition feeding regimen, patients should receive either a reduced rate of infusion or a lower strength formula for the first two or three days in an attempt to reduce the gastrointestinal complications. However, recent studies have demonstrated that this is not required and the nutritional support may commence using full strength feeds and at the desired rate. Another consideration is whether the feeding regimen should be given in bolus amounts (e.g. 200–400 ml at 3 or 4 hourly intervals), as a continuous infusion (50–125 ml h^{-1}) or as cyclical feeding. Recent studies have indicated that cyclical feeding (e.g. 16 hours feeding with a postabsorptive period of 8 hours) is optimal and more closely mimics the natural feeding cycle than do the other types of feeding regimens.[55] This leads to an improved nitrogen balance and ensures a period of time free from attachment to the enteral feeding system, which helps morale and allows improved mobilisation.

The enteral nutrition is administered through either a volumetric pump or, if this is not available, by drip flow via gravity. It is recommended in patients whose conscious level is impaired and in patients who are confined to bed, that their head should be elevated by approximately 25° so as to reduce their risks of pulmonary aspiration. Some clinicians prefer patients to be sitting upright when receiving enteral nutrition. It is also recommended that the patient's stomach contents should be aspirated every four hours during feeding and if there is a residual volume of more than 100 ml, enteral nutrition should be temporarily discontinued. The aspirate can be checked again after two hours and when satisfactory volumes are aspirated (<100 ml) then feeding can be instituted again. If more than 400 ml per 24 h is aspirated from the stomach then feeding should be discontinued. Gastric emptying may be improved by the administration of either cisapride or erythromycin, which may allow feeding to be continued.

Monitoring of enteral nutritional support

The patients receiving enteral nutritional support should be monitored by keeping an accurate recording of their fluid balance, and by daily weighing. The daily intake of calories and nitrogen should be documented. Biochemical assessments may include daily measurements of renal and liver function, and regular checks of phosphate, calcium, magnesium, albumin and protein levels and haematological indices, until the patient is stabilised. After stabilisation, once or twice weekly measurements only are necessary. Other methods of assessment may be used at regular intervals to ascertain patient progress (see Nutritional Assessment section). In addition, the routes of access should be regularly examined to ensure that the catheter is in the correct position and is mechanically satisfactory.

Complications of enteral nutritional support

Metabolic disturbances are less likely with enteral than parenteral feeding, although they do occur and are listed in Table 3.7. Hyperglycaemia, hypernatraemia and pre-renal uraemia are the most common. Also, abnormal liver function tests may occur as a result of a combination of factors; underlying disease, fatty infiltration of the liver or concomitant drug therapy. Nausea, vomiting, diarrhoea, dumping or abdominal distension may all occur, to a variable degree, but these usually respond to decreasing the rate of infusion of the enteral supplement. The other complications of enteral nutrition are those associated with the route of access to the gastrointestinal tract.

Parenteral nutritional support

Patients who require nutritional support, but in whom enteral feeding is contraindicated will require the provision of parenteral nutrition. These patients will usually have a non-functioning or inaccessible gastrointestinal tract. In patients with acute pancreatitis or high output enteric fistulae, where enteral nutrition would stimulate gastrointestinal secretion, parenteral nutrition is the preferred option.

Table 3.7 *Complications of enteral nutrition*

Type of complication	Constitutional disturbances
Gastrointestinal	Diarrhoea, nausea, vomiting, abdominal discomfort and bloating, regurgitation and aspiration of feed/stomach contents
Mechanical	Dislodgement of the feeding tube, blockage of the tube, leakage of stomach/small intestine contents onto the skin with the use of jejunostomies or gastrostomies.
Metabolic	Hyperkalaemia, hyperglycaemia, hyperphosphataemia, hypomagnesaemia, hypozincaemia, hypophosphataemia.
Infective	Local (e.g. diarrhoea, vomiting) or systemic effects (e.g. pyrexia, malaise etc.)

In addition, it may not be possible to provide sufficient intake of nutrients enterally, for example, because of a short segment of residual bowel or malabsorption. In these conditions, attempts to provide a sufficient intake by the enteral route may lead to diarrhoea or excessive losses in the stool. Therefore, parenteral nutritional supplementation may be required in addition to oral intake; this has the advantage of also maintaining intestinal stimulation for the reasons outlined earlier. In very catabolic situations, for example major burns and multiple trauma, the patients' nutritional demands may be so high as to require parenteral supplementation, in addition to enteral feeding. Detailed guidance for the administration of total parenteral nutrition (TPN) to hospitalised patients have been published by the ASPEN Board of Directors.[56]

Parenteral routes of access

Central venous access

Central venous access is obtained by positioning a catheter into the superior vena cava through the subclavian or internal jugular veins. The catheter either emerges through the skin (usually after being tunnelled in the subcutaneous fat for a short distance) or is connected to a port which is placed in the subcutaneous fat of the anterior chest wall. A variety of techniques for insertion of central venous lines are currently used in clinical practice. For example, catheters may be introduced into the subclavian vein either directly by 'blind' percutaneous puncture or by 'cut-down' techniques which utilise the cephalic vein to gain access to the subclavian vein.

The 'blind' percutaneous method, usually under local anaesthesia, is frequently employed by surgeons and anaesthetists (commonly utilising a Seldinger technique). The right subclavian vein is usually used, although some favour the left subclavian vein because it has a smoother and more gentle curve towards its junction with the superior vena cava than does the right subclavian vein. The procedure is carried out using a meticulous sterile technique and environment (operating theatre). The patient is positioned in the supine position, with a small rolled-up towel between the shoulder blades. The patient is then placed head down in the Trendelenberg position (thus filling and distending the subclavian vein), with the head turned to the opposite side. Using a 21G needle and syringe, local anaesthetic is infiltrated into the skin and subcutaneous tissues, approximately 1 cm below the clavicle at the junction of its medial two-thirds and lateral one-third. The index finger of the operator's other hand is then placed in the suprasternal notch. The needle is advanced below the clavicle (but above the first rib), then parallel to the skin, aiming towards the index finger in the suprasternal notch, with slight negative pressure (suction) as it proceeds. Usually the needle will enter the vein after advancing approximately two inches. Entry into the vein is easily recognised as there will be free aspiration of venous blood into the syringe.

The syringe is then detached from the needle and a guidewire passed through the needle (the patient should perform a Valsalva manoeuvre at this time so as to minimise the risks of air embolus). The guide wire should pass without resistance; approximately one half of the guide wire is inserted into the venous system before the needle is removed. In order to tunnel the catheter in the subcutaneous plane a second small stab incision is made under local anaesthesia approximately 5 cm below the exit point of the wire. A wide bore intravenous cannula is then passed up from this stab incision to emerge through the exit side of the guide wire. The guide wire is then repositioned through the intravenous cannula (with care) and emerges through the second stab incision below. The intravenous cannula is then withdrawn and the catheter positioned over the wire and passed distally to lie in the superior vena cava (determined either by radiological imaging at the time of insertion or by a chest radiograph taken subsequently after completion of the procedure). The catheter is attached to the skin by a suture, and then connected up to the infusion system. However, this technique has been criticised by some authors[57] because of the risks of inadvertent arterial puncture, of mediastinal haematomas (especially in patients with clotting defects), and a catheter-misplacement rate of approximately 5%. The complications of central venous catheter placement are summarised in Table 3.8.

In order to minimise these risks alternative techniques, such as direct insertion into the venous system through the cephalic or internal jugular veins, have been used. More recently, interventional radiologists have performed this procedure under local anaesthesia in an angiographic setting.[58] If fluoroscopic or ultrasound guidance is used

Table 3.8 *Complications of central venous catheter placement*

Type of complication	Incidence of occurrence
Catheter-related sepsis	Variable, but reported in up to 40% of catheters
Thrombosis of central vein	Variable, but reported in up to 20% of catheters
Pleural space damage	Pneumothorax (5–10%), haemothorax (2%)
Major arterial damage	Subclavian artery (1–2%)
Catheter problems	Thrombosis (1–2%), embolism (<1%), air embolism (<1%)
Miscellaneous problems	Brachial plexus (<1%), thoracic duct damage (<1%)

Adapted from The principles and scientific basis of surgical practice, Oxford University Press (in press).

then the risks of inadvertent arterial puncture are almost completely eliminated and the risks of pneumothorax or other complications may also be reduced.[57,59] Furthermore, the time required to insert the catheter and the necessity for the use of an operating theatre are obviated. In view of these aspects it has been suggested by some that venous access procedures should be carried out by radiologists. However, this has been rejected by many clinicians who have inserted such catheters using a variety of percutaneous 'blind' or cutdown procedures with great success.[60,61] Although meticulous technique and an experienced operator are of the utmost importance, adequate care of the line following insertion is also vital to reduce serious and life-threatening complications associated with the use of feeding catheters.

After connection of a feeding catheter to an infusion system, frequent and appropriate wound dressings are applied to the skin puncture site and frequent flushing of the catheter is performed to ensure that it remains patent. These necessary facets of catheter care may predispose to sepsis, may also be inconvenient for the patient and can interfere with normal daily activities. Therefore, subcutaneous port systems have recently become available for clinical use. The port is inserted into the subcutaneous tissue compartment in an accessible area (e.g. overlying a bony prominence) which is usually the anterior rib cage. The port (usually made of titanium or stainless steel) has on its anterior surface a self-sealing septum (silicone rubber), which can be pierced on more than 2000 occasions without any problems. The use of such port systems may result in a reduced incidence of line-sepsis, but large studies will be required to confirm this.

Technical aspects of feeding lines   Central lines are commonly manufactured from either polyurethane or silicone. Both of these materials are tolerated well in the body and have a low thrombogenic potential. However, polyurethane does have advantages. First, it is stiffer than silicone at room temperature, but at body temperature it becomes very pliable. Secondly, it has a higher tensile strength than silicone and is, therefore, less likely to fracture. Thirdly, polyurethane catheters have a smaller outside diameter thus making cannulation easier, as well as a greater resistance to the development of thrombus on their surfaces. Furthermore, some catheter manufacturers have also attempted to reduce the risks of bacterial colonisation of the line by bonding antiseptics (e.g. chlorhexidene) and antibiotics (e.g. silver sulphadiazine) into the fabric of the catheter. Some catheters also have an antimicrobial cuff, usually made of dacron, around their external surface. This is believed to act as a barrier to microorganisms which may otherwise migrate from the subcutaneous tissues along the external aspect of the catheter to its tip. Although some studies have suggested that the risks of septicaemia are reduced by using a cuff around the catheter, this does make the positioning of the catheter more difficult.

Catheter care   Care of the catheter is most important in preventing complications, in particular, in minimising the risk of infection. Appropriate dressings of the catheter are essential. For example, the dressing should normally be changed weekly; the skin exit site should be cleaned weekly with chlorhexidine using a sterile technique. A variety of dressings have also been used at the catheter exit site through the skin, but sterile gauze and a transparent, adherent type of dressings (e.g. Tegederm®) are used most commonly.

Infection of the catheter tip is the most serious type of infection that can occur. The patient usually has a pyrexia and may have systemic signs of sepsis. This may be diagnosed by taking blood cultures (at least three cultures one hour apart are taken) and catheter cultures.[62] Antibiotic therapy may result in eradication of the organism, but in some cases, the feeding line may have to be removed to eradicate the infection. However, less seriously, infection may occur at the exit site of the catheter in the skin. This is recognised by erythema of the surrounding skin, possibly associated with fluid exudate and pus.

Peripheral venous access

Peripheral venous cannulation, using a sterile technique, may be used to supply nutrients intravenously and avoids the hazards and complications associated with the insertion of central venous catheters. Peripheral intravenous nutrition is likely to be used in patients who do not require nutritional support for long enough to justify the risks and complications of central vein cannulation or in whom central vein cannulation is contraindicated (e.g. central line insertion sites are traumatised, increased risks of infective complications, if there is

Table 3.9 *Examples of Nutrient solutions available for use in patients receiving parenteral nutrition*

	Volume (ml)	Energy (kcal)	Nitro-gen (g)	Glucose (g)	Fat (g)	Na (mmol)	K (mmol)	Ca (mmol)	Mg (mmol)	Cl (mmol)
Vamin 9	1000	250	9.4			50	20	2.5	1.5	50
Vamin 14	1000	350	13.5			100	50	5	8	100
Vamin 9 glucose	1000	650	9.4	150		50	20	2.5	1.5	50
Vamin 18 EF[a]	1000	460	18							
Intralipid 10%	1000	1100			100					
Intralipid 20%	1000	2000			200					

[a]EF, electrolyte-free.

thrombosis of the central veins, or in the presence of significant clotting defects).

However, there are two main problems associated with the delivery of intravenous nutrition using the peripheral route: (1) there is a limit to the amount of nutrients which can be delivered, and (2) there is a high incidence of complications. Phlebitis occurs in up to 45%, and a subcutaneous perivascular infiltration in up to 60% of patients. The life-span of a peripheral intravenous cannula can be prolonged by treating it as one would a central line with regard to asepsis, and also by using a narrow gauge cannula which gives better mixing and flow characteristics of the nutrient solution. The risks of phlebitis can also be reduced by the following techniques: siting it in as large a vein as possible, by frequent changes of the infusion site, the use of ultrafine bore catheters, by adding heparin and a small dose of hydrocortisone to the infusion solution and by using solutions with osmolalities of less than $600\,\text{mosmol}\,\text{l}^{-1}$. Alternatively, the use of a vasodilator (e.g. transdermal glyceryl nitrate) may also increase the life span of a peripheral intravenous line.[63]

Nutrients used in parenteral feeding solutions

Some commercially available nutrient solutions (and their properties) that are commonly used in the provision of parenteral nutrition are listed in Table 3.9. A more complete list can be found in the British National Formulary.

Nitrogen sources

The nitrogen sources that are used are solutions of crystalline L-amino acids. It has been recommended that the amino acid solutions used for intravenous nutrition should contain all the essential and a balanced mixture of the non-essential amino acids required for protein synthesis. Approximately 40% of the total amino nitrogen should be in the form of essential amino acids. However, amino acids which are relatively insoluble (e.g. L-glutamine, L-arginine, L-taurine, L-tyrosine, L-methionine) may be absent or are present in what may be considered to be inadequate amounts.

In view of these difficulties, novel nitrogen sources are being developed and evaluated in clinical practice. In particular, attention has focused on the provision of L-glutamine because of its key roles in metabolism (discussed later). Glutamine may be supplied in the form of N-acetylglutamine (hydrolysed in the renal tubule to release free L-glutamine which is then reabsorbed into the systemic circulation) or as L-glutamine dipeptides such as alanylglutamine (which are also broken down to release free L-glutamine).[64]

An alternative approach has been to supplement parenteral nutrition solutions with ornithine α-ketoglutarate (OKG). Initial studies have shown that this will reduce the loss of skeletal muscle and nitrogen in patients who have undergone surgery.[65] It has been suggested that OKG may be a precursor for the synthesis of L-glutamine from α-ketoglutarate although other mechanisms may be involved. The results from studies evaluating these substances have been promising but further investigations are necessary to clarify their role before their routine introduction into parenteral nutrition solutions.

Energy sources

Energy is supplied as a balanced combination of dextrose and fat. Glucose is the primary carbohydrate source and the main form of energy supply to the majority of the body tissues. During critical illness (sepsis and trauma) the body's preferred calorie source is fat, both in the fasted state and during glucose feeding.[66–68]

However, glucose utilisation may be impaired in certain patients and glucose oxidation saturated, with a resultant hyperglycaemia. Glucose is then metabolised through other metabolic pathways resulting in an increased production of fatty acids (causing fatty infiltration of the liver, if excessive), and increased oxidation of fatty acids (this is less efficient than glucose oxidation and results in an increased amount of carbon dioxide that has to be excreted through the lungs). In addition, if glucose is the only calorie source, then patients may develop an essential fatty acid (linolenic, linoleic) deficiency. In view of these facts, therefore, fat (e.g. soyabean oil emulsions) is also given as an energy source. Usually, for most clinical circumstances, approximately 30–50% of the total calories are given as fat and the non-protein calorie to nitrogen ratio varies from 150:1 to 200:1 (this may be lower in hypercatabolic conditions). However, the provision of exogenous lipids has also been associated with certain problems. Intravenous fat emulsions have been shown to impair lung function,[69] to inhibit the reticuloendothelial system[70] and to modulate neutrophil function.[71]

Other nutrients

Commercially available preparations of trace elements (e.g. Addamel® or Additrace®) and water-soluble vitamins (e.g. Solivito®) can be used

Table 3.10 *Intravenous nutrition regimen suitable for most patients requiring parenteral support, but without abnormal metabolic demands (suitable for peripheral intravenous infusion)*

Constituent	Amount prescribed	Example of product	Volume	Comment
Macronutrients				
Nitrogen	9.4 g	Vamin 9 glucose® (V9G)	1000 ml	
Glucose	200 g	Dextrose 20%	500 ml	(100 g from V9G)
Fat	100 g	Intralipid® 20%	500 ml	
Electrolytes and minerals				
Sodium	120 mmol	Sodium chloride 30%	3.15 ml	(50 mmol from V9G, 42.5 as acetate, 7.5 from Addiphos®)
Potassium	70 mmol	Potassium chloride 20%	15.8 ml	(20 mmol from V9G, 7.5 from Addiphos®)
Acetate	42.5 mmol	Sodium acetate 4 mmol ml⁻¹	10.6 ml	
Calcium	5 mmol	Calcium gluconate 10%	11.2 ml	(2.5 mmol from V9G)
Magnesium	6 mmol	Magnesium sulphate 50%	2.25 ml	(1.5 mmol from V9G)
Phosphate	17.5 mmol	Addiphos®	5 ml	(7.5 mmol from Intralipid®)
Vitamins				
Water soluble	RDA	Solivito N®	1 vial	[a]
Fat soluble	RDA	Vitlipid N Adult®	10 ml	[a]
Trace elements				
	RDA	Additrace®	10 ml	[a]
Zinc	100 μmol	Zinc sulphate 40 μmol ml⁻¹	nil	(100 μmol included in 10 ml Additrace®)

®These samples use Pharmacia Upjohn products for illustration. A wide variety of products are made by this and other companies, hence a prescription may be prepared in a number of different ways. Differences in other constituents (such as sodium), have to be taken into account when calculating amounts of the other additives.

[a]Recommended daily allowance (RDA) not established for all constituents of the micronutrient additive mixtures.

Table 3.11 *Intravenous nutrition regimen for patients in catabolic state*

Constituent	Amount prescribed	Example of product	Volume	Comment
Macronutrients:				
Nitrogen	13.5 g	Vamin 14® (V14)	1000 ml	
Glucose	250 g	Dextrose 50%	500 ml	
Fat	100 g	Intralipid® 20%	500 ml	
Electrolytes and minerals				
Sodium	120 mmol	Sodium chloride 30%	1.97 ml	(100 mmol from V14, 7.5 from Addiphos®)
Potassium	80 mmol	Potassium chloride 20%	8.36 ml	(50 mmol from V14, 7.5 from Addiphos®)
Acetate	135 mmol	Sodium acetate 4 mmol ml^{-1}	nil	(135 mmol in V14)
Calcium	5 mmol	Calcium gluconate 10%	nil	(5 mmol in V14)
Magnesium	8 mmol	Magnesium sulphate 50%	nil	(8 mmol in V14)
Phosphate	17.5 mmol	Addiphos®	5 ml	(7.5 mmol from Intralipid®)
Vitamins				
Water soluble	RDA	Solivito N®	1 vial	[a]
Fat soluble	RDA	Vitlipid N Adult®	10 ml	[a]
Trace elements				
Zinc	RDA	Additrace®	10 ml	[a]
	200 μmol	Zinc sulphate 40 μmol ml^{-1}	2.5 ml	(100 μmol included in 10 ml Additrace®)

®These samples use Pharmacia Upjohn products for illustration. A wide variety of products are made by this and other companies, hence a prescription may be prepared in a number of different ways. Differences in other constituents (such as sodium), have to be taken into account when calculating amounts of the other additives.

[a]Recommended daily allowance (RDA) not established for all constituents of the micronutrient additive mixtures.

Table 3.12 *Intravenous nutrition regimen for patients in renal failure (undergoing regular haemodialysis)*

Constituent	Amount prescribed	Example of product	Volume	Comment
Macronutrients				
Nitrogen	18 g	Vamin 18	1000 ml	
Glucose	250 g	Dextrose 50%	500 ml	
Fat	100 g	Intralipid® 20%	500 ml	
Electrolytes and minerals				
Sodium	30 mmol	Sodium chloride 30%	1.97 ml	(3.25 from Addiphos®)
Potassium	3.25 mmol	Potassium chloride 20%	nil	(3.25 from Addiphos®)
Acetate	30 mmol	Sodium acetate 4 mmol ml^{-1}	7.5 ml	
Calcium	4 mmol	Calcium gluconate 10%	18 ml	
Magnesium	3 mmol	Magnesium sulphate 50%	1.5 ml	
Phosphate	12.5 mmol	Addiphos®	2.5 ml	(7.5 mmol from Intralipid®)
Vitamins				
Water soluble	RDA	Solivito N®	1 vial	[a]
Fat soluble	RDA	Vitlipid N Adult®	10 ml	[a]
Trace elements				
Zinc	RDA	Additrace®	10 ml	[a]
	100 μmol	Zinc sulphate 40 μmol ml^{-1}	nil	(100 μmol included in 10 ml Additrace®)

®These samples use Pharmacia Upjohn products for illustration. A wide variety of products are made by this and other companies, hence a prescription may be prepared in a number of different ways. Differences in other constituents (such as sodium), have to be taken into account when calculating amounts of the other additives.

[a]Recommended daily allowance (RDA) not established for all constituents of the micronutrient additive mixtures.

Table 3.13 *Intravenous nutrition regimen for patients with major burns (e.g. 50% full thickness), nursed in high temperature environment*

Constituent	Amount prescribed	Example of product	Volume	Comment
Macronutrients				
Nitrogen	9.4 g	Vamin 9 glucose® (V9G)	1000 ml	
Glucose	200 g	Dextrose 20%	500 ml	(100 g from V9G)
Fat	100 g	Intralipid® 20%	500 ml	
Electrolytes and minerals				
Sodium	100 mmol	Sodium chloride 30%	nil	(50 mmol from V9G, 47.75 as acetate, 3.25 from Addiphos®)
Potassium	40 mmol	Potassium chloride 20%	15.8 ml	(20 mmol from V9G, 3.25 from Addiphos®)
Acetate	47.75 mmol	Sodium acetate 4 mmol ml⁻¹	10.6 ml	
Calcium	4 mmol	Calcium gluconate 10%	6.75 ml	(2.5 mmol from V9G)
Magnesium	3 mmol	Magnesium sulphate 50%	0.75 ml	(1.5 mmol from V9G)
Phosphate	12.5 mmol	Addiphos®	2.5 ml	(7.5 mmol from Intralipid®)
Vitamins				
Water soluble	RDA	Solivito N®	1 vial	a
Fat soluble	0.5×RDA	Vitlipid N Adult®	5 ml	a
Trace elements				
	0.5×RDA	Additrace®	5 ml	a
Zinc	100 μmol	Zinc sulphate 40 μmol ml⁻¹	nil	(100 μmol included in 10 ml Additrace®)

Two of these bags would be given daily. The compounded bag degrades rapidly at the higher ambient temperature, hence should be changed more frequently than normal. ®These samples use Pharmacia Upjohn products for illustration. A wide variety of products are made by this and other companies, hence a prescription may be prepared in a number of different ways. Differences in other constituents (such as sodium), have to be taken into account when calculating amounts of the other additives.

aRecommended daily allowance (RDA) not established for all constituents of the micronutrient additive mixtures.

to supply the daily requirements of these micronutrients. In addition, the total fluid volume and the amounts of electrolytes can be modified on a daily basis to meet the particular needs of any patient.

Delivery and administration of TPN – 'all-in-one' bags

In clinical practice, the commercially available solutions for parenteral infusion are mixed together under sterile conditions in a laminar flow facility. The feeding regimen is made up in a 3-litre bag (made of ethyl vinyl acetate) and comprises amino acids, dextrose, lipid, vitamins, trace elements and electrolytes, which can be stored for up to a week prior to use, depending on the stability of the formulation. In addition, certain drugs may also be added to the bags (e.g. ranitidine, heparin or insulin). However, it is important to remember that insulin may 'bind' to the bag and giving set and the dose actually received by the patient may not necessarily be the same as that added to the bag. Also, it is important to consider the compatibilities of the different constituents used to make up the feeding solution. The expertise of the clinical pharmacist is invaluable for these reasons.

The advantages of the 3-litre bags have been documented previously[72] and include: cost effectiveness, reduced risks of infection, a more uniform administration of a balanced solution over a prolonged period, decreased lipid toxicity as a result of the greater dilution of the lipid emulsion and the longer duration of its infusion, ease of delivery and storage, reduced long-term accumulation of triglycerides (which can occur with glucose-based TPN). The parenteral nutrition is infused through the cannula at a given rate using one of the commercially available infusion pumps. Examples of some currently used feeding regimens for different clinical situations are shown in Tables 3.10–3.13.

Monitoring patients receiving parenteral nutrition

Patients receiving parenteral nutrition require careful monitoring, both clinically and by using laboratory indices. The patient's clinical condition should be evaluated daily (daily weighing, signs of fluid depletion or overload). Various biochemical indices should be monitored; serum electrolytes, urea, creatinine and glucose are checked daily, whilst serum albumin, protein, calcium, magnesium, phosphate and liver function tests are checked twice per week, and haematological indices (haemoglobin, white blood cell count, haematocrit) are checked twice weekly. The circulating glucose level should be monitored four times per day initially in case the patient becomes hyperglycaemic.

Other assessments, such as muscle function, nitrogen balance, measurement of trace elements and vitamins, may also be performed, if required. In addition, the catheter, its site of access and the equipment infusing the feeding solution must also be carefully examined for any possible complications or dysfunction.

Table 3.14 *Metabolic complications of parenteral nutrition*

Complication	Causes(s)
Glucose disturbances	
Hyperglycaemia	Excessive administration of glucose, inadequate insulin, sepsis
Hypoglycaemia	Rebound hypoglycaemia occurs if glucose stopped abruptly but insulin levels remain high
Lipid disturbances	
Hyperlipidaemia	Excess administration of lipid, reduced metabolism (e.g. renal failure, liver failure)
Fatty acid deficiency	Essential fatty acid deficiency – hair loss, dry skin, impaired wound healing
Nitrogen disturbances	
Hyperammonaemia	Occurs if deficiency of L-arginine, L-ornithine, L-aspartate or L-glutamate in infusion. Also occurs in liver diseases
Metabolic acidosis	Due to excessive amount of chloride and monochloride amino acids
Electrolyte disturbances	
Hyperkalaemia	Excessive potassium administration or reduced losses
Hypokalaemia	Inadequate potassium administration or excessive loss
Hypocalcaemia	Inadequate calcium replacement, losses in pancreatitis, hypoalbuminaemia
Hypophosphataemia	Inadequate phosphorus supplementation, also tissue compartment fluxes
Liver disturbances	
	Elevations in aspartate aminotransferase, alkaline phosphatase and γ-glutamyl transferase may occur because of enzyme induction secondary to amino acid imbalances or deposition of fat and/or glycogen in liver
Ventilatory problems	
	If excessive amounts of glucose are given, the increased production of CO_2 may precipitate ventilatory failure in non-ventilated patients

Complications of parenteral nutritional support

The instant availability of nutrients provided by the intravenous route can lead to metabolic complications if the composition or flow rate are inappropriate. Rapid infusion of high concentrations of glucose can precipitate hyperglycaemia which may be further complicated by lactic acidosis. Electrolyte disturbances may present problems, not least because the intravenous feeding regimen is usually prescribed in advance for a 24 h period. Prediction of the patient's nutrient requirements must be complemented by frequent monitoring, as described above. The provision of nutrients may lead to further electrolyte abnormalities when potassium, magnesium and phosphate enter the intracellular compartment. This is particularly noticeable in patients whose previous nutrient intake was especially poor. Other complications of TPN are shown in Table 3.14.

Nutritional support teams

It has become clear that for the optimal provision of nutritional support, a multidisciplinary nutritional support team is required. This may comprise a clinician with a special interest in the provision of nutrition and understanding of metabolic pathways, a biochemist, pharmacist, dietician and nursing specialist. It has been demonstrated that the provision of nutritional support by such a team results in the most cost-effective use of nutritional support and is associated with the least risk of infective, metabolic and feeding line complications.[73]

Nutritional support in defined clinical situations

Perioperative nutritional support

In 1936, Studley demonstrated the importance of weight loss in patients undergoing surgery.[1] He documented that in patients undergoing elective peptic ulcer surgery who had a weight loss of 20% or more there was an eightfold increase in postoperative mortality, when compared with patients who had lost less than 20% of their body weight (Fig. 3.6).

It has also been reported that up to 60% of patients with diseases of the gastrointestinal tract are malnourished at the time of surgery.[74] In view of this, therefore, many studies have evaluated the role of nutritional support given in the perioperative period to patients undergoing major surgery. These studies of nutritional support, administered either by the oral or parenteral routes, have yielded variable results.

Holter and Fischer[75] reported the findings of the first randomised trial designed to evaluate the role of perioperative nutritional support. In this study, 56 patients with upper gastrointestinal malignancies who had lost weight (greater than 10 lbs (4.5 kg) in the three-month period prior to surgery), were randomised to receive either 80 g of protein and 2000 kcal day^{-1} intravenously, commencing 72 h before surgery and continuing for 10 days after surgery, or no nutritional support. In addition, there was a group of patients with no weight loss who served as controls. The mortality was the same between the groups, but major postoperative complications occurred more frequently in the group not receiving nutritional support. Intravenous nutrition reduced (but not significantly) the major complication rate from 19% to 13%. A randomised study was also carried out in patients with oesophageal carcinoma undergoing surgical resection of the tumour through a thoracic approach.[76] This was a small study of 15 patients, with ten being randomised to receive 5–7 days of pre-

Figure 3.6 *The effect of weight loss on mortality in patients following surgery for chronic peptic ulcer disease (data from ref. 1).*

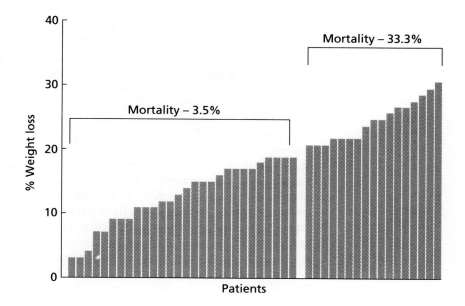

operative parenteral nutrition (35 kcal kg^{-1} body weight and 0.2 g kg^{-1} body weight of nitrogen per day), and this was continued for 6–7 days after surgery. The control group of five patients were given an oral diet plus intravenous dextrose/saline (6 kcal kg^{-1} body weight per day) over the same period. The patients who received parenteral nutrition had a positive nitrogen balance following surgery, whereas those patients in the control group had a negative nitrogen balance. Furthermore, an increased morbidity was reported in the control group, with impaired wound healing occurring in four of these five patients.

The first study to show a significant benefit of nutritional support in patients undergoing surgery was reported by Heatley *et al.*[77] In this study, 75 patients with malignant disease of the stomach or oesophagus were randomised to one of two study groups: (1) intensive oral feeding or (2) combined oral and intravenous feeding, for 10 days prior to surgery. The results of this study revealed that there was a significant reduction in wound infections in the patients receiving combined oral and intravenous feeding. However, this benefit was found to occur in those patients whose serum albumin concentration was initially less than 35 g l^{-1}. Another study also showed a benefit of perioperative nutritional support.[78] In this study, patients who were undergoing laparotomy for intra-abdominal malignancy were evaluated and were randomised to receive either 10 days of TPN or a standard hospital diet. The main findings in this study were that patients who received TPN had a significant reduction in both morbidity and mortality. Similarly, Muller *et al.*[79] evaluated 125 patients with gastric and oesophageal cancer who were undergoing surgery. Patients were randomised to receive either 10 days of TPN or to receive a standard hospital diet. This study showed that patients in the TPN group had a significant reduction in postoperative mortality (three-fold) and anastomotic breakdown, when compared with a control group of 59 patients not receiving supplementation.

Clinical benefit with supplemental nutrition has not been a consistent finding and other studies have failed to show significant benefit from nutritional support. This may have been because these were often small studies, frequently without proper randomisation or allowance for the nutritional status of the patients prior to commencing the study. A meta-analysis of trials of perioperative nutritional support has revealed that nutritional supplementation reduced morbidity by 21% and mortality by 32% following major surgery, but it was not possible to clearly identify which particular patients would benefit.[80] Furthermore, it was also of concern that major iatrogenic complications occurred in 7% of the patients receiving TPN.

More recently, two large trials of perioperative nutritional support have been reported by the Veteran Affairs (VA) Total Parenteral Nutrition Cooperative Study group[81] and by Fan *et al.*[82] The VA study[81] was a randomised trial performed to assess the efficacy of perioperative TPN in malnourished patients undergoing major intrathoracic (non-cardiac) or intra-abdominal surgery. A total of 395 malnourished patients (approximately two-thirds had malignant disease) were randomised to receive either TPN for 7–15 days before surgery and 3 days postoperation or an oral intake, as clinically indicated. The patients were followed up for 90 days after surgery. The results of this study revealed that the major complication rates were comparable between the two groups. However, there was an increased incidence of infectious complications in the TPN group, when compared with the control group (14% versus 6%). Also, there was a small, but non-significant, increase in the incidence of non-infectious complications in the control group (17% versus 22%). Further subgroup analyses were carried out in an attempt to define which patients were most likely to benefit from perioperative nutrition in this study. This revealed that in the severely malnourished group of patients (as defined by using a 'Nutrition Risk Index'), the incidence of non-infectious complications and major complications for the TPN and control groups were 5% versus 43%, and 21% versus 47%, respectively. However, it should be noted that only 50 patients fell into this severely malnourished category.

Fan *et al.*[82] also documented beneficial effects of perioperative nutritional support in patients with hepatocellular carcinoma undergoing hepatectomy. In this study, 124 patients with hepatocellular carcinoma were randomised to receive either perioperative intravenous nutrition (35% branched-chain amino acids, dextrose and lipid emulsion) for seven days prior to and seven days after surgery. The patients in the control group received their usual oral intake prior to surgery and intravenous fluids and electrolytes in the immediate postoperative period. The two groups of patients were well matched for nutritional status, but only 15% of patients had lost greater than 10% of their usual body weight.

The results of this study revealed that patients receiving TPN had a reduction in the overall postoperative morbidity rate (34% versus 55%) and a reduction in the risk of infectious complications (17% versus 37%), when compared with the control patients. In addition, patients in the TPN group also had benefits in terms of a reduced requirement for diuretics to control ascites, less weight loss post-operatively and less deterioration in liver function. There were also fewer deaths in the TPN group, but this did not achieve statistical significance. This study also attempted to identify which patients benefited most from nutritional support. It was found that in those patients who had cirrhosis (approximately half of all patients), TPN supplementation resulted in a lowering of the postoperative morbidity by almost 50%, when compared with patients in the control group. In addition, in those patients undergoing a 'major' hepatectomy, TPN also resulted in a significant reduction in postoperative morbidity.

From these various studies it can be deduced that the following groups of patients may benefit from perioperative nutritional support; (1) severely malnourished prior to surgery, (2) well nourished prior to surgery, but have complications that result in 10–14 days of inadequate nutritional intake, and (3) well nourished prior to surgery, but expected to have inadequate intake for 10–14 days because of the nature of their surgery (Table 3.15).

Nutritional support in patients with burns

Major burns induce severe hypermetabolic and hypercatabolic states. There is increased skeletal muscle breakdown, with nitrogen losses of 15 g N day^{-1} or more and up to a doubling of the metabolic rate. In patients with burns of greater than 20% of their body surface areas, nutritional support is required, either orally or by nasoenteric feeding. If these routes are not possible, as occurs in the presence of gastric stasis, ileus or other co-existent injuries, then parenteral nutrition is required.

Several formulae exist for calculating the protein and calorie requirements of the individual patient (see ref. 84 for summary), and an example is shown in Table 3.16. However, up to 20–25 g of nitrogen per day may be required initially, with a non-protein calorie to nitrogen ratio of 100–200 being advocated. In a study of children with substantial burns, it was found that a high protein diet with a calorie to nitrogen ratio of 100:1 resulted in better survival than in children receiving a ratio of 150:1.[85] Energy is provided as carbohydrate and lipids, with the calorie requirement being 35–50% as lipid (minimising the problems associated with a high glucose load).

Table 3.15 *Studies showing clinical benefits from nutritional supplementation*

Reference	Patient group	No. of patients	Study plan	Results
77	Stomach, oesophageal cancer	75	Patients received either TPN and oral diet or an oral diet for 7–10 days prior to surgery	Wound infections less in TPN group compared with the orally fed patients (mainly in patients with albumin <35 g l⁻¹)
79	Gastrointestinal tract cancers	125	Patients randomised to either TPN or a standard oral diet for 10 days before surgery	Reduction of mortality (3% versus 11%) in patients receiving TPN compared with those receiving oral nutrition; also reduction in morbidity in TPN group
81	Thoracotomy or laparotomy	395	Patients received either TPN for 7–15 days before surgery and 3 days after surgery or an oral diet	'Severely' malnourished patients had reduced risk of complications (21% versus 47%). No differences in mortality or morbidity when all patients analysed together
75	Upper gastro-intestinal tract cancers	30	Patients received either TPN or no nutritional support for 3 days before and 10 days after surgery	Reduced incidence of major complications in patients receiving TPN (13% versus 19%). No difference in mortality between the two groups
78	Intra-abdominal cancers	145	Patients received either TPN for 10 days before surgery or a standard oral diet	Significant reduction in the risk of major complications in the TPN group of patients. No difference in mortality
83	Benign gastro-intestinal surgery	28	Patients received either enteral feeding or intravenous fluids after laparotomy	Patients receiving enteral nutrition had reduced incidence of complications
82	Hepatocellular carcinoma	125	Patients randomised to receive TPN for 7 days before and 7 days after hepatic resection, or an oral diet	TPN group had reduced postoperative morbidity compared with oral group (34% versus 55%); patients with underlying cirrhosis or those undergoing major hepatic resections benefited most

Modified with permission from: Heys SD, Park KGM, Garlick PJ, Eremin O. Nutrition and malignant disease: implications for surgical practice. Br J Surg 1992; 79: 614–23

Table 3.16 *Estimated nutritional requirements of adult patients with burns*

Basal energy requirements (BEE) per Harris–Benedict equation
Male BEE = 66 + (13.7 × Wt) + (5 × Ht) − (6.8 × age)
Female BEE = 655 + (9.6 × Wt) + (1.9 × Ht) − (4.7 × age)

Adjustments for burn severity

Extent of burn	BEE	Protein	NPCN ratio
Moderate burn (15–30% TBSA)	1.5 × normal	1.5 g kg^{-1} day^{-1}	100–120:1
Major burn (31–49% TBSA)	1.5–1.8 × normal	1.5–2 g kg^{-1} day^{-1}	100:1
Massive burn (50%+TBSA)	1.8–2.1 × normal	2–2.3 g kg^{-1} day^{-1}	100:1

Wt = weight in kg; Ht = height (cm); TBSA = total body surface area; NPCN = non-protein calorie to nitrogen ratio.

Reproduced from: Deitch EA. Nutritional support of the burn patient. Crit Care Clin 1995; 11: 735–50, with permission.

Nutritional support and pancreatitis

Severe pancreatitis produces a major catabolic stress, with a rapid loss of muscle proteins. Enteral support through the nasogastric route is contraindicated in the early phase of the disease, as this would stimulate pancreatic activity. The nitrogen requirements of such patients are higher than normal, reaching 1.2–2.0 g kg^{-1} day^{-1} protein (0.2–0.3 g kg^{-1} day^{-1} nitrogen). Energy requirements also increase with disease severity and are in the range of 28–35 kcal kg^{-1} day^{-1}. Up to half of this requirement may be given as fat. Intravenous lipids do not stimulate pancreatic secretion, nor cause hypertriglyceridaemia, although caution is required where lipaemia pre-exists. Exogenous insulin is frequently required and should be infused intravenously according to a sliding scale, with continuation of the nutrition over 24 h. Appropriate electrolytes and minerals should be added, with particular attention to calcium and magnesium as their levels are often low. The calcium and magnesium supplementation required to correct hypocalcaemia and hypomagnesaemia may have to be given separately because the quantities required can cause instability of the parenteral nutrition emulsion.

Nutritional support in liver disease

The liver plays a crucial role in many homeostatic mechanisms. In particular, it controls the supply of the energy substrate, glucose, to the tissues. In patients with liver disease, both the storage of glucose (through glycogen and fatty acid synthesis) and the synthesis of glucose (gluconeogenesis), may be impaired. In addition, the control of amino acid, protein and lipid metabolism may also be altered. Patients with liver disease may also have a reduction in the availability of bile in the intestinal lumen. This will cause fat malabsorption and a resultant reduction in calorie availability for the body tissues. Nutritional support is widely advocated, therefore, in patients with acute liver disease and also as a supportive measure in patients awaiting hepatic transplantation. If oral intake is insufficient, enteral feeding should be employed where possible because the risk of sepsis and other complications of the intravenous route are increased in these patients. Protein requirements are in the order of $1 \, g \, kg^{-1} \, day^{-1}$ (0.16 g nitrogen $kg^{-1} \, day^{-1}$), possibly higher in severe illness.[86] However, hepatic encephalopathy may restrict protein intake in some patients. Energy requirements will be around $25 \, kcal \, kg^{-1} \, day^{-1}$ (non-protein) with one third of these calories being provided as fat. Medium-chain triglycerides have also been advocated, as they are thought to be easier to metabolise, although evidence as to their efficacy is conflicting. Rates of glucose infusion higher than $16 \, kcal \, kg^{-1} \, day^{-1}$ should be avoided because of the risk of developing a 'fatty liver'. In those patients who are being fluid restricted (e.g. patients with ascites or hepatorenal failure), more concentrated enteral or parenteral feeds should be used. Electrolytes should be tailored to requirements as assessed clinically and biochemically. Generally, less sodium and more potassium than normal will be required, especially in the presence of ascites. Normal amounts of mineral and vitamin supplements should be used, although isolated deficiencies (especially magnesium, phosphate and B group vitamins) are particularly common in alcoholic liver disease, and feeds should be supplemented accordingly.

Nutritional supplements enriched with branched-chain amino acids have been suggested to reduce muscle breakdown, especially in liver disease where pre-supplementation levels are low. However, although some studies have suggested that branched-chain amino acid enriched formulations will improve hepatic encephalopathy, larger analyses have still not confirmed that this is so. Furthermore, the effects of branch-chain amino acid enriched solutions in lowering mortality have not, as yet, been established.[87]

Nutritional supplementation in inflammatory bowel disease

A significant number of patients with Crohn's disease and ulcerative colitis, especially during acute exacerbations, can become malnourished. The reasons for this include a decreased nutrient intake, malabsorption by the small intestine (decreased length, bacterial overgrowth, protein-losing enteropathy) and possibly increased calorie and nitrogen requirements if there is co-existent sepsis. Furthermore, there may also be deficiencies of specific vitamins and trace elements in these patients.

Nutritional support in such patients may have two roles; the first is to provide the nutritional requirements and correct any nutritional deficiencies that the patient may have, and the second is the possibility that the provision of TPN with bowel rest may itself be therapeutically beneficial. The results of studies that have addressed this latter point have been disappointing.[88–90] These investigations have suggested that parenteral nutrition itself does not have a therapeutic effect in patients with inflammatory bowel disease. Furthermore, there is evidence to show that enteral nutritional support is as effective as TPN in these patients,[91] and this has the added benefits of maintaining the integrity of the gut mucosa and stimulating the production of gut hormones necessary for gut function.

Nutritional support in enterocutaneous fistulae

Nutritional support has an important role to play in the management of patients with enterocutaneous fistulae. It has been shown that up to 50% of patients with fistulae are malnourished. The importance of adequate nutritional support in these patients was demonstrated by Chapman *et al.* in 1964.[92] They found that if patients with fistulae received nutritional support with TPN and enteral feeding (>3000 kcal day^{-1}), then spontaneous fistula healing with a reduced mortality occurred, when compared with patients with fistulae who received less than 1000 kcal day^{-1}. The management of patients with fistulae commences with correction of any fluid and electrolyte deficits and elimination of any foci of sepsis. TPN is required to correct any nutritional deficits and to provide maintenance requirements when the patient is stabilised. However, if the fistula output is low, then enteral nutritional support should be considered because of the benefits already outlined.

Nutrition in acute renal failure

In patients with acute renal failure, energy requirements are the same as those that would be required for a similar underlying condition, before developing renal failure. Most patients require at least 30 kcal kg^{-1} day^{-1} (non-protein) increasing to 50 kcal kg^{-1} day^{-1}, depending on the severity of the underlying illness. Approximately one third of the calories should be as fat (to reduce the osmolarity of the supplementation), the remainder being as glucose. However, achieving a positive nitrogen balance in these patients is very unlikely because increasing intake simply results in increasing the nitrogen losses. Approximately 0.9 g protein kg^{-1} day^{-1} (0.15 g nitrogen kg^{-1} day^{-1}) should avoid unwanted accumulation of metabolites, and result in an acceptable nitrogen balance in most patients. Lower amounts of nitrogen may be provided so as to reduce dialysis requirements for short periods (larger amounts may be required in very catabolic patients). Overall fluid requirements vary with the type of dialysis and phase of the renal failure.

In mild disease, fluid volume (and hence nutrients) may be kept to a minimum to reduce the requirements for dialysis. To maximise nutrient intake for a minimal supply of water, highly concentrated enteric nutritional supplements should be used. However, the high osmolarity of these supplements may cause significant diarrhoea. For parenteral nutrition, glucose solutions of 50% (or greater) are utilised, with fat solutions of up to 30%. In this way, 2000 kcal (non-protein) and more than 10 g nitrogen can be given in a total fluid volume of 1.3 litres. In general, reduced quantities of electrolytes and minerals are required, but their circulating blood levels should be monitored and adjustments made as necessary. Water-soluble vitamins are given in normal amounts and trace elements and fat-soluble vitamins in usual doses, although some advocate providing reduced amounts of the latter two nutrient groups.

Recent advances in dialysis techniques include the use of 'biocompatible' membranes which are thought to reduce catabolic stress. These also are less affected by lipid emulsions than conventional membranes. Continuous haemofiltration allows removal of more fluid than conventional intermittent dialysis, and although some nutrients will be lost, this is thought to be small. In some cases the dialysis fluid contains glucose (nutritional dialysis); this itself can provide some 200–800 kcal, which should be taken into account when prescribing daily requirements.

Nutritional support during chemotherapy and radiotherapy

Chemotherapy

Nutritional intake is often reduced in patients who are receiving intensive chemotherapy or radiotherapy. There are many reasons why this may occur, including anorexia, altered perception of taste, diarrhoea and malabsorption. In view of this, patients undergoing chemotherapy or radiotherapy have been given nutritional support.

Two analyses of the effects of parenteral nutritional support in patients undergoing chemotherapy have been reported.[93,94] These studies concluded that patients given nutritional support were less likely to survive or achieve a therapeutic response than patients not receiving nutritional supplementation. Those patients who received nutritional support had a fourfold increase in the risk of sepsis, compared with patients not receiving nutritional supplementation. As a result of these studies the American College of Physicians recommended that parenteral nutritional support should not be used in patients receiving chemotherapy.[95] Similarly, there is no evidence that

Table 3.17 *Studies of nutritional support in patients receiving radiotherapy for malignant disease*

Reference	Nutritional support (no. of patients)	Malignancy	Improvement with nutritional support	Mortality
97	TPN v standard oral diet (81)	Ovarian and GI tract	Fewer side-effects with therapy, increased weight	No difference
98	TPN v standard oral diet (81)	Ovarian	Less 'malnutrition'	No difference
99	Oral supplements v roughage (47)	Bladder and prostate	None	No difference
100	TPN v standard oral diet and supplements (20)	Abdominal and pelvic	Increased body weight and increased serum transferrin	No difference
101	TPN v standard oral diet (32)	GU tract	Increased weight	No difference
102	Standard diet v supplementation with elemental diet (30)	GI tract	None	No difference

GI tract, gastrointestinal tract; GU tract, genitourinary tract; TPN, total parenteral nutrition.

Reproduced with permission from: Heys SD, Park KGM, Garlick PJ, Eremin O. Nutrition and malignant disease: implications for surgical practice. Br J Surg 1992; 79: 614–623.

enteral nutritional support increases the effectiveness of chemotherapy or reduces the treatment-associated toxicities.[96] Therefore, nutritional support is not generally indicated in such patients, although there might be subgroups (e.g. severely malnourished patients) who might benefit from supplemental nutrition.

Radiotherapy

Nutritional support has also been given to patients undergoing radiotherapy and these studies have been outlined in Table 3.17 which shows that there is no convincing evidence that patients having radiotherapy will benefit from nutritional support. Therefore, in the absence of such benefits, it is not possible to make recommendations for the use of nutritional supplementation in patients undergoing radiotherapy.

Recent interest, however, has focused on the role of glutamine supplementation and its effects on the intestine following radiotherapy. These effects are discussed more fully below.

Nutritional support and modulation of tumour growth

Studies in experimental animals have investigated what effects nutritional support can have on growth of a tumour. These have, however, revealed conflicting results, with some studies finding no stimulation of tumour growth, and others showing a selective enhancement of tumour growth. Previous investigations in man have shown that in patients with gastrointestinal cancer and sarcomas there was no difference in indices of tumour growth in patients receiving nutritional support. More recently, however, studies have found that the provision of nutritional support may increase the fractional rate of protein synthesis of human colorectal cancers *in vivo*, and that this effect was mediated through a selective stimulation of the malignant cells themselves.[103,104]

Nutritional pharmacology in the management of the surgical patient

Certain nutrients can have marked effects on the function of normal cells and tissues, as well as on tissues involved in various pathological processes. Furthermore, some of these nutrients can also modulate immune and inflammatory responses, if given in excess of normal intake or requirements. The use of nutrients in this way has been termed 'nutritional pharmacology'. Nutrients that are attracting interest are certain amino acids (L-arginine, L-glutamine, branched-chain amino acids), essential fatty acids and polyribonucleotides. The effects of these nutrients on metabolism and the immune system and their current application to clinical practice is offering novel approaches in the management of patients with many diseases.

L-Arginine

L-Arginine is essential for growth and nitrogen balance in many young animals but does not appear to be an essential amino acid in healthy children and adults.[105] It may become essential in conditions such as stress, sepsis and trauma. A standard diet contains approximately 5 g of L-arginine (meat, fish, poultry and dairy produce). However, following injury there is an increased requirement for L-arginine to maintain optimal metabolic functions. Studies in patients undergoing surgery have demonstrated that dietary supplementation with L-arginine (in doses of 15–30 g day^{-1}) can reduce nitrogen excretion and improve nitrogen balance.[106,107] L-Arginine supplementation has also been shown to have beneficial effects on wound healing. For example, Barbul *et al.*[108] have demonstrated that in healthy volunteers, two weeks of dietary supplementation with L-arginine (25 g day^{-1} orally), resulted in an increase in collagen synthesis, when compared with those not receiving an L-arginine supplemented diet.

L-Arginine has been shown to have important effects on various aspects of the immune system, including macrophages, lymphocytes and natural killer (NK) cells. Studies in man have shown that the addition of various concentrations of L-arginine to lymphocytes *in vitro* resulted in an increase in proliferation in response to mitogens. Also if L-arginine was given to volunteers for seven days (25 g day^{-1}) there was an increased response *in vitro* of peripheral blood lymphocytes with mitogens.[108] Daly *et al.*[107] demonstrated a similar stimulation of the immune system in patients with gastrointestinal cancer. The *in vitro* supplementation with L-arginine of peripheral blood lymphocytes resulted in an enhancement of NK and lymphokine-activated killer (LAK) cell cytotoxicities (cells which are believed to be important in the destruction of malignant cells).[109] These effects on NK and LAK cells have also been shown to occur *in vivo* in patients with breast cancer receiving 3 days of L-arginine supplementation[110] and in those receiving chemotherapy.[111] In addition to its effects on lymphocytes, L-arginine has been shown to activate macrophage antitumour cytotoxic effector mechanisms. The exact mechanisms by which L-arginine mediates these immunostimulatory effects are not known but may include increased production of hormones, enhanced polyamine synthesis, release of cytokines and production of nitric oxide.

L-Glutamine

L-Glutamine is a non-essential amino acid under normal circumstances and is synthesised in skeletal muscle from other amino acids, mainly the branched chains, by transamination (requiring glutamine synthetase). L-Glutamine comprises 50–60% of the intracellular free amino acid pool[112] and is the predominant amino acid in the circulation. The functions of L-glutamine are shown in Table 3.18. In certain conditions, e.g. severe sepsis, major burns and multiple trauma there is an increased efflux of amino acids, including L-glutamine, from skeletal muscle.[113] There is a resultant fall in intracellular L-glutamine concentration, and although the plasma concentration may be maintained at first, a continuing demand results in a fall in plasma levels.

Table 3.18 *Functions of L-glutamine*

Acts as a nitrogen shuttle between tissues
Is a precursor for the synthesis of purines, pyrimidines and amino acids
Essential for normal cellular proliferation and tissue growth and development
Controls protein synthesis in skeletal muscle (as yet not established unequivocally)
An important fuel for the gastrointestinal tract (enterocytes and colonocytes), lymphocytes and fibroblasts
Key fuel for lymphocytes and macrophages; important for lymphocyte proliferation and macrophage function

Furthermore, it has been demonstrated that the reduction in free intracellular L-glutamine concentration in septic patients correlated with poorer survival.[114] Attempts have, therefore, been made to correct these pathophysiological disturbances by provision of L-glutamine supplementation to patients (in particular, to modulate nitrogen metabolism and enhance host defences). However, L-glutamine itself is relatively insoluble and also forms pyroglutamic acid with heat sterilisation and, therefore, is not usually present in solutions for parenteral administration. In order to overcome these difficulties L-glutamine has been provided by using glutamine analogues or dipeptides (e.g. alanyl-glutamine, ornithine-α-ketoglutarate) which are hydrolysed in the body to L-glutamine. The results from studies evaluating the role of L-glutamine supplementation have demonstrated that various aspects of immune function can be enhanced and nitrogen balance improved.[115–118]

An important study has evaluated dietary supplementation with L-glutamine in patients undergoing bone marrow transplantation.[117] The patients were randomised to receive a standard parenteral nutritional regimen or one supplemented with L-glutamine ($0.57\,g\,kg^{-1}$ body weight per day) starting on the first day after transplantation and continuing for approximately 28 days. The results of this study demonstrated that L-glutamine supplementation resulted in clinically beneficial effects. Another possible role for L-glutamine supplementation is in the protection of the bowel following radiotherapy and/or chemotherapy. In animal studies the administration of an oral diet supplemented with L-glutamine resulted in better intestinal healing, a decreased rate of bacterial translocation and an improved survival, when compared with animals not receiving a supplemented diet.[119,120] However, further studies are required to determine if these protective effects occur in man.

A further interesting application of L-glutamine is in the treatment of short bowel syndrome. A recent study has evaluated the effects of a glutamine-supplemented diet (high carbohydrate, low fat) in combination with growth hormone in patients with short-bowel who required TPN maintenance.[121] The patients were given this therapy for 28 days and then received only the L-glutamine supplementation and diet. There was an increase in protein absorption by approximately 40% together with a reduction in stool output by one third. Furthermore, 40% of the patients remained off TPN and a further 40% had reduced TPN requirements with a mean follow-up of 12 months and a maximum follow-up of 60 months.

Branched-chain amino acids (BCAA)

The BCAAs (L-leucine, L-isoleucine, L-valine) are essential amino acids. They have several important properties which distinguish them from other amino acids: (1) they are metabolised extensively in peripheral tissues, especially skeletal muscle, (2) they may modulate tissue protein synthesis and/or breakdown (especially leucine), (3) they are transported into brain tissue using the same mechanisms that transport aromatic amino acids.

The effects of BCAAs on protein synthesis in skeletal muscle has been extensively studied. Some investigators have shown that the BCAA (or L-leucine alone) can stimulate protein synthesis *in vitro* but others have failed to demonstrate this effect *in vivo*. Investigations of the administration of BCAA to patients with cancer have compared BCAA-enriched solutions and 'standard' amino acid solutions. Tayek *et al.*[122] found that in malnourished cancer patients, administration of a 50% BCAA-enriched solution resulted in significant increases in the rate of whole body protein synthesis and in the fractional rate of albumin synthesis. Some studies have demonstrated that BCAA supplementation can result in an improved whole body nitrogen balance in traumatised or septic patients. In contrast, others have failed to demonstrate that BCAA supplementation can modulate skeletal muscle protein synthesis *in vivo* in man. However, although biochemical advantages have been demonstrated in some studies, no clinically beneficial effects of BCAA supplementation have been documented and the conclusion of the Workshop on Clinical Uses of BCAA, that there is no evidence to support the routine use of BCAA supplemented regimens, published 10 years ago,[123] is still valid. However, in severely traumatised patients BCAA supplementation may be indicated and may have beneficial effects on nitrogen balance.

Essential fatty acids

Essential fatty acids (EFAs) cannot be synthesized by mammals and, therefore, must be present in the diet for maintenance of normal health and body function. These EFAs are important constituents of cell membranes and their metabolites are key second messengers in controlling various aspects of cellular metabolism. The *n*-6 series of EFAs are derived from linoleic acid (e.g. γ-linolenic acid (GLA) and arachidonic acid (AA)), the *n*-3 series are derived from α-linolenic acid (e.g. eicosapentaenoic acid (EPA) and docosahexaenoic acid (DHA)). GLA is found in oats, barley, some meats and particularly in plant seed oils, whereas EPA and DHA are found predominantly in fish.

The EFAs have been shown to have cytotoxic effects against malignant cells and to modulate immune reactivity.[124] Studies have shown that the addition of GLA to a range of malignant cells *in vitro* resulted in cell death within 5–10 days. Normal cells, however, were not affected by GLA. Animal studies have also found that GLA supplementation in the diet resulted in an inhibition of tumour growth. In man, pilot studies have been carried out evaluating the role of dietary supplementation with EFAs in patients with several different types of tumours. Another possible role for EFAs in the treatment of malignancy is in combination with cytotoxic drug therapy as studies in cell lines have shown that the preincubation of tumour cells with EFAs increased substantially the subsequent cytotoxic effect.

Dietary supplementation with n-3 EFAs leads to the synthesis of the 3 series of prostaglandins (PGs) rather than those of the 2 series. The PG_3 compounds have been demonstrated to be less immunosuppressive than PG_2 compounds. However, *in vivo* studies of dietary supplementation with EFAs have revealed interesting findings. In patients with colorectal cancer, prolonged dietary supplementation (up to 6 months) with high doses of EFAs (containing both n-3 and n-6 series) significantly reduced the activity of peripheral blood lymphocytes[125] and natural cytotoxicity.[126] This was accompanied by reduced serum levels of interleukins 1, 2, 4, 6, tumour necrosis factor (TNF) alpha, and interferon (IFN) gamma.[127] These changes were not observed in control patients with advanced and progressive colorectal cancer. These effects on cytokine production may have important implications for weight-losing cachectic patients. This is because some of the key cytokines, e.g. TNFα, IL6 and IL1, may be important factors in the pathogenesis of cachexia. Animal studies have evaluated this possibility further by demonstrating that dietary EFA supplementation can reverse weight loss associated with malignant disease, but further studies are required to determine if this will also occur in man.

Polyribonucleotides

Interest in the role of ribonucleotides as modulators of the immune system began over 30 years ago. Initial studies demonstrated that the administration of nucleic acid-rich material could restore immune function in irradiated animals. Subsequently, synthetic double-stranded polyribonucleotides were developed for clinical use (single-stranded polyribonucleotides were ineffective). Examples of such agents are, polyadenylic polyuridylic acid (PAPU) and polyinosinic polycytidylic acid (PIPC). PAPU has been most used in clinical practice and will be discussed in more detail.

PAPU modulates cell-mediated and humoral immunity, possibly through alteration in the production of cytokines such as IFNγ. A wide range of effects of PAPU on various aspects of immunity have been demonstrated in animal studies.[128] In human studies, the administration of PAPU will enhance macrophage function, augment or suppress antibody production, induce cytokine release (e.g. IL1β, IL2, IL6, TNFα and IFNγ) and stimulate both NK and LAK cell cytotoxicity.[129,130] Other studies have investigated if these apparently beneficial effects on the immune system are translated into clinical benefits, in patients with cancer. Substantial numbers of patients with breast, stomach and colon cancer have been treated. Clinical benefits have been demonstrated in patients with breast and stomach cancer, with a prolongation in disease-free and overall survival in patients receiving PAPU, particularly in those patients with nodal involvement by tumour. In patients with breast cancer PAPU was as effective as chemotherapy, in terms of prolonging overall survival.[131–133] However, these benefits were not demonstrated in patients with colorectal cancer;[134] the reasons for this are not clear.

Nutrient combinations in clinical practice

Dietary supplementation with single nutrients has been discussed above and although beneficial effects on the immune system and/or metabolism have been demonstrated, the clinical benefits have not been so readily demonstrated. Recent interest has, therefore, focused on evaluating the use of combinations of key nutrients in clinical practice. A combination of L-arginine, n-3 EFAs and ribonucleic acid is commercially available (e.g. Impact®; Sandoz Nutrition, Minneapolis, MN).

The effects of this combination of nutrients on immune function on patients in intensive care units was first reported by Cerra et al. in 1990.[135] They evaluated 20 patients who had either undergone elective general surgery or who had experienced trauma and/or sepsis which necessitated admission to the intensive care unit. Patients were randomised to receive either the supplemented diet (Impact®) or a standard diet for up to 10 days. Patients receiving Impact® had enhanced responses of peripheral blood lymphocytes to mitogenic stimulation, but there were no clinical benefits demonstrated in this small study. However, it was subsequently demonstrated that such a nutritional regimen could have clinically beneficial effects.[136] 85 patients who were undergoing major abdominal surgery for upper gastrointestinal malignancies were studied. A supplemented diet (L-arginine, up to 34 g day^{-1}; RNA, up to 3 g day^{-1}; n-3 fatty acids, up to 5.3 g day^{-1}) was compared with an isocaloric enteral regimen given for the first seven days postoperatively. The patients receiving the supplemented diet had a reduced incidence of wound complications and wound infections. Furthermore, there was a significant reduction in the mean hospital stay, when compared with the non-supplemented group (10 days versus 15 days, respectively). However, it should be noted that the patients receiving the supplemented diet had a substantially increased nitrogen intake.

A larger, multicentre trial has also investigated the effects of supplementation with L-arginine, RNA and n-3 EFAs (Impact®) in 326 patients who had undergone surgery, trauma or sepsis and required admission to an intensive care unit.[137] All patients had an Acute Physiology and Chronic Health Evaluation II (APACHE II) score of equal to or greater than 10 or a Therapeutic Intervention Scoring System score of 20 or more. Patients were stratified according to age and disease (septic or systemic inflammatory response syndrome) and then randomised to receive either a standard diet (Osmolite HN®) or a diet supplemented with L-arginine, n-3 EFAs and RNA (Impact®), given enterally. The results from this study demonstrated that the patients receiving the supplemented diet had a median reduction in hospital stay of 8 days

Table 3.19 *Nutrient combinations in clinical practice*

Reference	Patients studied	Numbers	Regimen	Effects observed (clinical, immunological)
136	Oesophageal, gastric, pancreatic cancers	85	Randomised to receive enteral diet (Osmolite HN®) or diet supplemented with L-arginine, n-3 EFAs, ribonucleotides (Impact®), for first seven days postoperatively	Supplementation resulted in improved nitrogen balances, stimulation of immunity, reduction in wound infections and complications, reduced hospital in-patient stay
138	Gastro-intestinal malignancies	42	Patients received either a standard diet or diet supplemented with L-arginine, n-3 EFAs, ribonucleotides (Impact®), for 10 days following surgery	Supplementation resulted in immune stimulation (numbers of T cells, T helper and activated T cells; increased antibody levels (IgM, IgG) and increased cytokines (IFN$_\gamma$)). Clinically beneficial effects unknown
139	Upper gastro-intestinal and pancreatic cancers	60	Patients randomised to receive either standard enteral nutrition (Traumacal®) or enteral nutrition supplemented with L-arginine, n-3 EFAs and ribonucleotides (Impact®)	Supplementation resulted in reduction in wound infections and/or complications and shorter hospital stay

Table 3.19 *Continued*

Reference	Patients studied	Numbers	Regimen	Effects observed (clinical, immunological)
135	Sepsis, trauma, elective general surgery	20	Patients randomised to receive either an enteral diet supplemented with L-arginine, n-3 EFAs, ribonucleotides (Impact®), or a standard diet (Osmolite HN®), given for 7–10 days	*In vitro* tests of immune function (*in vitro* lymphocyte responses to mitogens) were enhanced in the supplemented group of patients; no differences in clinical outcome or length of intensive care unit stay
140	Major trauma (abdomen/chest)	98	Patients randomised to either Immun-Aid® (supplemented with L-glutamine, L-arginine, BCAAs, n-3 EFAs, vitamin E, zinc) or Vivonex T.E.N.®	Patients receiving supplemented diet had increases in total lymphocyte count and T helper cells. Clinical benefits of supplementation were fewer intra-abdominal abscesses (0% vs 11%) and less multiple organ failure (0% vs 11%), when compared with non-supplemented patients
137	Sepsis, trauma or following surgery	326	Patients randomised to receive either Impact® or Osmolite HN®, given enterally.	Supplementation resulted in a median reduction in hospital stay for all patients of 8 days, for septic patients of 10 days. Significantly fewer nosocomial infections in the nutritionally supplemented patients. No difference in mortality between the two groups

(P<0.05), but for septic patients the median reduction in hospital stay was 10 days (P<0.05). Furthermore, there was a significant reduction in the development of nosocomial infections in the nutritionally supplemented patients (P<0.01). There was no difference, on the other hand, in mortality rates between the two groups of patients. However, the supplemented diet had (1) β-carotene and higher levels of vitamin E and selenium (known to have immune enhancing properties), (2) contained less total fat, and (3) received more nitrogen, than patients receiving the standard diet. Other studies evaluating these nutrient combinations are summarised in Table 3.19.

In summary, therefore, the use of specific combinations of nutrients seems to offer the most promise in translating the benefits documented on the immune system and metabolic processes into clinically relevant effects. Further studies are now required to define the optimal combinations of nutrients for use in critically ill patients.

Acknowledgements

We are grateful to Dr J Broom MRCP, MRCPath for his helpful comments and for reading the manuscript.

References

1. Studley HO. Percentage of weight loss. A basic indicator of surgical risk in patients with chronic peptic ulcer. JAMA 1936; 106: 458–60.
2. Detsky AS, Baker JP, O'Rourke K et al. Predicting nutrition-associated complications for patients undergoing gastrointestinal surgery. JPEN 1987; 11: 440–6.
3. Lentner C. Geigy scientific tables, 8th edn. Volume 1: Units of measurement, body fluids, composition of the body, nutrition. Ciba Geigy, Basle, 1981.
4. McNeil G. Energy. In: Garrow JS, James WPT (eds) Human nutrition and dietetics 9th edn. Edinburgh: Churchill Livingstone, 1993, pp. 24–37.
5. Demling RH, DeBiasse MA. Micronutrients in critical illness. Crit Care Clin 1995; 11: 651–73.
6. White MF. The transport of cationic amino acids across the plasma membrane of mammalian cells. Biochim Biophys Acta 1985; 822: 355–74.
7. Cuthbertson DP. Observations on the disturbances of metabolism produced by injury to the limbs. Q J Med 1932; 1: 233–46.
8. O'Keefe SJD, Sender PM, James WPT. Catabolic loss of body nitrogen in response to surgery. Lancet 1974; ii: 1035–8.
9. Bergstrom J, Furst P, Noree L-O et al. Intracellular free amino acid concentration in human muscle tissue. J Appl Physiol 1973; 36: 693–8.
10. Essen P, Wernerman J, Ali MR et al. Changes in concentrations of free amino acids in skeletal muscle during 24 hr immediately following elective surgery. Clin Nutr 1988; 7(Suppl): 67.
11. Calder PC. Glutamine and the immune system. Clin Nutr 1994; 13: 2–8.
12. McLennan PA, Brown RA, Rennie MJ. A positive relationship between protein synthetic rate and intracellular glutamine concentration in perfused rat skeletal muscle. FEBS Lett 1987; 215: 187–191.

13. Woolfe RR, Shaw JHF, Durkot MJ. Effect of sepsis on VLDL kinetics: responses in basal state and during glucose infusion. Am J Physiol 1985; 248: 732–40.

14. Nordenstrom J, Carpentier YA, Askanazi J *et al*. Free fatty acid mobilisation and oxidation during total parenteral nutrition in trauma and infection. Ann Surg 1983; 198: 725–35.

15. Stoner HB. Studies on the mechanism of shock. The quantitative aspects of glycogen metabolism after limb ischaemia in the rat. Br J Exp Pathol 1958; 39: 635–51.

16. Allsop JR, Wolfe RR, Burke JF. Glucose kinetics and responsiveness to insulin in the rat injured by burn. Surg Gynecol Obstet 1978; 147: 565–73.

17. Carpentier YA, Askanazi J, Elwyn DH *et al*. Effects of hypocaloric glucose infusion on lipid metabolism in injury and sepsis. J Trauma 1979; 19: 649–54.

18. Burns HJG. The metabolic and nutritional effects of injury and sepsis. In: Burns HJG (ed.) Clinical gastroenterology. London: Ballière Tindall, 1988, pp. 849–67.

19. Broom J. Sepsis and trauma. In: Garrow JS, James WPT (eds) Human nutrition and dietetics, 9th edn. Edinburgh: Churchill Livingstone, 1993, pp. 456–64.

20. Rich AJ, Wright PD. Ketosis and nitrogen excretion in undernourished surgical patients. JPEN 1979; 3: 350–4.

21. Metropolitan Life Assurance Company. Statistical Bulletin 1959; 40: 1.

22. Pettigrew RA. Assessment of malnourished patients. In: Burns HG (ed.) Clinical gastroenterology. London; Ballière Tindall, 1988, pp. 729–49.

23. Durnin JVGA, Womersley J. Body-fat assessed from total body density and its estimation from skin-fold thickness: measurements on 481 men and women aged from 16 to 72 years. Br J Nutr 1974; 32: 77–97.

24. Bistrian BR, Blackburn GL, Hallowell E, Heddle R. Protein status of general surgical patients. JAMA 1974; 230: 858–60.

25. Lukaski HC. Methods for the assessment of human body composition. Am J Clin Nutr 1987; 46: 537–56.

26. Kushner RE, Kunigk A, Alspaugh M *et al*. Validation of bioelectrical-impedance analysis as a measurement of change in body composition in obesity. Am J Clin Nutr 1990; 52: 219–23.

27. Ancell H. Course of lectures on the physiology and pathology of the blood and other animal fluids. Lancet 1939; i: 222–31.

28. Ryan JA, Taft DA. Preoperative nutritional assessment does not predict morbidity and mortality in abdominal operations. Surg Forum 1980; 31: 96–8.

29. McFarlane H, Ogbeide MI, Reddy S *et al*. Biochemical assessment of protein-calorie malnutrition. Lancet 1969; i: 392–5.

30. Rothschild MA, Oratz M, Schreiber SS. Albumin metabolism. Gastroenterology 1973; 64: 324–37.

31. Fleck A, Raines G, Hawker F *et al*. Increased vascular permeability: a major cause of hypoalbuminaemia in disease and injury. Lancet 1985; i: 781–4.

32. Cruikshank AM, Hansell DT, Burns HJG *et al*. Effect of nutritional status on acute phase protein response to elective surgery. Br J Surg 1989; 76: 165–7.

33. Bistrian BR, Blackburn GL, Sherman M, Scrimshaw NS. Therapeutic index of nutritional depletion in hospitalised patients. Surg Gynecol Obstet 1975; 512–16.

34. Eremin O, Broom J. Nutrition and the immune response. In: Eremin O, Sewell HF (eds) The immunological basis of surgical science and practice. Oxford: Oxford University Press, 1992, pp. 133–44.

35. Seltzer MH, Bastidas JA, Cooper DM *et al*. Instant nutritional assessment. JPEN 1979; 3: 157–9.

36. Heys SD, Khan AL, Eremin O. Immune suppression in surgery. Postgrad Surg 1995; 5: 62–7.

37. Russel DM, Walker PM, Leiter LA *et al*. Metabolic and structural changes in skeletal muscle during hypocaloric dieting. Am J Clin Nutr 1984; 39: 503–513.

38. Klidjian AM, Foster KJ, Kammerling RM, Cooper A, Karran SJ. Anthropometric and dynamometric variables to predict serious postoperative complications. Br Med J 1980; 281: 899–901.

39. Lopes J, Russke DM, Whitwell J *et al*. Skeletal muscle function in malnutrition. Am J Clin Nutr 1982; 36: 602–10.

40. Daley BJ, Bistrian BR. Nutritional assess-

ment. In: Zaloga GP (ed.) Nutrition in critical care. St Louis: Mosby Year Book Inc, 1994, p. 28.

41. Mullen JL, Buzby GP, Waldman MT, Gertner MH, Hobbs CL, Rosato EF. Prediction of operative morbidity and mortality by pre-operative nutritional assessment. Surg Forum 1979; 30: 80–2.

42. Mullen JL, Buzby GP, Matthews DC, Smale BF, Rosato EF. Reduction of operative morbidity and mortality by combined pre-operative and post-operative nutritional support. Arch Surg 1980; 192: 604–13.

43. Detsky AL, McLaughlin JR, Baker JP et al. What is subjective global assessment of nutritional status? JPEN 1987, 11: 8–13.

44. Baker JP, Detsky AS, Wesson DE et al. Nutritional assessment. A comparison of clinical judgement and objective measurements. N Engl J Med 1982; 306: 969–72.

45. Hill G, Windsor JA. Nutritional assessment in clinical practice. Nutrition 1995; 11(Suppl): 198–201.

46. Johnson LR, Copeland EM, Dudrick SJ et al. Structural and hormonal alterations in the gastrointestinal tract of parenterally fed rats. Gastroenterology 1975; 68: 1177–83.

47. Levine GM, Deren JJ, Steiger E et al. Role of oral intake in maintenance of gut mass and disaccharide activity. Gastroenterology 1974; 67: 975–82.

48. Wilmore D, Smith R, O'Dwyer S et al. The gut: a central organ after sepsis. Surgery 1988; 104: 917–23.

49. Fong Y, Marano MA, Barber A et al. Total parenteral nutrition and bowel rest modify the metabolic response to endotoxin in humans. Ann Surg 1989; 210: 449–56.

50. Gauderer MWL, Ponsky JL, Izant RJ. Gastrostomy without laparotomy: a percutaneous endoscopic technique for feeding gastrostomy. J Pediatr Surg 1980: 15: 872–5.

51. Hicks ME, Surratt RS, Picus D, Marx MV, Lang EV. Fluoroscopically guided percutaneous gastrostomy and gastroenterostomy: analysis of 158 consecutive cases. AJR 1990; 154: 725–728.

52. Halkier BK, Ho C-S, Yee ACN. Percutaneous feeding gastrostomy with the Seldinger technique: Review of 252 patients. Radiology 1989; 171: 359–62.

53. Grimble GK, Payne-James JJ, Rees RGP, Silk DBA. Nutrition support. London: Medical Tribune UK Ltd, 1989, pp. 32–51.

54. Meguid MM, Campos ACL. Peri-operative feeding. In: Heatley RV, Green JH, Losowsky MS (eds) Consensus in clinical nutrition. Cambridge: Cambridge University Press, 1994, pp. 256–306.

55. Gayle D, Pinchcofsky-Devlin RD, Kaminski MV. Visceral protein increase associated with interrupt versus continuous enteral hyperalimentation. JPEN 1985; 9: 474–6.

56. ASPEN Board of Directors. Guidelines for the use of total parenteral nutrition in the hospitalised adult patient. JPEN 1987; 10: 441–5.

57. Adam A. Insertion of long term central venous catheters: time for a new look. Br Med J 1995; 311: 341–2.

58. Robertson LJ, Mauro MA, Jaques PF. Radiologic placement of Hickman catheters. Radiology 1989; 170: 1007.

59. Lameris JS, Post PJM, Zonderland HM, Gerritsen PG, Kappers-Klunne MC, Schutte HE. Percutaneous placement of Hickman catheters: comparison of sonographically guided and blinded techniques. AJR 1990; 155: 1097–9.

60. Young D, Kettlewell M, Hamilton H. Case for angiographically guided placement is not proved. Br Med J 1995; 311: 1090.

61. Richards DM, Hill J, Scott NA, Bancewicz J, Irving M. Open technique has lower evidence of complications. Br Med J 1995; 311: 1090.

62.. Maki DG, Ringer M. Evaluation of dressing regimens for prevention of infection with peripheral intravenous catheters. JAMA 1987; 258: 2396–403.

63. Khawaja HT, Campbell MJ, Weaver PC. Effect of transdermal glyceryl trinitrate on the survival of peripheral intravenous infusions: a double-blind prospective clinical study. Br J Surg 1988; 75: 1212–15.

64. Furst P, Albers D. Stehle P. Stress-induced intracellular glutamine depletion. The potential use of glutamine containing peptides in parenteral nutrition. In: Adibi SA, Fekl W, Oehmke M (eds) Dipeptides as new substrates in nutrition therapy. Munich: Karger, 1987, pp. 117–36.

65. Wernerman J, Hammarqvist F, von der Decken A, Vinnars E. Ornithine-alpha-

ketoglutarate improves skeletal muscle protein synthesis as assessed by ribosome anal,sis and nitrogen use after surgery. Ann Surg 1987; 206: 674–8.

66. Nanni G, Siegl JH, Coleman B *et al.* Increased lipid fuel dependence in the critically ill septic patient. J Trauma 1984; 24: 14–30.

67. Levinson MR, Groeger JS, Jeevanandam M *et al.* Free fatty acid turnover and lipolysis in septic mechanically ventilated cancer-bearing humans. Metabolism 1988; 37: 618–25.

68. Shaw JHF, Woolfe RR. Energy and protein metabolism in sepsis and trauma. Aust NZ J Surg 1987; 57: 41–7.

69. Venus B, Patel CB, Mathru M *et al.* Pulmonary effects of lipid infusion in patients with acute respiratory failure. Crit Care Med 1984; 12: 293(abstract).

70. Seidner DL, Mascioli EA, Istfan NW *et al.* Effects of long chain triglyceride emulsions on reticuloendothelial system function in humans. JPEN 1989; 13: 614–19.

71. Nordenstrom J, Jarstrand C, Wiernik A. Decreased chemotactic and random migration of leucocytes during intralipid infusion. Am J Clin Nutr 1979; 32: 2416–22.

72. Meguid MM, Campos ACL. Peri-operative feeding. In: Heatley RV, Green JH, Losowsky MS (eds) Consensus in clinical nutrition. Cambridge: Cambridge University Press, 1994, pp. 286.

73. Shanbhogue LKR, Chawls WJ, Weintraub M, Blackburn GL. Parenteral nutrition in the surgical patient. Br J Surg 1987; 74: 172–80.

74. Meguid MM, Campos AC, Hammond WG. Nutritional support in surgical practice: Part I. Am J Surg. 1990; 159: 345–58.

75. Holter AR, Fischer JE. The effects of perioperative hyperalimentation on complications in patients with carcinoma and weight loss. J Surg Res 1977; 23: 31–4.

76. Moghissi K, Hornshaw J, Teasdale PR, Dawes EA. Parenteral nutrition in carcinoma of the oesophagus treated by surgery: nitrogen balance and clinical studies. Br J Surg 1977; 64: 125–8.

77. Heatley RV, Williams RHP, Lewis MH. Preoperative intravenous feeding – a controlled trial. Postgrad Med J 1979, 55: 541–5.

78. Mullen JL, Buzby GP, Matthews DC, Smale BF, Rosato EF. Reduction of operative morbidity and mortality by combined perioperative and postoperative nutritional support. Ann Surg 1980; 192: 604–13.

79. Muller JM, Dients C, Brenner U, Pichlmaier H. Perioperative parenteral feeding in patients with gastrointestinal carcinoma. Lancet 1982, i: 68–71.

80. Detsky AS, Baker JP, O'Rourke K, Goel V. Perioperative parenteral nutrition: a meta-analysis. Ann Intern Med 1987; 107: 196–203.

81. The Veterans Affairs Total Parenteral Nutrition Cooperative Study Group. Perioperative total parenteral nutrition in surgical patients. N Engl J Med 1991; 325: 525–32.

82. Fan S-T, Lo C-M, Lai ECS, Chu K-M, Liu C-L, Wong J. Perioperative nutritional support in patients undergoing hepatectomy for hepatocellular carcinoma. N Engl J Med 1994; 1547–52.

83. Carr CS, Ling KDE, Boulos P, Singer M. Randomised trial of safety and efficacy of immediate post-operative enteral feeding in patients undergoing gastric resection. Br Med J 1996; 312. 869–70.

84. Chiarelli A, Siliprandi L. Burns. In: Zagola GP (ed.) Nutrition in critical care. St Louis: Mosby-Year Book Inc, 1994, pp. 587–97.

85. Deitch EA. Nutrition support of the burn patient. Crit Care Clin 1995; 11: 735–50.

86. McCullough AJ, Tavill AS. Disordered energy and protein metabolism in liver disease. Semin Liver Dis 1991; 11: 265–77.

87. D'atellis N, Skeie B, Kvetan V. Branched chain amino acids. In: Zaloga GP (ed.) Nutrition in critical care. St Louis: Mosby, 1994, pp. 81–106.

88. Dickinson RJ, Ashton MG, Axon ATR, Smith RC, Yeung CK, Hill GL. Controlled trial of intravenous hyperalimentation as an adjunct to the routine therapy of acute colitis. Gastroenterology 1980; 79: 1199–204.

89. McIntyre PB, Powell-Tuck J, Wood SR *et al.* Controlled trial of bowel rest in the treatment of severe acute colitis. Gut 1976; 27: 481–5.

90. Muller JM, Keller HW, Erasmi H, Pichlmaier H. Total parenteral nutrition as sole therapy in Crohn's disease – a prospective study. Br J Surg 1983; 70: 40–3.

91. Jones VA. Comparison of total parenteral

nutrition and enteral diet in induction of remission in Crohn's disease: long term maintenance of remission by personalised food exclusion. Dig Dis Sci 1987; 32(Suppl): 1005–75.

92. Chapman R, Foran R, Dunphey JE. Management of intestinal fistulas. Am J Surg 1964; 108: 157–64.

93. Koretz RL. Nutritional support: how much for how much? Gut 1986; 27(Suppl 1): 85–95.

94. Klein S, Simes J, Blackburn GL. Total parenteral nutrition and cancer clinical trials. Cancer 1986; 58: 1378–86.

95. McGeer AJ, Detsky AS, O'Rourke K. Parenteral nutrition in patients receiving cancer chemotherapy. Ann Intern Med 1989; 110: 734–5.

96. Bozetti F. Is enteral nutrition a primary therapy in cancer patients? Gut 1994; S1: S65–S68.

97. Solassol CI, Joyeux H. Artificial gut with complete nutritive mixtures as a major adjuvant therapy in cancer patients. Acta Chir Scand 1979; 494S: 186–7.

98. Solassol CI, Joyeux H, Dubois J-B. Total parenteral nutrition (TPN) with complete nutritive mixtures: an artificial gut in cancer patients. Nutr Cancer 1979; 1: 13–17.

99 Brown MS, Buchanan RB, Karran SJ. Clinical observations on the effects of elemental diet supplementation during irradiation. Clin Radiol 1980; 31: 19–20.

100. Valerio D, Overett L, Malcolm A et al. Nutritional support of cancer patients receiving abdominal and pelvic radiotherapy: a randomized prospective clinical experiment of intravenous feeding. Surg Forum 1978; 29: 145–8.

101. Kinsella TJ, Malcolm AW, Bothe A. et al. Prospective study of nutritional support during pelvic irradiation. Int J Radiat Oncol Biol Phys 1981; 7: 543–8.

102. Douglass HO, Milliron S, Nava H et al. Elemental diet as an adjuvant for patients with locally advanced gastrointestinal cancer receiving radiation therapy: a prospectively randomized study. JPEN 1978; 2: 682–6.

103. Heys SD, Park KGM, McNurlan MA et al. Stimulation of protein synthesis in human tumours: evidence for modulation of tumour growth. Br J Surg 1991; 78: 483–7.

104. McNurlan MA, Heys SD, Park KGM et al. Tumour and host tissue responses to branched chain amino acid supplementation in patients with cancer. Clin Sci 1994; 86: 339–45.

105. Nakagawa J, Takahashi T, Suzuki T et al. Amino acid requirements of children: minimal needs of tryptophan, arginine, histidine based on nitrogen balance. J Nutr 1963; 80: 305–10.

106. Elsair J, Poey J, Isaad J et al. Effect of arginine chlorhydrate on nitrogen balance during the three days following surgery in man. Biomedicine 1978; 29: 312–17.

107. Daly JM, Reynolds J, Thom A et al. Immune and metabolic effects of arginine in the surgical patient. Ann Surg 1988; 208: 513–23.

108. Barbul A, Lazarou SA, Efron DT, Wasserkrug HL, Efron G. Arginine enhances wound healing and lymphocyte immune responses in humans. Surgery 1990; 108: 331–7.

109. Park KGM, Hayes PD, Garlick PJ et al. Stimulation of lymphocyte natural cytotoxicity by L-arginine. Lancet 1991; 337: 645–6.

110. Brittenden J, Park KGM, Heys SD et al. L-Arginine stimulates host defenses in patients with breast cancer. Surgery, 1994; 115: 205–12.

111. Brittenden J. Heys SD, Ross J, Park KGM, Eremin O. Natural cytotoxicity in breast cancer patients receiving neoadjuvant chemotherapy: effects of L-arginine supplementation. Eur J Surg Oncol 1994; 20: 467–72.

112. Bergstrom J, Furst P, Noree L-O, Vinnars E. Intracellular free amino acid concentration in human muscle tissue. J Appl Physiol 1974; 36: 693–6.

113. Aulick LH, Wilmore DM. Increased peripheral amino acid release following burn surgery. Surgery 1979; 85: 560–5.

114. Roth E, Furnovics J, Muhlbacher F et al. Metabolic disorders in severe abdominal sepsis: glutamine deficiency in skeletal muscle. Clin Nutr 1982; 1: 25–41.

115. Hammarqvist F, Wernerman J, Ali R, von der Decken A, Vinnars E. Addition of glutamine to total parenteral nutrition after elective abdominal surgery spares free glutamine in muscle, counteracts the fall in muscle protein synthesis, and improves

nitrogen balance. Ann Surg 1989; 209: 455–61.

116. Stehle P, Mertes N, Puchstein Ch, Zander J, Albers S, Lawin P. Effect of parenteral glutamine peptide supplements on muscle glutamine loss and nitrogen balance after major surgery. Lancet 1989; 1: 231–3.

117. Ziegler TR, Young LS, Benfell K *et al.* Clinical and metabolic efficacy of glutamine-supplemented parenteral nutrition after bone marrow transplantation. Ann Intern Med 1992; 16: 821–8.

118. O'Riordain MG, Fearon KCH, Ross JA *et al.* Glutamine-supplemented total parenteral nutrition enhances T-lymphocyte response in surgical patients undergoing colorectal resection. Ann Surg 1994; 220: 212–21.

119. Klimberg CS, Salloum RM, Kasper M *et al.* Oral glutamine accelerates healing of the small intestine and improves outcome after whole abdominal radiation. Arch Surg 1990; 125: 1040–5.

120. Souba WW, Klimberg VS, Copeland EM. Glutamine nutrition in the management of radiation enteritis. JPEN 1990; 14(suppl 4): 106–8.

121. Byrne TA, Persinger RL, Young LS, Ziegler TR, Wilmore DW. A new treatment for patients with short-bowel syndrome. Ann Surg 1995; 222: 243–55.

122. Tayek JA, Bistrian BR, Hehir DJ, Martin R, Moldawer L, Blackburn GL. Improved protein kinetics and albumin synthesis by branched chain amino acid-enriched total parenteral nutrition in cancer cachexia. Cancer 1986; 58: 147–57.

123. Brennan MF, Cerra F, Daly JM *et al.* Branched chain amino acids in stress and injury. JPEN 1986; 10: 446–52.

124. Heys SD, Gough DB, Khan AL, Eremin O. Nutritional pharmacology and malignant disease: a therapeutic modality in patients with cancer. Br J Surg, 1996; 83: 608–19.

125. Purasiri P, Ashby J, Heys SD, Eremin O. Effect of essential fatty acids on circulating T cell subsets in patients with colorectal cancer. Cancer Immunol Immunother 1994; 39: 217–22.

126. Purasiri P, Ashby J, Heys SD, Eremin O. Effect of essential fatty acids on natural cytotoxicity in patients with colorectal cancer. Eur J Surg Oncol 1995; 21: 254–60.

127. Purasiri P, Murray A, Richardson S, Heys SD, Horrobin D, Eremin O. Modulation of cytokine production in vivo by dietary essential fatty acids in patients with colorectal cancer. Clin Sci 1994; 87: 711–17.

128. Braun W, Ishizuka M, Yajima Y *et al.* Spectrum and mode of actions of poly A:U in the stimulation of immune responses. In: Beers RF, Braun W (eds) Biological effect of polyribonucleotides. New York: Springer, 1971, p. 139.

129. Khan AL, Richardson S, Drew J. *et al.* Polyadenylic-polyuridylic acid (PAPU) enhances natural cell-mediated cytotoxicity in patients with breast cancer undergoing mastectomy. Surgery, 1995; 118: 531–8.

130. Khan AL. Heys SD, Eremin O. Synthetic polyribonucleotides: current role and potential use in oncological practice. Eur J Surg Oncol 1995; 21: 224–7.

131. Lacour J, Lacour F, Spira A *et al.* Adjuvant treatment with polyadenylic-polyuridylic acid (polyA.polyU) in operable breast cancer. Lancet 1980; i: 161–4.

132. Lacour J, Lacour F, Spira A *et al.* Adjuvant treatment with polyadenylic polyuridylic acid in operable breast cancer: updated results of a randomised trial. Br Med J 1984; 288: 589–92.

133. Lacour J, Laplanche A, Delozier T *et al.* Polyadenylic-polyuridylic acid plus loco-regional and pelvic radiotherapy versus chemotherapy with CMF as adjuvants in operable breast cancer. Breast Cancer Res Treat 1991; 19: 15–21.

134. Lacour J, Laplanche A, Malafosse M *et al.* Polyadenylic-polyuridylic acid as an adjuvant in resectable colorectal carcinoma: a 6½ year follow-up analysis of a multicentre double blind randomized trial. Eur J Surg Oncol 1992; 18: 599–604.

135. Cerra FB, Lehman S, Konstantinides N, Konstantinides F, Shronts EP, Holman R. Effect of enteral nutrition on in vitro tests of immune function in ICU patients: a preliminary report. Nutrition 1990; 6: 84–7.

136. Daly JM, Lieberman MD, Goldfine J *et al.* Enteral nutrition with supplemental arginine, RNA, and omega-3 fatty acids in patients after operation: Immunologic, metabolic, and clinical outcome. Surgery 1992; 112: 56–67.

137. Bower RH, Cerra FB, Berdashadsky B *et al.*
Early enteral administration of a formula
(Impact®) supplemented with arginine,
nucleotides, and fish oil in intensive care
patients: results of a multicenter, prospective, randomized, clinical trial. Crit Care
Med 1995; 23: 436–9.

138. Kemen M, Senkal M. Homann H-H *et al.*
Early post-operative enteral nutrition with
arginine-ω-3 fatty acids and ribonucleic
acid-supplemented diet versus placebo in
cancer patients: An immunologic evaluation
of impact. Crit Care Med 1995; 23: 652–9.

139. Daly JM, Weintraub FN, Shou J, Rosato EF,
Lucia M. Enteral nutrition during multi-
modality therapy in upper gastrointestinal
cancer patients. Ann Surg 1995; 221:
327–38.

140. Moore FA, Moore EE, Kudsk K *et al.* Clinical
benefits of an immune-enhancing diet for
early postinjury enteral feeds. J Trauma
1994; 37: 607–15.

4 The treatment of non-variceal upper gastrointestinal bleeding

Robert J. C. Steele

Introduction

Non-variceal upper gastrointestinal bleeding remains a significant problem in the Western World. A recent population based audit of upper gastrointestinal bleeding (the first in 25 years)[1] gives the incidence of acute bleeding as 103 cases per 100 000 adults per year. Of this variceal bleeding accounted for only 4% of the total. Overall mortality was 14% (11% in emergency admissions and 33% among inpatients who began bleeding).

It is interesting to compare these figures with those from two previous studies from the 1960s,[2,3] where mortality was 10% and 14% respectively. It is important to note, however, that 27% of patients from the recent audit were over the age of 80 years, as compared with less than 10% in the earlier studies, and that both incidence and mortality increased markedly with age.

Thus, although there has been little improvement in mortality over the years, this observation must be set against a dramatic shift in the age of the population at risk.

There is no room for complacency, however, and there is little doubt that the formation of specialist gastrointestinal bleeding units can minimise the morbidity and mortality of gastrointestinal bleeding.[4] Many of the therapeutic advances described in this chapter have been shown to have a significant effect, but it must be stressed that they can only be useful when employed by enthusiastic, dedicated and properly trained personnel.

Aetiology

Peptic ulcer remains by far the most common cause for upper gastrointestinal haemorrhage in the Western World. The recent audit reported by Rockall and others[1] found that peptic ulcer accounted for

Figure 4.1
Frequency of causes for upper gastro-intestinal bleeding in the United Kingdom. (From Rockall et al.[1])

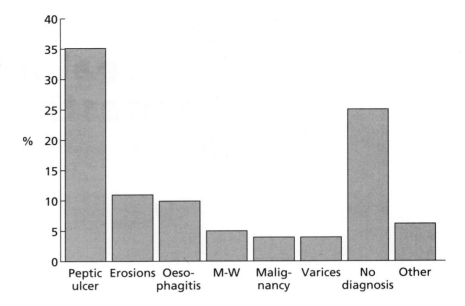

35% of cases (Fig. 4.1), and the rest of this chapter is therefore largely devoted to the management of this problem. Peptic ulcers bleed because of erosion of blood vessels, and the severity of the bleed is dependent on the size of the vessel affected. Simple oozing is caused by damage to small submucosal vessels less than 0.1 mm in diameter, but the more important arterial bleeding indicates a large vessel (between 0.1 and 2 mm in diameter) in the base of the ulcer which has been eroded by the inflammatory process.

In this case, the vessel tends to loop up to the base of the ulcer (Fig. 4.2), and when the apex of this loop becomes eroded, haemorrhage occurs. This defect in the artery may become plugged by a sentinel clot or thrombus, and it is this which is usually interpreted as a visible vessel by the endoscopist. In ulcers on the posterior wall of the duodenum or the lesser curve of the stomach the gastroduodenal or left gastric arteries can be involved, and these lesions are particularly prone to massive haemorrhage and rebleeding after initial stabilisation.[5]

Other less common but appreciably frequent causes of non-variceal upper gastrointestinal bleeding include erosions, oesophagitis, Mallory–Weiss tears and malignancy.

Erosions

Acute erosive gastritis must be distinguished from the chronic forms of gastritis as these do not bleed. Haemorrhagic gastritis is often caused by stressful stimuli such as head injury, burns, shock or hepatic failure and is probably related to impaired mucosal blood flow. Drugs may also be responsible, and the agents which are commonly

Figure 4.2 *Vessel looping up to the ulcer base.*

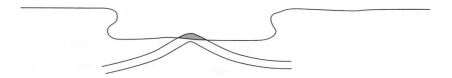

implicated include steroids, non-steroidal inflammatory agents and alcohol.

Oesophagitis

Oesophagitis is a form of peptic ulcer disease, but usually only causes minor acute bleeding. Occasionally, however, a significant vessel may be involved with consequent massive arterial haemorrhage which must be distinguished from variceal bleeding.

Mallory–Weiss tear

The Mallory–Weiss (M-W) tear occurs in the region of the gastro-oesophageal junction as a result of severe vomiting or retching, often after excessive alcohol intake. The tear is mostly in the gastric mucosa, but may extend into the oesophagus, and although bleeding is profuse, it usually stops spontaneously. Very occasionally repeated vomiting may result in a full thickness tear, 'Boerhaave's syndrome' and this is inevitably associated with sudden onset of severe pain in the upper abdomen or chest.

Malignancy

Carcinoma and lymphoma of the stomach, when at an advanced ulcerated stage, commonly bleed. This usually results in occult blood loss, but will occasionally present with acute haemorrhage.

Other diagnoses

There are several other conditions which may present as upper gastrointestinal haemorrhage and these are listed in Table 4.1.

Presentation and assessment

Patients with acute gastrointestinal haemorrhage present with haematemesis, melaena or frank rectal bleeding plus the signs and symptoms of hypovolaemia in varying degrees. Haematemesis implies vomiting of blood, either in a recognisable form or as dark brown grainy material ('coffee grounds') if the blood has been in the stomach long enough for acid to convert the haemoglobin into methaemoglobin.

Table 4.1 *Causes of upper gastrointestinal bleeding*

	Oesophagus	Stomach	Duodenum	Small bowel
Inflammation	Oesophagitis Barret's ulcer	Peptic ulcer Gastritis Dieulafoy lesion	Peptic ulcer	Peptic ulcer at stoma or Meckel's diverticulum Crohn's disease
Vascular abnormalities	Varices Aortic aneurysm	Varices Vascular malformation	Aorto-duodenal fistula	Vascular malformation
Neoplasia	Carcinoma	Carcinoma Leiomyoma Lymphoma Polyp	Carcinoma of ampulla Carcinoma of pancreas	Tumour
Other	Mallory–Weiss tear		Haemobilia Pancreatitis Post ERCP	Diverticulum

Melaena is the passage of altered blood per rectum. This is recognised as jet black liquid stool, sometimes tinged red when very fresh, which has a characteristic, pungent smell. It results from the oxidation of haem by intestinal and bacterial enzymes, and indicates that the site of bleeding is probably from the upper gastrointestinal tract, and almost certainly proximal to the ileocaecal junction. It is important to appreciate that melaena can persist for several days after the cessation of active bleeding, and its continued appearance may be misleading. It is also very important to distinguish between melaena and other causes of dark stool. Simple constipation tends to be associated with hard, dark faeces, and oral iron results in a sticky but relatively solid grey–black motion.

Fresh rectal bleeding immediately suggests a site within the colon, rectum or anal canal, but it must be remembered that brisk bleeding from the upper gastrointestinal tract can easily present in this way. Thus, in the patient with massive fresh rectal bleeding, particularly when there are signs of hypovolaemia, urgent steps must be taken to exclude bleeding from the stomach or duodenum.

When the patient with acute gastrointestinal bleeding has been identified from one of the above symptoms, the following assessment and management plan should be instituted.

1. Assess the patient rapidly to ascertain airway patency, conscious level and external signs of blood loss.

2. Measure pulse and blood pressure.
3. Establish venous access and cross-match blood.
4. If the patient is haemodynamically stable, obtain a full history, carry out a full examination and proceed with investigations promptly but within normal working hours.
5. If the patient is haemodynamically unstable, fluid resuscitation must start immediately. If an adequate pulse and blood pressure are achieved rapidly and can be maintained without aggressive fluid replacement, then it is possible to proceed as for the stable patient. However, if any difficulty is encountered in stabilisation, it is necessary to investigate the patient rapidly, often with *simultaneous* resuscitation.

Investigation

The mainstay of the investigation of acute upper gastrointestinal bleeding is flexible endoscopy. Accordingly, this section concentrates mostly on endoscopy and is divided into the following sections: (1) endoscopy equipment, (2) technique in acute bleeding; (3) endoscopic appearances in acute bleeding and (4) other diagnostic techniques.

Endoscopy equipment

Most modern endoscopy units have videoendoscopy equipment, and for routine gastrointestinal endoscopy this has major advantages. First, it affords an excellent view to all the members of the team, which is of great importance for endoscopic intervention where the assistant has to coordinate with the endoscopist, and it greatly facilitates teaching. Secondly, the head of the endoscope is held away from the endoscopist's face, which reduces the risk of blood or secretions splashing into the eyes.

Unfortunately, even the latest generation of videoendoscopy equipment is not ideal for examining the bleeding patient. In the presence of large amounts of blood the image can become very dark and fuzzy owing to saturation of the 'red channel' of the chip camera, and this can seriously hamper both diagnosis and therapy. Thus, although videoendoscopy is often suitable for upper gastrointestinal haemorrhage, it is useful to have a direct-viewing instrument to hand for the demanding situation.

The endoscope itself must be chosen with some care for the particular circumstances. The slim or 'paediatric' instrument is very manoeuvrable, but its 2.8 mm working or biopsy channel limits the use of therapeutic accessories, and does not allow good suction. The big double-channel endoscope allows good suction and washing through the unoccupied channel when an accessory is in use, but it is uncomfortable for the patient and cumbersome when trying to reach relatively inaccessible lesions. The best compromise is an endoscope with a single wide (3.7 mm) working channel, and a separate forward washing channel which allows good suction and the passage of a wide range of therapeutic instruments.

Other pieces of equipment which are important in the acute bleeding situation include a lavage tube, a pharyngeal overtube, washing devices and therapeutic accessories. *The lavage tube* is occasionally required when the stomach is full of clot, and the most useful device is a wide bore (40 Fr if possible), soft tube with an open end as well as side holes. *The pharyngeal overtube* is a 30 cm tube with a flange at one end to prevent it slipping into the mouth. This can be passed over the endoscope when lavage is needed; it both facilitates repeated changes between the endoscope and the lavage tube, while at the same time protecting the airway. The simplest *washing method* is to insert the nozzle of a 20 ml syringe filled with water directly into the working or washing channel of the endoscope and to empty its contents in one rapid action. A useful alternative is to use a dental irrigator (water toothbrush) modified by the provision of a foot switch and by attaching the outlet to the working or washing channel. Finally it is important to have all the therapeutic accessories that might be required immediately to hand; these will be described in a later section.

Endoscopy technique in acute bleeding

Even when not urgent as a life-saving procedure, endoscopy should take place within 24 h of admission, as the chances of making a diagnosis diminish rapidly after this time.[6] Usually the endoscopy will take place in the endoscopy room under benzodiazepine sedation, but in the patient who is vomiting copious quantities of blood, general anaesthesia with cuffed endotracheal intubation should be considered. When sedation is considered adequate, careful monitoring is still required, and the patient's pulse and blood pressure should be measured regularly, preferably using an automatic device. Pulse oximetry should also be regarded as mandatory, as arterial desaturation is a particular risk during a prolonged procedure with a large diameter endoscope. For this reason it is also wise to administer oxygen throughout the procedure, either nasally or by means of a specially designed mouth guard.

The endoscopy should take place on a bed or trolley which can tip into either the head-up or head-down position. The examination should start with the patient in the strict left lateral position, as this encourages blood to pool in the fundus of the stomach where ulcers are uncommon (Fig. 4.3). If it becomes necessary to view the fundus, this can be done by turning the patient on to the right side, and tipping the trolley head-up so that the blood falls into the antrum. When the endoscope has been passed beyond the gastro-oesophageal junction, it is not uncommon to encounter a seeming impenetrable mass of blood and clot. However, as long as the stomach is given long enough to distend and the above guidelines are followed, a moderate amount of blood in the stomach rarely prevents adequate visualisation of the responsible lesion. Often clot will be seen overlying an ulcer, and it is

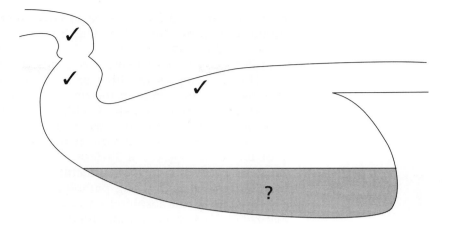

Figure 4.3 *Pooling of blood in the stomach in the left lateral position. This leaves the lesser curve, antrum and duodenum clear of blood. ✓, indicates areas visible; ?, indicates area of uncertainty.*

important to wash this to ascertain whether or not it is adherent; this has implications for prognosis and treatment, and gentle washing will rarely precipitate haemorrhage.

Occasionally, however, there will be too much blood in the stomach to allow an adequate examination, and lavage will be necessary. The 40 Fr lavage tube, ideally with a pharyngeal overtube in place, is passed into the stomach and direct suction is applied. This will often clear enough blood and clot to allow the examination to proceed. If not, it then becomes necessary to carry out a formal lavage, by rapidly pouring in a litre of water via a funnel. This will break up the clot, which can then be siphoned out by placing the tube in a dependent position.

Endoscopic appearances of the bleeding ulcer

The endoscopic appearance of a peptic ulcer which has bled or is still bleeding provides valuable prognostic information which can be used to predict outcome and risk of rebleeding.[7–10] Various classification systems have been used, and possibly the most popular has been that proposed by Forrest and others which distinguishes between active bleeding, a non-bleeding visible vessel and adherent clot.[6] Unfortunately, however, there is considerable interobserver variation in the interpretation of these appearances[11–13] indicating that the descriptive terms commonly employed lack sufficient precision. It is nonetheless important to have some means of describing the 'stigmata of recent haemorrhage', and the categories given below are widely recognised.

Active arterial bleeding indicates erosion of an artery or arteriole, and although studies have indicated that this type of bleeding may stop in up to 40% of cases[14], it is regarded as a clear indication for intervention.

Active non-pulsatile bleeding or oozing from the base of an ulcer implies ongoing bleeding from a partially occluded vessel and is associated with a 20–30% chance of continued bleeding. It must be distinguished from contact bleeding from the edge of an ulcer which is of no significance.

A visible vessel is best defined as a raised lesion in the base of an ulcer. This may represent either an exposed vessel or an organised thrombus plugging a hole in the underlying vessel, and is important as it carries a significant risk of rebleeding if untreated. The precise risk is difficult to ascertain because there is considerable disagreement among endoscopists as to what constitutes a visible vessel,[11–13] but it is probably in the region of 30–50%.

Adherent blood clot may be difficult to distinguish from a visible vessel, but as the underlying pathology is usually identical, making the distinction is not absolutely necessary.

Flat red or *black spots* indicate dried blood in the slough of the ulcer base, and are of little significance, with a rebleeding rate of less than 5%.

These stigmata change fairly rapidly, and a recent study from China has indicated that visible vessels disappear in a mean of four days.[15] Given the sinister implications of a visible vessel, it is unwise to discharge a patient from hospital until endoscopic evidence of fading is seen, regardless of whether or not endoscopic therapy has been delivered.

Other diagnostic techniques

When upper gastrointestinal endoscopy by an experienced endoscopist fails to provide the diagnosis, other approaches are required. If blood is not seen in the stomach, and the patient is haemodynamically unstable with continuing signs of bleeding, it is usually best to move immediately to mesenteric angiography.[16] With fresh melaena or rectal bleeding, colonoscopy is usually fruitless, and if the blood loss is more than $0.5 \, ml \, min^{-1}$, on angiography the bleeding site will be seen as contrast entering the bowel lumen.

If the bleeding site is in the colon, its anatomical position will be obvious. However, when it is in the small bowel localisation can be a problem, and it is helpful for the radiologist to leave a super-selective angiogram catheter as close as possible to the lesion so that at laparotomy the affected segment of bowel can be identified by injection of methylene blue.

When the patient is bleeding intermittently, angiography may not be able to detect the blood loss, and in this case labelled red call scanning may provide useful information.[17] A blood sample is taken, the red cells labelled with an isotope such as ^{99m}Tc-methyl diphosphonate or Indium-111 and re-injected into the patient. When the bleeding occurs, a proportion of the cells will enter the gut and be seen as a distinct 'blush' on the gamma-camera image. Unfortunately, once blood has entered the intestine it rapidly moves along making localisation of the lesion imprecise. For this reason it is important for the

Figure 4.4
Algorithm for the investigation of massive rectal bleeding.

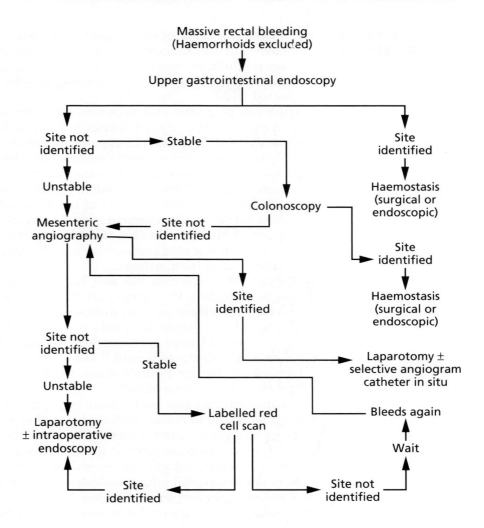

patient to have regular, frequent scans over a prolonged period, and this is often not feasible.

Occasionally it will be impossible to localise the site of bleeding, and the surgeon will be forced into an exploratory operation. At laparotomy it is usually possible to determine whether the bleeding is originating from the small or large bowel, and an appropriate intra-operative endoscopy can be performed to pin-point the lesion.[18,19] This is done either per anuum after antegrade lavage of the colon with warm saline, or through a small bowel enterotomy at the most convenient site. An algorithm for the investigation of massive melaena or rectal bleeding is given in Fig. 4.4.

Medical treatment

The majority of cases of upper gastrointestinal bleeding will resolve spontaneously, and supportive care will be all that is necessary. There is, however, little evidence that specific pharmacological intervention has any effect on peptic ulcer bleeding despite a number of well conducted trials.

Reduction of gastric acid secretion might be expected to help, as an acid environment impairs platelet function and haemostasis, and a meta-analysis of trials of H_2 receptor antagonists has suggested that such therapy might reduce mortality, especially for gastric ulcer bleeding.[20] Meta-analysis has its limitations, however, and more important data come from two large independent placebo-controlled randomised trials. The first examined the effect of the powerful H_2 receptor antagonist famotidine,[21] and the second looked at the proton pump inhibitor omeprazole.[22] Neither was able to demonstrate any effect, and it has to be concluded that acid suppression has little influence on the course of gastrointestinal haemorrhage.

Inhibition of fibrinolysis has also been explored, and in one large trial of tranexamic acid, a significant 50% reduction in mortality was seen.[23] However, there were no differences in rebleeding or operation rates, and for this reason the study has been criticised. All the trials of tranexamic acid have been put together in a meta-analysis which suggests that patients do benefit,[24] but as this conclusion was greatly influenced by the one positive study the use of fibrinolysis therapy cannot be firmly recommended.

Somatostatin has also been tested in peptic ulcer bleeding on the basis of its ability to reduce both acid secretion and splanchnic blood flow, but apart from some evidence that it may be useful in torrential bleeding from gastric erosions,[25] the trials have been disappointing. The prostaglandin analogue misoprostol appears to be promising, and there is one small trial which indicates that it may reduce the need for emergency surgery in peptic ulcer bleeding.[26]

Overall, therefore, the evidence indicates that pharmacological treatment makes little difference to the outcome in non-variceal upper gastrointestinal haemorrhage. Further studies are underway, however, and the results are awaited with interest.

Endoscopic treatment

Endoscopic haemostasis for peptic ulcer bleeding is now well established, and many randomised trials testify to the ability of several treatment modalities in reducing rebleeding and the need for emergency surgery. In this section, the various available methods will be described, and evidence relating to their efficacy will be reviewed.

Techniques of endoscopic haemostasis

Currently, the main endoscopic techniques available for controlling peptic ulcer bleeding are laser photocoagulation, bipolar diathermy, heater probe, injection sclerotherapy and adrenaline injection. Each of these will now be considered in turn.

Laser photocoagulation

Laser photocoagulation is essentially a method of delivering energy which is converted into heat on contact with tissue. The laser which is now used almost exclusively for peptic ulcer bleeding is the neodymium yttrium aluminium garnet (Nd-YAG), as this appears to achieve sufficient tissue penetration to coagulate vessels of reasonable size. A suitable laser unit has to be capable of delivering 60–100 watts, and it is best used with a double-channel endoscope. This allows adequate venting which prevents overdistension of the stomach and permits escape of the smoke generated by vaporisation of tissue.

When an ulcer is to be treated by laser therapy, it is washed clear of blood and loose clot so that the bleeding point can be clearly seen. A red helium neon aiming beam is then activated, and a test 0.5 s 70 watt pulse of the invisible Nd-YAG laser delivered to the edge of the ulcer. If the settings are correct, this should cause blanching of the mucosa but no ulceration. Ideally, the fibre should be 1 cm from the ulcer when the laser is activated.

The aim is then to coagulate the feeding vessel, but it is impossible to be sure of the course of this vessel from the external appearance of the ulcer (Fig. 4.5). For this reason it is necessary to surround the bleeding point or visible vessel with a tight ring of pulses. This will maximise the chances of delivering heat both upstream and downstream of the exposed portion of the vessel.

The main reported dangers of laser therapy are perforation of the stomach or duodenum and exacerbation of the bleeding, but these can be minimised by good technique. The laser is also hazardous for staff, and it is important for everyone involved to wear specific filter goggles to prevent possible retinal damage; the room used also has to be specifically modified. These problems, together with the cost of the

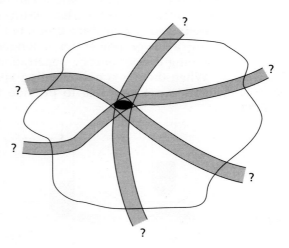

Figure 4.5 *Diagram illustrating the unpredictability of the course of a vessel which becomes visible in an ulcer base.*

laser unit, its relative immobility and the rather indifferent results achieved in randomised trials, have resulted in laser therapy being superseded by the simpler methods described below.

Bipolar diathermy

Diathermy also relies on the generation of heat, this time by electrical current flowing through tissue near an electrode. This can be achieved by a monopolar or a bipolar system, but the former causes an unpredictably deep thermal injury and adherence of coagulated tissue to the probe can be a problem. Bipolar diathermy avoids these disadvantages to a greater extent, and has now superseded the monopolar equipment.

All contact probes, including bipolar diathermy and heat probes, rely on coaptive coagulation to achieve optimum results (Fig. 4.6). This implies that the walls of the vessel to be treated are brought into close apposition by external pressure while heat is applied. This has two advantages. First, if the pressure stops active bleeding, it means that the probe must be correctly positioned. Second, the dissipation of heat by the flow of blood ('heat sink') is minimised so that the heat has maximum effect.

The bipolar device which is now most widely used is the BICAP® probe which consists of three pairs of bipolar electrodes arranged radially around the tip. This allows current to pass into the tissue regardless of the angle of the probe tip relative to the surface of the ulcer. The current delivered to tissue is dependent on electrical resistance, and as this increases with desiccation, the current flow is decreased as the tissue heats up and dries out, thus limiting damage. The probes come in various sizes, but the best results have been reported with the largest (3.2 mm).

As for laser therapy, the ulcer must be washed to obtain a good view of the bleeding point, and if there is active bleeding this should be compressed firmly in order to obtain as much control as possible. The power and pulse length can be varied considerably, and there is some debate as to the ideal settings. Conventionally, a 50 W 2 s pulse is delivered two or three times, but it has recently been suggested that using a lower power for a longer time produces better results by allowing deeper energy penetration of the tissue.

When there is a non-bleeding visible vessel tamponade of haemorrhage is not available to provide the clue as to where to place the

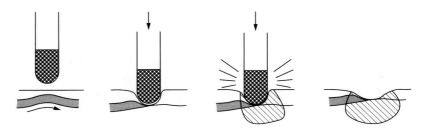

Figure 4.6 *Coaptive coagulation.*

probe, and it is then necessary to produce a ring of coagulation around the vessel as for laser treatment. When this has been done it is usual to treat the vessel itself in order to flatten any protruding lesion.

Heat probe

The principles of using the heat probe are very similar to that of the BICAP® device, but there are two theoretical advantages. First, because no electrical energy has to pass into the tissue, the probe can be coated by non-stick material which prevents adherence to coagulated tissue. Second, because the temperature developed is independent of tissue desiccation, the delivery of energy is not impeded by coagulum and tissue bonding may therefore be greater.

The heat probe consists of a coated hollow metal tip containing an inner heater coil which can rapidly generate a temperature of 150°C. This temperature is effective for coagulation, but avoids excessive vaporisation. The probe also incorporates channels for washing which allows better visualisation during coaptation and coagulation. As with BICAP®, the largest available probe (3.2 mm) is preferable.

The technique for using the heat probe is almost identical to that for the BICAP® device with the exception that the energy settings are graded as joules rather than watts and duration. The probe is positioned with firm pressure, and three to four pulses of around 30 J are delivered.

Both heat probe and bipolar diathermy are relatively safe, but both have been reported as causing perforations and reactivation of bleeding. It is therefore important to exercise great care in their use.

Adrenaline injection

Adrenaline injection probably achieves immediate haemostasis by virtue of the tamponade effect of the injected fluid, but the permanent effect depends on vasospasm and platelet activation encouraging the formation of platelet and fibrin thrombus within the vessel lumen.[27] A solution of 1 in 10 000 is most often used, delivered by means of endoscopic injection needle of the type used for sclerotherapy for oesophageal varices.

When an active bleeding point is identified, the ulcer is washed and the needle assembly, already flushed through with the adrenaline solution, is passed through the working channel of the endoscope with the point withdrawn into the sheath. As soon as the needle is seen emerging from the endoscope, the assistant is asked to push out the needle point. The needle is then advanced into the base of the bleeding point, and the assistant injects 0.5 ml of the adrenaline solution. A fair degree of force is required, and if the injection is very easy, the needle is probably not in the tissue. If the bleeding does not stop immediately, a further 0.5 ml should be injected at the same site and the needle moved to a slightly different site to repeat the process. When the bleeding has stopped more adrenaline should be injected around the bleeding point in four to six 0.5 ml aliquots. The non-bleeding visible vessel can be treated in the same manner.

One situation where injection therapy is particularly useful is where adherent clot obscures the bleeding point. This makes thermal coagulation difficult, but it is quite easy to pass a needle through the clot to allow injection of the ulcer base. Exacerbation of the bleeding is not a significant problem, presumably due to the combined tamponade and vasoconstriction.

Adrenaline injection appears to be very safe, with no recorded instances of perforation. Tachycardia and hypertension can occur, however, and although fatal arrhythmias have not been reported, it is a sensible precaution to use ECG monitoring in addition to pulse and blood pressure recording during the procedure.

Injection sclerotherapy

The sclerosants which have been used in non-variceal haemorrhage include absolute alcohol, 1% polidocanol, 5% ethanolamine and 3% sodium tetradecyl sulphate (STD). Alcohol acts by dehydration and fixation of tissue whereas the others are detergents which cause endothelial damage; the intended end result is obliteration or thrombosis of the feeding vessel.

If there is active bleeding it is usual to control this with adrenaline injection as above, and then to surround the bleeding point with aliquots of sclerosant – 0.1 ml for alcohol or 0.5 ml for the other sclerosants. Sclerotherapy of a non-bleeding vessel will not require adrenaline injection unless the injection precipitates active bleeding. As for adrenaline, sclerotherapy appears to be safe, although there have been a few cases of extensive necrosis of the stomach wall after injection of the left gastric artery.[28]

Results of endoscopic treatment

Because most upper gastrointestinal bleeding stops without intervention it is important for techniques of endoscopic therapy to be subjected to randomised trials before they are accepted as effective. Before drawing conclusions from these trials, however, it is important to be clear about the end points which are being studied.

Mortality is obviously the most important, but as this is likely to be around 5% in interested centres, it would take a very large trial to demonstrate a convincing improvement in death rate.[29] The next most important is probably need for emergency surgery; this can be associated with a mortality of up to 20%,[30] and any intervention which can reduce urgent operation rates is likely to be translated into a reduction in morbidity and mortality. Rebleeding is less reliable as an end point as it does not necessarily represent a clinically significant outcome if it does not result in surgery or death. In many trials, however, rebleeding is the only end point which is affected.

The available trials can be delivered into those which have compared a specific form of endoscopic haemostasis with no endoscopic therapy, and those which have compared different techniques. In the remainder of this section, the trials which have examined the efficacy of each of the commonly used methods against conventional treatment will be considered, and this will be followed by an appraisal of the comparative trials.

Laser photocoagulation

Laser photocoagulation was first used for bleeding peptic ulcer in the 1970s, and since then there have been at least 12 randomised controlled trials comparing it with no endoscopic therapy.[31,32] Both the Nd-YAG and the argon laser have been used, but the former has superseded the latter owing to its superior tissue penetration qualities.

Of the nine trials of the Nd-YAG laser, four were poorly designed or were not based on sufficiently accurate definitions of the lesions being treated. Of the five remaining studies, four produced favourable results.[33-36] In the first, from Rutgeerts and colleagues, significant reduction in clinical rebleeding was seen among those who had active bleeding, but there were no differences in mortality or need for surgery.[33] Two studies have shown a reduction in the need for emergency surgery,[34,35] and one of these showed a reduction in mortality in a high-risk subgroup.[35] In both of these studies, however, relatively large numbers of patients were excluded prior to randomisation usually because of difficulties in aiming the laser beam. In another study, no benefit whatsoever was seen from laser therapy,[37] but this may have been related to selection of low-risk patients and relative lack of experience among the endoscopists.

Bipolar diathermy

Of six controlled trials of bipolar diathermy, three have been unable to demonstrate any benefit.[38-40] One showed a reduction in clinical rebleeding, but no difference in the need for emergency surgery.[41] The most impressive studies, however, were carried out by Loren Laine who performed one trial in patients with active bleeding[42] and one in patients whose ulcers exhibited non-bleeding visible vessels;[43] in both studies a reduction in the need for emergency surgery was seen. It is significant that in both of these studies the large 10 Fr probe was used and, perhaps more importantly, all the therapy was delivered by Laine himself.

Heat probe

In heat probe therapy, there have been four randomised controlled trials with 'no endoscopic treatment' arms. Two of these showed no benefit,[36,44] and one demonstrated a reduction in rebleeding but no effect on surgery rates.[45] In the 'CURE' study, however, Jensen's group demonstrated significant reduction in both rebleeding and the need for emergency surgery in high risk patients with arterial bleeding or

Table 4.2 *Comparative trials of different techniques for endoscopic haemostasis in non-variceal haemorrhage. A best result is only indicated where there was a statistically significant difference*

Study	Methods compared	Best result
Johnston *et al.* (1985)[59]	Laser vs heat probe	Heat probe
Goff *et al.* (1986)[60]	Laser vs BICAP®	No difference
Rutgeerts *et al.* (1989)[61]	Laser vs BICAP®	No difference
Rutgeerts *et al.* (1989)[62]	Laser vs adrenaline vs adrenaline + sclerosant	Adrenaline + sclerosant
Chiozzini *et al.* (1989)[63]	Ethanol vs adrenaline	No difference
Matthewson *et al.* (1990)[36]	Laser vs heat probe	No difference
Loizou *et al.* (1991)[64]	Laser vs adrenaline	No difference
Hui *et al.* (1991)[65]	Laser vs heat probe vs BICAP®	No difference
Lin *et al.* (1990)[66]	Heat probe vs alcohol	Heat probe
Jensen *et al.* (1990)[46]	Heat probe vs BICAP®	Heat probe
Laine (1990)[67]	BICAP® vs alcohol	No difference
Chung *et al.* (1991)[68]	Heat probe vs adrenaline	No difference
Waring *et al.* (1991)[69]	BICAP® vs alcohol	No difference
Choudari *et al.* (1992)[70]	Heat probe vs adrenaline	No difference
Chung *et al.* (1993)[71]	Adrenaline vs adrenaline + sclerosant	No difference
Lin *et al.* (1993)[72]	Alcohol vs glucose vs saline	No difference
Choudari *et al.* (1994)[73]	Adrenaline vs adrenaline + sclerosant	No difference
Jensen *et al.* (1994)[74]	Heat probe vs adrenaline + heat probe	No difference
Chung *et al.* (1994)[49]	Adrenaline vs adrenaline + heat probe	No difference

visible vessels.[46] In this report, the need for the large (3.2 mm) probe, firm tamponade of the vessel and the use of four 30 J pulses was stressed.

Adrenaline injection

Adrenaline injection of actively bleeding ulcers has been widely used in conjunction with other forms of treatment including laser, heat probe and injection sclerotherapy.[47-49] The rationale has been twofold: first to facilitate the delivery of the main therapeutic modality by stopping any active bleeding and secondly to reduce the heat sink effect (*vide supra*). It is now clear, however, that adrenaline injection can be effective on its own.

There has been one randomised trial of 1:10 000 adrenaline versus no endoscopic treatment in actively bleeding ulcers which showed reductions in the need for emergency surgery, blood transfusion and hospital stay in the treated group.[50] Furthermore, there have been several studies comparing adrenaline alone with adrenaline plus another form of treatment, and none of these has shown the supplementary therapy to have been of any value (Table 4.2).

Injection sclerotherapy

Although the use of absolute alcohol is very popular, especially in Japan,[51] there have been no true trials comparing it with no treatment. However, there has been one comparative study which has suggested that it can reduce emergency surgery rates,[52] and a trial which indicated that it produces better results than spraying with adrenaline and thrombin in gastric ulcers with non-bleeding visible vessels.[53]

The sclerosant polidocanol has also been widely used, and it has been tested in two randomised trials, both utilising pre-injection with adrenaline. One showed a reduction in the need for emergency surgery,[54] although the other was only able to show an effect on rebleeding.[55] In addition there have been two trials of adrenaline followed by 5% ethanolamine which showed reductions in rebleeding and non-significant trends towards less emergency surgery.[56,57]

Comparison between different methods

There is now little doubt that endoscopic haemostasis should be employed. It is effective in producing initial control of active bleeding, reducing clinical rebleeding and reducing the need for emergency or urgent surgical intervention. Whether or not it saves lives is more contentious, but a meta-analysis by Cook *et al.*[58] has indicated that endoscopic therapy can significantly reduce mortality (odds ratio 0.55; confidence interval 0.40–0.76).

Making a decision as to which type of endoscopic therapy to use is more difficult, however, and when appraising the different trials it is very important to take account of the type of lesions which have been treated. When trials in which the control patients were treated non-surgically until they fulfilled criteria which were independent of endoscopic appearances are studied, it is found that patients with active arterial bleeding came to surgery in about 60% of cases.[14] Those with active oozing or non-bleeding visible vessel required surgery in about 25% and 40%, respectively. When the results of adequately documented trials are put together, it becomes clear that whereas laser photocoagulation for active arterial bleeding is associated with an emergency surgery rate of about 40%, diathermy and injection techniques can reduce it to around 15%.[14]

In addition to this type of analysis, there have now been a very large number of trials comparing one method of endoscopic therapy with another, and these are summarised in Table 4.2. It can be seen that very few of the trials showed any difference between the techniques studied with the exception that laser therapy seems to be the least favourable. It would therefore seem that the choice of therapeutic modality remains largely personal based on training and experience. The current author's preference and reasons for his choice are given in the section on overall recommendations.

Surgical treatment

Despite the important advances in endoscopic intervention outlined above, there remains a small group of patients who will require surgical intervention as a life-saving procedure. This is becoming a major problem, as few surgeons in this country now have extensive experience of operating for peptic ulcer disease, and the emergency which does not respond to endoscopic treatment usually represents a significant surgical challenge. It is therefore vital that surgery for upper gastrointestinal bleeding is carried out by an experienced surgeon who is used to operating on the stomach and duodenum, and is not delegated to a junior member of staff.

This section looks at the indications for surgery in peptic ulcer bleeding and then examines specific techniques for dealing with duodenal, gastric and oesophageal ulcers, respectively. Finally, the role of vagotomy and the choice of procedure is considered.

Indications for surgery

Before the introduction of endoscopic haemostasis the decision whether or not to operate for bleeding peptic ulcer could be difficult. When active bleeding was seen at the time of endoscopy this was usually taken as an absolute indication to proceed. However, it was more common to find that the patient had stopped bleeding at the time of endoscopy, and the surgeon had to decide between waiting for clinical evidence of rebleeding and performing 'prophylactic' surgery.

The most important factors in predicting rebleeding appeared to be the presence of significant endoscopic stigmata of recent haemorrhage, an ulcer on the posterior wall of the duodenum or high on the lesser curve of the stomach, age over 60 years and shock or anaemia on admission.[75,76] In 1984, Morris and others published the results of a randomised study comparing a policy of delayed surgery with early surgery.[77] The criteria for early surgery were one rebleed in hospital, four units of plasma expander or blood in 24 hours, endoscopic stigmata or a previous history of peptic ulcer with bleeding. In the delayed group the criteria consisted of two rebleeds in hospital or eight units of blood or plasma expander in 24 hours. For patients over the age of 60 years, early surgery was associated with a lower mortality, and despite doubts as to the appropriateness of the endoscopic stigmata chosen and the very high operation rate, this study did emphasise the need for prompt surgical intervention in high-risk elderly patients.

Since the widespread adoption of endoscopic haemostasis, it can be argued that the decision as to when to operate has become easier to make. If initial control of active bleeding is impossible endoscopically then surgery is mandatory. If re-bleeding occurs after successful delivery of endoscopic treatment then immediate surgery should be undertaken unless the patient is deemed unfit. Some endoscopists consider that re-treatment after clinical rebleeding is safe,[78] but good evidence for this is lacking. In this author's experience such a policy can be very dangerous, not infrequently leading to a patient being presented for surgery in less than optimal condition.

Some endoscopists follow a policy of routine re-endoscopy within 24 hours of endoscopic haemostasis with retreatment if indicated.[51] This policy has been tested in a small randomised trial which showed a non-significant benefit,[79] and it is possible that this approach might improve the results of endoscopic treatment. This must not, however, be confused with the re-treatment of overt clinical rebleeding.

If clinical rebleeding is to be used as an indication for surgery, it is very important to have clear definitive criteria, especially as melaena can continue for several days following a major bleed. If a patient remains haemodynamically stable without aggressive fluid replacement and does not have a fresh haematemesis or a substantial drop in haemoglobin after initial resuscitation, then rebleeding can be discounted. If there is any doubt as to whether or not a patient has rebled, then a check endoscopy should be carried out before committing the patient to surgery.

Techniques

The bleeding duodenal ulcer

The majority of bleeding duodenal ulcers which require surgery are chronic posterior wall ulcers involving the gastroduodenal artery. The first step is to make a longitudinal duodenotomy immediately *distal* to the pyloric ring, and if there is active arterial bleeding, to obtain immediate haemostasis with finger pressure. It may then be necessary to extend the duodenotomy proximally through the pyloric ring in order to obtain adequate access, but unless a vagotomy is to be carried out (see below), the pylorus should be preserved if possible.

The next stage is to clear the stomach and duodenum of blood and clot with suction to obtain an optimal view of the bleeding site. If access is still difficult, mobilisation of the duodenum laterally (Kocher's manoeuvre) may help, and taking a firm grasp of the posterior duodenal mucosa distal to the ulcer with Babcock's forceps can allow the ulcer to be drawn up into the operative field.

Regardless of whether there is active bleeding or a non-bleeding exposed artery it is then important to obtain secure control of the vessel. This is best achieved using a small (1 cm diameter), heavy, round-bodied or taper-cut semicircular needle with 0 or No. 1 size suture material. This type of needle is ideal for the relatively restricted space and the tough fibrous tissue encountered at the base of a chronic ulcer. The material can be absorbable, but of reasonable strength duration (e.g. Vicryl or Dexon). The vessel must be under-run using two deeply placed sutures – one above the bleeding point and one below (Fig. 4.7). Use of the small needle suggested above will minimise the risk of damaging underlying structures such as the bile duct.

Figure 4.7
Placement of sutures above and below a visible vessel in a posterior duodenal ulcer.

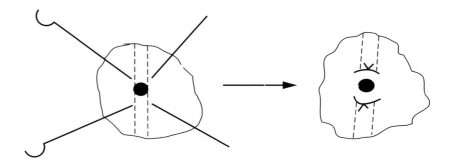

The duodenotomy may then be closed in the same direction as it was made, but if a truncal vagotomy has been performed, then a pyloroplasty should be constructed. This involves dividing the pyloric ring, if this has not already been done, and closing the defect transversely in the Heineke–Mickulicz fashion. If, however, a very long duodenotomy has been necessary, this may be impossible to achieve safely. In this case, the duodenotomy can be closed longitudinally and a gastrojejunostomy performed. Alternatively, a Finney pyloroplasty can be fashioned by approximating the adjacent walls of the first and second parts of the duodenum as the posterior wall of the new lumen (Fig. 4.8).

Occasionally, the first part of the duodenum will be virtually destroyed by a giant ulcer, and once opened, it will be impossible to repair. In this case it is necessary to proceed to a partial gastrectomy once the vessel has been secured. The right gastric and gastro-epiploic vessels are ligated and divided, and the stomach is separated from the ulcer with a combination of sharp and blunt dissection. The stomach is then divided at a level which will represent an antrectomy, and continuity restored by a gastrojejunostomy. The difficulty then lies in closing the duodenal stump.

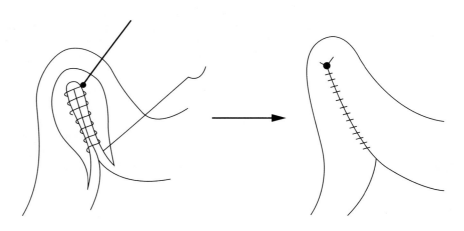

Figure 4.8 *A Finney pyloroplasty.*

Figure 4.9 *The Nissen method for closing a difficult duodenal stump.*

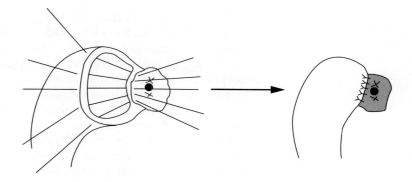

Although this may be achieved by pinching the second part of the duodenum away from the ulcer to allow conventional closure, this is generally hazardous and should not be attempted. Rather, it is preferable to employ Nissen's method where the anterior wall of the duodenum is sutured on to the edge of the fibrotic ulcer base with interrupted sutures. A second layer of sutures is then inserted in the same way, rolling the anterior wall of the duodenum on to the ulcer base (Fig. 4.9). Drainage of the blind duodenal stump is then advisable, and this is most conveniently achieved by means of a T-tube brought out through the healthy side wall of the second part of the duodenum (Fig. 4.10).

The bleeding gastric ulcer

Conventionally, the bleeding gastric ulcer is treated by means of a partial gastrectomy, and for a sizeable antral ulcer this is often the best approach. However, with effective endoscopic haemostasis, by far the commonest situation requiring surgery is the chronic high lesser curve ulcer involving the left gastric artery. The important part of the procedure is then excision of the lesser curve (Pauchet's manoeuvre), and, for secure haemostasis, a formal gastrectomy may be unnecessary.

For the high lesser curve ulcer, therefore, simple ulcer excision is often the treatment of choice. This is not, however, a minor procedure, and has to be carried out with great care. The lesser curve has to be mobilised completely, often pinching the ulcer off the posterior

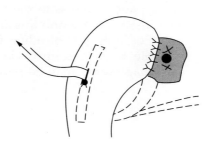

Figure 4.10 *The use of a T-tube for draining the duodenal stump.*

abdominal wall, and dividing the left gastric vessels. The stomach wall is then divided around the ulcer, making the incision in healthy tissue. If an anterior gastrotomy has to be made initially in order to find the ulcer or to obtain initial haemostasis, it should be made so that it can be incorporated in the excision. The defect in the lesser curve can then be closed with a continuous suture, and this is best achieved with an initial mucosal suture to obtain secure haemostasis followed by a separate serosubmucosal suture.

In a patient with a large gastric ulcer with a visible vessel, it is often tempting to merely under-run the vessel. Unless the patient will be put at risk by ulcer excision, this should be resisted as it is associated with a high risk of rebleeding. On the other hand, the tiny ulcer with an exposed vessel – the 'Dieulafoy Lesion' – can be treated very adequately in this way. In this latter condition, the ulcer can be very difficult to find at operation, even if it has been well seen at endoscopy. Rather than trying to see the lesion, it is better to feel the suspicious area with the tips of the fingers and the vessel will usually declare itself as a distinct 'bristle'.

Occasionally, with multiple erosions throughout the stomach, it will be necessary to carry out a total gastrectomy. In this case the site of bleeding is unclear, and it is important to reduce gastric blood flow as quickly as possible. The first steps should therefore be to ligate and divide the right gastric and gastro-epiploic vessels, divide the duodenum, lift up the stomach and ligate and divide the left gastric vessels. The rest of the operation can then be done at relative leisure.

The bleeding oesophageal ulcer

Arterial bleeding from the oesophagus is usually due to reflux oesophagitis or a Mallory–Weiss tear. It is very unusual for either of these to come to surgery as both tend to settle spontaneously, and even if they do not, adrenaline injection almost always achieves permanent haemostasis.[80]

However, if a Mallory–Weiss tear does require surgery, it is nearly always possible to gain access through the abdomen, certainly in a thin patient. The oesophagus is mobilised, and the gastro-oesophageal junction is opened anteriorly by means of a longitudinal incision. It is then possible to see and under-run the tear in the mucosa. In the obese patient, access to the lower oesophagus may be easier through a left thoracotomy, and this approach should certainly be used for true lower oesophageal bleeding from oesophagitis. In this case it may be possible to gain control via an oesophagotomy, but in some cases oesophagectomy may be necessary.

Choice of procedure

Vagotomy

For many years the standard treatment for a bleeding duodenal ulcer was truncal vagotomy and drainage, and when a gastrectomy was necessary, a vagotomy was often added. The rationale behind this approach was to provide definitive therapy and thereby minimise the risk of life-threatening recurrence. Over the past ten years or so, however, changes in the management of peptic ulcer disease have brought about a sea-change in attitude to this problem.

Firstly, the side effects of truncal vagotomy prompted the development of the highly selective vagotomy (HSV),[81] and it has been suggested that after local control of bleeding, HSV should be the definitive procedure.[82] However, the results of HSV are highly operator dependent, and few surgeons now have extensive experience of the operation. This, along with the time-consuming nature of the operation makes it impractical in most emergency situations.

More importantly, the medical treatment of peptic ulcer has improved immeasurably over the years. Although ineffective in stopping bleeding, anti-secretory therapy in the form of the H_2 receptor antagonists or the proton-pump inhibitors is highly effective in securing ulcer healing. In addition, the pathogenic role of *Helicobacter pylori* is now firmly established, in duodenal ulcer at least, and successful eradication therapy reduces the risk of recurrent ulcer to very acceptable levels.[83]

For these reasons, the use of truncal vagotomy in acute bleeding may now be seriously questioned. It is this author's view that secure haemostasis is sufficient in the majority of patients in the acute situation. Of course it is then mandatory to ensure that the patient is properly treated and investigated postoperatively; this implies an immediate course of H_2 receptor antagonist or proton pump inhibitor followed by check endoscopy. It is then important to establish the *Helicobacter pylori* status, but this must be done when the patient is off all medication as anti-secretory agents can lead to false-negative results. The urea breath test is convenient and obviates the need for another endoscopy.

Occasionally, the surgeon will encounter the patient who has had multiple courses of treatment and attempts at *H. pylori* eradication who then bleeds from an ulcer. In this case a vagotomy is definitely indicated, but should only be carried out by a surgeon who is experienced in the technique.

Control of ulcer bleeding

In the duodenum, this inevitably involves under-running of the bleeding vessel, and, vagotomy aside, the only choice then is between closure of the duodenotomy and gastrectomy. The ideal course of action is usually obvious and determined by the size of the ulcer as outlined above. In gastric ulcer the decision can be more difficult. Two groups have found that simple under-running for bleeding gastric ulcer produced satisfactory results.[84,85] However, in a randomised trial comparing minimal surgery with conventional ulcer surgery, Poxon and others found that patients treated by under-running alone were more likely to suffer fatal rebleeding.[86]

The ideal operation for bleeding peptic ulcer is highly individual, and must vary with the clinical situation and the experience of the surgeon. The main aim is to save life; this requires secure haemostasis by whatever means are appropriate, and all other considerations are secondary.

Overall recommendations

The reasons for the following recommendations are elaborated in the main text of this chapter, but a brief outline is given with each one.

1. *A Gastrointestinal Bleeding Unit should be formed in all acute hospitals.* Interested surgeons, gastroenterologists and radiologists should be prepared to work closely together. Only in this way will patients receive optimal care, and there is good evidence that this approach reduces mortality.

2. *The patient with upper gastrointestinal bleeding should have prompt endoscopy.* This maximises the change of making a diagnosis, provides prognostic information and allows endoscopic treatment. In the high risk patient, it is very important to document the precise location of the ulcer; ideally, the endoscopy should be carried out by the surgeon who will be operating if it becomes necessary. If videoendoscopy is available, a record of the exact ulcer location can be taken.

3. *In massive bleeding where endoscopy fails to provide a diagnosis, urgent mesenteric angiography should be arranged.* It is very important to have a clear idea of the source of bleeding before embarking on a laparotomy.

4. *Medical therapy should not be relied on for control of bleeding.* Good supportive care is obviously very important, but there is no good evidence that specific pharmacological treatment has any effect on the outcome.

5. *For active ulcer bleeding and visible vessels, endoscopic haemostasis with injection of 1:10 000 adrenaline is recommended.* Although heat probe, BICAP® and injection sclerotherapy have all been shown to be effective, adrenaline is often used with these modalities, and the available trials indicate that adrenaline alone is equally effective. In addition, adrenaline appears to be associated with the lowest incidence of adverse effects. Laser therapy cannot now be recommended.

6. *A patient with a visible vessel in an ulcer should not be discharged from hospital without endoscopic evidence of fading.* A resolving visible vessel takes about four days to disappear, and it is recommended that repeat endoscopy should provide definite evidence that the vessel

is fading before the patient is discharged from hospital. Massive rebleeding at home is more likely to be fatal.

7. *Surgical intervention is indicated when endoscopic therapy fails to control active bleeding, or at the first clinical rebleed after apparently successful endoscopic treatment.* Although routine repeat endoscopy within 24 hours with re-injection if appropriate may be of value, multiple re-injections for clinical rebleeding should be avoided if at all possible.

8. *The aim of surgery is to obtain secure haemostasis.* Unless the patient has a long history of failed medical management including attempted *H. pylori* eradication, vagotomy should be avoided. For gastric ulcer, the ideal treatment is often formal ulcer excision.

Future directions

The aims of future developments in the management of non-variceal upper gastrointestinal bleeding are to improve mortality rates and to reduce the need for emergency surgery. To this end, it is possible that improved medical treatment and new methods of endoscopic haemostasis may make contributions.

However, perhaps the most pressing immediate need is to improve the definition of stigmata of recent haemorrhage. Several studies have demonstrated that, apart from active arterial (spurting) bleeding, there is huge variation in the interpretation of the endoscopic appearances of the peptic ulcer which has bled, even among very experienced endoscopists.[11-13] This makes the results of many of the trials of endoscopic haemostasis difficult to assess, and the true value of treating a

Table 4.3 *Descriptive definitions for the endoscopic appearances of the bleeding peptic ulcer*

Definitions

Arterial bleeding – spurting blood

Oozing – blood trickling from the ulcer base

Visible vessel – a protruding discoloured lesion arising from the ulcer base, but not fleshy clot

Adherent clot – fleshy clot on the ulcer base which cannot be washed away

Stigmata
1. Arterial bleeding
2. Visible vessel with oozing
3. Adherent clot with oozing
4. Non-bleeding visible vessel
5. Non-bleeding adherent clot

NB: other appearances *not* included as too vague and of doubtful prognostic significance non-bleeding lesion is therefore still unclear. A simple, purely descriptive classification is given in Table 4.3; this has proved to be useful and reasonably reproducible, but the only way to ensure uniformity world-wide is to initiate coordinated, international consensus panels and training schemes.

Another difficult and related area is the problem of identifying those lesions which are at high risk of rebleeding after apparently successful endoscopic haemostasis. This can be fully resolved only when agreement is reached on endoscopic appearances, but there is now evidence that Doppler ultrasound may be useful in indicating the persistence of a large vessel in an ulcer.[87] This might provide a more objective measure of risk, and could be used to identify those patients who should go for early surgery.

Real improvements in the care of patients with upper gastrointestinal haemorrhage have been seen in recent years, particularly in centres which have developed bleeding units. There can be no substitute for enthusiasm and dedication in the management of this demanding problem, and the real challenge for the future is to ensure widespread cooperation between interested specialists in acute hospitals. Only in this way can a coordinated and effective response to gastrointestinal bleeding be achieved.

References

1. Rockall TA, Logan RFA, Devlin HB, Northfield TC. Incidence of and mortality from acute upper gastrointestinal haemorrhage in the United Kingdom. Br Med J 1995; 311: 222–6.

2. Schiller KFR, Truelove SC, Williams DG. Haematemesis and melaena, with special reference to factors influencing the outcome. Br Med J 1970; ii: 7–14.

3. Johnston SJ, Jones PF, Kyle J, Needham CD. Epidemiology and course of gastrointestinal haemorrhage in North-East Scotland. Br Med J 1973; iii: 655–60.

4. Dronfield MW. Special units for acute upper gastrointestinal bleeding. Br Med J 1987; 294: 1308–9.

5. Swain CP, Salmon PR, Northfield TC. Does ulcer position influence presentation or prognosis of upper gastrointestinal bleeding? Gut 1986; 27:A632.

6. Forrest JAH, Finlayson NDC, Shearmen DJV. Endoscopy in gastrointestinal bleeding. Lancet 1974; 11:394–7.

7. Foster DN, Miloszewski KJ, Losowsky MS. Stigmata of recent haemorrhage in diagnosis and prognosis of upper gastrointestinal bleeding. Br Med J 1978; i: 1173–7.

8. Griffiths WJ, Neumann DA, Welsh JD. The visible vessel as an indicator of a controlled or recurrent gastrointestinal haemorrhage. N Engl J Med 1979; 300: 1411-13.

9. Storey DW, Bown SJ, Swain CP, Salmon PR, Kirkham JS, Northfield TC. Endoscopic prediction of recurrent bleeding in peptic ulcers. N Engl J Med 1981; 305: 915–16.

10. Wara P. Endoscopic prediction of major rebleeding – a prospective study of stigmata of haemorrhage in bleeding ulcer. Gastroenterology 1985; 88: 1209–14.

11. Lau YWJ, Sung JYJ, Chan CWJ et al. Stigmata of haemorrhage in bleeding peptic ulcers: an inter-observer agreement study among international experts. In press

12. Laine L, Freeman M, Cohen H. Lack of uniformity in evaluation of endoscopic prognostic features of bleeding ulcers. Gastrointest Endosc 1994; 40: 411–17.

13. Moorman PW, Siersema PD, van Ginneken AM. Descriptive features of gastric ulcers: do endoscopists agree on what they see?

Gastrointest Endosc 1995; 42: 555–9.

14. Steele RJC. Endoscopic haemostasis for non-variceal upper gastrointestinal haemorrhage. Br J Surg 1989; 76: 219–25.

15. Yang CC, Shin JS, Lin XZ, Hsu PI, Chen KW, Lin CY. The natural history (fading time) of stigmata of recent haemorrhage in peptic ulcer disease. Gastrointest Endosc 1994; 40: 562–6.

16. Thomson JN, Salem RR, Hemingway AP et al. Specialist investigation of obscure gastrointestinal bleeding. Gut 1987; 28: 47–51.

17. Winzelberg GG, McKusick KA, Froelich JW et al. Detection of gastrointestinal bleeding with 99Tm-labelled red blood cells. Semin Nucl Med 1982; 12: 126–38.

18. Desa LA, Ohri SK, Hutton KAR, Lee H, Spencer J. Role of intraoperative enteroscopy in obscure gastrointestinal bleeding of small bowel origin. Br J Surg 1991; 78: 192–5.

19. Berry AR, Campbell WB, Kettlewell MGW. Management of major colonic haemorrhage. 1988; 75: 637–40.

20. Collins R, Langman M. Treatment with histamine H_2 antagonists in acute upper gastrointestinal haemorrhage. Implications of randomised trials. N Engl J Med 1985; 313: 660–6.

21. Walt RP, Cottrell J, Mann SG et al. Randomised, double blind, controlled trial of intravenous famotidine infusion in 1005 patients with peptic ulcer bleeding. Gut 1991; 32: A571–2.

22. Daneshmend TK, Hawkey CJ, Langman MJS et al. Omeprazole versus placebo for acute upper gastrointestinal bleeding. Results of a randomised, double-blind controlled trial. Br Med J 1992; 304: 143–8.

23. Barer D, Ogilvie A, Henry D et al. Cimetidine and tranexamic acid in the treatment of acute upper gastrointestinal tract bleeding. N Engl J Med 1983; 308: 1571–5.

24. Henry DA, O'Connell DL. Effects of fibrinolytic inhibitors on mortality from upper gastrointestinal haemorrhage. Br Med J 1989; 298: 1142–6.

25. Jenkins SA, Taylor BA, Nott DM et al. Management of massive upper gastrointestinal haemorrhage from multiple sites of peptic ulceration with somatostatin and octreotide – a report of five cases. Gut 1992; 33: 404–7.

26. Birnie GC, Fenn GC, Shield MJ et al. Double blind comparative study of Misoprostol with placebo in acute upper gastrointestinal bleeding. Gut 1991; 32: A1246.

27. Pinkas H, McAllister E, Norman J, Robinson B, Brady PG, Dawson PJ. Prolonged evaluation of epinephrine and normal saline solution injections in an acute ulcer model with a single bleeding artery. Gastrointest Endosc 1995; 41: 51–5.

28. Levy J, Khakoo S, Barton R, Vicary R. Fatal injection sclerotherapy of a bleeding peptic ulcer. Lancet 1991; 37: 504.

29. Fromm D. Endoscopic coagulation for gastrointestinal bleeding. N Engl J Med 1987; 316: 1652–4.

30. Welch CE, Rodkey GV, von Ryll-Gryska P. A thousand operations for ulcer disease. Ann Surg 1986; 204: 454–67.

31. Laurence BH, Cotton PB. Bleeding gastroduodenal ulcers: nonoperative treatment. World J Surg 1987; 11: 295–303.

32. Matthewson K, Swain CP, Bland M, Kirkham JS, Bown SG, Northfield TC. Randomised comparison of NdYAG laser, heater probe and no endoscopic therapy for bleeding peptic ulcers. Gastroenterology 1990; 98: 1239–44.

33. Rutgeerts P, Van Trappen G, Broeckaert L et al. Controlled trial of YAG laser treatment of upper digestive haemorrhage. Gastroenterology 1982; 83: 410–16.

34. MacLeod IA, Mills PR, MacKenzie JF et al. Neodymium yttrium aluminium garnet laser photocoagulation for major haemorrhage from peptic ulcers and single vessels: a single double blind controlled study. Br Med J 1983; 286: 345–8.

35. Swain CP, Kirkham JS, Salmon PR et al. Controlled trial of Nd-YAG laser photocoagulation in bleeding peptic ulcers. Lancet 1986; i: 1113–16.

36. Matthewson K, Swain CP, Bland M et al. Randomised comparison of NdYAG laser, heater probe and no endoscopic therapy for bleeding peptic ulcers. Gastroenterol 1990; 98: 1239–44.

37. Krejs GJ, Little KH, Westergaard H et al. Laser photocoagulation for the treatment of acute peptic-ulcer bleeding. N Engl J Med 1987; 316: 1618–21.

38. Goudie BM, Mitchell KG, Birnie GC et al.

Controlled trial of endoscopic bipolar electrocoagulation in the treatment of bleeding peptic ulcers. Gut 1984; 25: A1185.

39. Kernohan RM, Anderson JR, McKelvey STD et al. A controlled trial of bipolar electrocoagulation in patients with upper gastrointestinal bleeding. Br J Surg 1984; 71: 889–91.

40. Brearly S, Hawker PC, Dykes PW et al. Perendoscopic bipolar diathermy coagulation of visible vessel using a 3.2 mm probe – a randomised clinical trial. Endoscopy 1987; 19: 160–3.

41. O'Brien JD, Day SJ, Burnham WR. Controlled trial of small bipolar probe in bleeding peptic ulcers. Lancet 1986; i: 464–7.

42. Laine L. Multipolar electrocoagulation in the treatment of active upper gastrointestinal haemorrhage. N Engl J Med 1987; 316: 1613–17.

43. Laine L. Multipolar electrocoagulation for the treatment of ulcers with non-bleeding visible vessels: a prospective, controlled trial. Gastroenterology 1988; 94: A246.

44. Avgerinos A, Rekoumis G, Argirakis G et al. Randomised comparison of endoscopic heater probe electrocoagulation, injection of adrenaline and no endoscopic therapy for bleeding peptic ulcers. Gastoenterology 1989; 98: A18.

45. Fullarton GM, Birnie GC, MacDonald A et al. Controlled trial of heater probe treatment in bleeding peptic ulcers. Br J Surg 1989; 76: 541–4.

46. Jensen DM. Heat probe for haemostasis of bleeding peptic ulcers: techniques and results of randomised controlled trials. Gastrointest Endosc 1990; 36: S42–9.

47. Rutgeerts P, Van Trappen G, Brieckaert L et al. A new and effective technique of Yag laser photocoagulation for severe upper gastrointestinal bleeding. Endoscopy 1984; 16: 115–17.

48. Soehendra N, Grimm H, Stenzel M. Injection of nonvariceal bleeding lesions of the upper gastrointestinal tract. Endoscopy 1985; 17: 129–32.

49. Chung SCS, Sung JY, Lai CW, Ng EKW, Chan KL, Yung MY. Epinephrine injection alone or epinephrine injection plus heater probe treatment for bleeding ulcers. Gastrointest Endosc 1994; 40: A271.

50. Chung SCS, Leung JWC, Steele RJC et al.

Endoscopic adrenaline injection for actively bleeding ulcers: a randomised trial. Br Med J 1988; 296: 1631–3.

51. Asaki S. Endoscopic haemostasis by local absolute alcohol injection for upper gastrointestinal tract bleeding – a multicentre study. In: Okabe H, Honda T, Ohshiba S (eds) Endoscopic surgery. New York: Elsevier, pp. 105–16.

52. Pascu O, Draghici A, Acalovachi I. The effect of endoscopic haemostasis with alcohol on the mortality rate of nonvariceal upper gastrointestinal haemorrhage: a randomised prospective study. Endoscopy 1989; 36: S53–5.

53. Koyama T, Fukimoto K, Iwakiri R et al. Prevention of recurrent bleeding from gastric ulcer with a nonbleeding visible vessel by the endoscopic injection of absolute ethanol: a prospective, controlled trial. Gastrointest Endosc 1995; 42: 128–31.

54. Panes J, Viver J, Forne M et al. Controlled trial of endoscopic sclerosis in bleeding peptic ulcers. Lancet 1987; ii: 1292–4.

55. Balanzo J, Sainz S, Such J et al. Endoscopic haemostasis by local injection of epinephrine and polidocanol in bleeding ulcer. A prospective, randomised trial. Endoscopy 1988; 20: 298–291.

56. Rajgopal C, Palmer KR. Endoscopic injection sclerosis: effective therapy for bleeding peptic ulcer. Gut 1991; 32: 727–9.

57. Oxner RBG, Simmonds NJ, Gertner DJ, Nightingale JMD, Burnham WR. Controlled trial of endoscopic injection treatment for bleeding from peptic ulcers with visible vessels. Lancet 1992; 339: 966–8.

58. Cook DJ, Guyatt GH, Salena BJ et al. Endoscopic therapy for acute non-variceal upper gastrointestinal haemorrhage: a meta-analysis. Gastroenterology 1992; 102: 139–48.

59. Johnston JH, Sones JQ, Long BW, Posey LE. Comparison of heater probe and YAG laser in endoscopic treatment of major bleeding from peptic ulcers. Gastrointest Endosc 1985; 31: 175–80.

60. Goff JS. Bipolar electrocoagulation versus Nd-YAG laser photocoagulation for upper gastrointestinal bleeding lesions. Dig Dis Sci 1986; 31: 906–10.

61. Rutgeerts P, Van Trappen G, Van Hootegem P et al. Neodymium-YAG laser photocoagulation versus multipolar electrocoagulation

for the treatment of severely bleeding peptic ulcers: a randomised comparison. Gastrointest Endosc 1987; 33: 199–202.

62. Rutgeerts P, Van Trappen G, Broechaert L, Coremans G, Janssens J, Hiele M. Comparison of endoscopic polidocanol injection and YAG laser therapy for bleeding peptic ulcers. Lancet 1989; 1: 1164–7.

63. Chiezzini G, Bortoluzzi F, Pallin D et al. Controlled trial of absolute ethanol vs epinephrine as injection agent in gastrointestinal bleeding. Gastroenterology 1989; 96: A86.

64. Loizou LA, Bown SG. Endoscopic treatment for bleeding peptic ulcers: randomised comparison of adrenaline injection and adrenaline injection + Nd:YAG laser. Gut 1991; 32: 1100–3.

65. Hui Wm, Ng MMT, Lok ASF, Lai CL, Lau YN, Lam SK. A randomised comparative study of laser photocoagulation, heater probe and bipolar electrocoagulation in the treatment of actively bleeding ulcers. Gastrointest Endosc 1991; 37: 299–304.

66. Lin HJ, Lee FY, Kang WM, Tsai YT, Lee SD, Lee CH. Heat probe thermocoagulation and pure alcohol injection in massive peptic ulcer haemorrhage: a prospective, randomised controlled trial. Gut 1990; 31: 753–7.

67. Laine L. Multipolar electrocoagulation versus injection therapy in the treatment of bleeding peptic ulcers. Gastroenterology 1990; 99: 1303–6.

68. Chung SCS, Leung JWC, Sung JY, Lo KK, Li AKC. Injection or heat probe for bleeding ulcer. Gastroenterology 1991; 100: 30–7.

69. Waring JP, Sanowski RA, Sawyer RL, Woods CA, Foutch PG. A randomised comparison of multipolar electrocoagulation and injection sclerosis for the treatment of bleeding peptic ulcer. Gastrointest Endosc 1991; 37: 295–8.

70. Choudari CD, Rajgopal C, Palmer KR. Comparison of endoscopic injection therapy versus the heater probe in major peptic ulcer haemorrhage. Gut 1992; 33: 1159–61.

71. Chung SCS, Leung JWC, Leong HT, Lo KK, Li AKC. Adding a sclerosant to endoscopic epinephrine injection in actively bleeding ulcers: a randomised trial. Gastrointest Endosc 1993; 39: 611–15.

72. Lin HJ, Perng CL, Lee FY. Endoscopic injection for the arrest of peptic ulcer haemorrhage: final results of a prospective, randomised comparative trial. Gastrointest Endosc 1993; 39: 15–19.

73. Choudari CP, Palmer KR. Endoscopic injection therapy for bleeding peptic ulcer; a comparison of adrenaline alone with adrenaline plus ethanolamine oleate. Gut 1994; 35: 608–10.

74. Jensen DM, Kovacs T, Randall G, Smith J, Freenan M, Jutabha R. Prospective study of thermal coagulation (gold probe-GP) vs combination injection and thermal (Ing + GP) treatment of high risk patients with severe ulcer or Mallory Weiss (MW) bleeding. Gastrointest Endosc 1994; 40: A42.

75. Clason AE, Macleod DAD, Elton RA. Clinical factors in the prediction of further haemorrhage or mortality in acute upper gastrointestinal haemorrhage. Br J Surg 1986; 73: 985–7.

76. Hunt PS. Bleeding gastroduodenal ulcers: selection of patients for surgery. World J Surg 1987; 11: 289–94.

77. Morris DL. Hawker PC, Brearley S et al. Optimal timing of operation for bleeding peptic ulcer: prospective randomised trial. Br Med J 1984; 288: 1277–80.

78. Palmer KR, Choudari CP. Endoscopic intervention in bleeding peptic ulcer. Gut 1995; 37: 161–4.

79. Villanueva C, Balanzo J, Torras X, Soriano G, Sainz S, Vilardell F. Value of second-look endoscopy after injection therapy for bleeding peptic ulcer: a prospective and randomised trial. Gastrointest Endosc 1994; 40: 34–9.

80. Park KGM, Steele RJC, Masson J. Endoscopic adrenaline injection for benign oesophageal ulcer haemorrhage. Br J Surg 1994; 81: 1317–18.

81. Johnston D. Operative mortality and postoperative morbidity of highly selective vagotomy. Br Med J 1975; 4: 545–7.

82. Miedema BW, Torres PR, Farnell MB et al. Proximal gastric vagotomy in the emergency treatment of bleeding duodenal ulcer. Am J Surg 1991; 162: 64–7.

83. Moss S, Calam J. Helicobacter pylori and peptic ulcers: the present position. Gut 1992; 33: 289–92.

84. Teenan RP, Murray WR. Late outcome of undersewing alone for gastric ulcer haemorrhage. Br J Surg 1990; 77: 811–12.

85. Schein M, Gecelter G. Apache II score in massive upper gastrointestinal haemorrhage from peptic ulcer: prognostic value and potential clinical applications. Br J Surg 1989; 76: 733–6.

86. Poxon VA, Keighley MRB, Dykes PW *et al.* Comparison of minimal and conventional surgery in patients with bleeding peptic ulcer: a multicentre trial. Br J Surg 1991; 78: 1344–5.

87. Fullarton GM, Murray WR. Prediction of rebleeding in peptic ulcers by visual stigmata and endoscopic doppler ultrasound criteria. Endoscopy 1990; 22: 68–71.

5 Acute conditions of the large intestine

Kenneth L. Campbell
Alexander Munro

Volvulus of the colon

Sigmoid volvulus

Introduction

There is a marked variation in the incidence of sigmoid volvulus throughout the world. In industrialised countries typical incidence figures are 1.7 per 100 000 in the Lothians of Scotland[1] and 1.47 per 100 000 in Olmsted County, Minnesota.[2] In contrast, in the Brong Ahafo region of Ghana the incidence rises to 12 per 100 000 of the population.[3] The patients who develop sigmoid volvulus in the industrialised world tend to be older and a third of patents either have mental illness or are institutionalised.[4] This is not a feature of patients with sigmoid volvulus in Africa.[5]

The sigmoid colon rotates through 180–720° in either a clockwise or anticlockwise direction to produce the volvulus.[6] A narrowed sigmoid mesocolon is a predisposing factor because it provides a pedicle for rotation. The condition is occasionally associated with Chagas' disease and Hirschprung's disease in which redundancy of the colon is a feature. Non-specific motility disorders of the colon may be a significant predisposing factor.[4]

Presentation

A typical patient with sigmoid volvulus presents with abdominal pain, constipation and bloating. On examination there is marked distension which is often asymmetrical. Severe pain and tenderness associated with tachycardia and hypotension may suggest colonic ischaemia. There is a history of previous attacks in around 50% of cases. Ileosigmoid knotting is a variant of sigmoid volvulus in which the ileum twists around the base of the sigmoid mesocolon. It is most common in countries where sigmoid volvulus is prevalent. At the time of presentation there is less distension than in patients with sigmoid volvulus but signs of peritonitis are common due to gangrene of both the sigmoid and small bowel loops.

Figure 5.1 *Plain abdominal radiograph of sigmoid volvulus.*

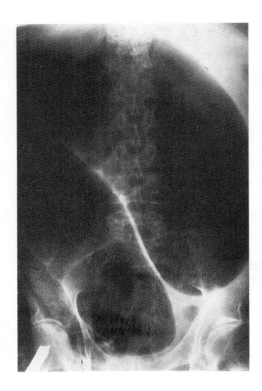

Radiological diagnosis

Findings on the plain abdominal radiograph are often characteristic. Massive distension of the sigmoid loop is visible; the bowel loses its haustrations and extends in an inverted U from the pelvis to the right upper quadrant of the abdomen (Fig. 5.1). Wide fluid levels are seen in both limbs of the loop on the erect film, commonly at different levels ('pair of scales').[7] In one-third of patients the appearances are not typical and an emergency contrast enema should be carried out. This may demonstrate narrowing of the contrast column at the point of twisting. This appearance has been described as resembling the beak of a bird of prey.[8]

Management options

A nasogastric tube should be inserted to decompress the stomach and small bowel. Intravenous fluids will usually be required. It is important to stress that in spite of the fact that many of these patients can be managed conservatively there may still be considerable fluid and electrolyte disturbance which requires careful management.

Non-operative decompression

Since Bruusgaard in 1947 reported sigmoidoscopic decompression in 124 cases of sigmoid volvulus, the endoscopic route became firmly established as the treatment of choice.[9] If this method is to be used it is important that the patient does not have clinical features suggestive of colonic strangulation. The technique involves pushing a soft catheter through the twisted segment into the sigmoid loop using a rigid sigmoidoscope. When the sigmoid loop decompresses is usually derotates. Success has been reported in more than 80% of cases.[9,10] Most surgeons suggest that the catheter should be left *in situ* for 24–72 h secured in place by a suture to the perineal skin to prevent immediate recurrence.

There are limitations and disadvantages to this technique however, First, there is the risk of reduction of gangrenous sigmoid colon.[11] This risk may be minimised by performing laparotomy when (a) the bowel content draining through the rectal catheter is blood-stained or (b) gangrenous patches are seen on the mucosa of the sigmoid colon. Secondly there is a small risk of perforation of the colon.[12]

The endoscopic method of decompression has been refined by the use of the flexible fibreoptic colonoscope instead of the rigid sigmoidoscope.[13] The potential advantages are that decompression can be done under vision and the accuracy of insertion through the twisted segment in the sigmoid colon is thereby increased. In addition the mucosa of the whole sigmoid loop can be visualised directly. The experience of colonoscopic reduction of sigmoid volvulus has been encouraging. A report from Nigeria on 92 patients with sigmoid volvulus has shown that decompression was achieved in 83 patients using colonoscopy. The remaining nine patients were noted to have ischaemic changes and were therefore operated on. All patients in this series survived.[14]

Operative management

If symptoms and signs at the time of presentation suggest ischaemia of the colon, laparotomy should be undertaken when the patient is adequately resuscitated (see Chapter 2). Likewise the patient who has unsuccessful non-operative treatment and those who have clinical features suggestive of colonic ischaemia at endoscopy should have emergency laparotomy. Since it is likely that colonic resection will be required, the patient should be placed in the lithotomy–Trendelenberg position on the operating table. If colonic distension makes it difficult to handle the colon, a needle inserted obliquely through a taenia attached to a suction apparatus will aid decompression (Fig. 5.2). If the colon is gangrenous it should be resected with as little manipulation as possible; the most widely recommended procedure is a Hartmann's operation with end colostomy and closure of the rectal stump.[1,3]

A small number of surgeons have described resection and primary anastomosis with good results. A recent study from Ghana reported 21 patients with acute sigmoid volvulus treated by single-stage resection and anastomosis; 15 of these had gangrene of the bowel.[15] Only one patient had a minor anastomotic leak which responded to conservative management. Intraoperative colonic irrigation may

Figure 5.2 *Needle decompression of the colon. A size 14 or 16 gauge needle attached to suction tubing is inserted obliquely through the taenia of the colon. The transverse colon is usually decompressed but the technique is also suitable for decompression of sigmoid colon or caecum.*

(Reproduced with permission from Williamson RJ, Cooper MJ (eds). In: Emergencies of Abdominal Surgery. Edinburgh: Churchill Livingstone, 1990.)

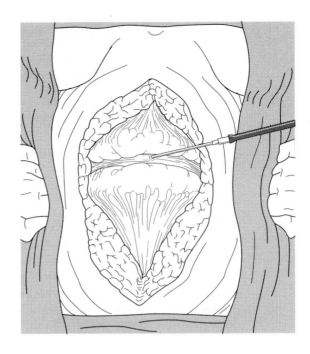

facilitate primary anastomosis in patients with sigmoid volvulus who require emergency operation since faecal loading proximal to the volvulus may increase the risk of anastomotic dehiscence. Although there is an increased trend towards primary resection with anastomosis, it is still important that only patients who are generally fit (without features of systemic sepsis and peritoneal contamination) are selected for this procedure. It is also crucial that the surgeon responsible for the procedure is experienced in emergency colonic surgery.

Elective resection

Because the risk of recurrent volvulus after decompression and derotation has been reported to be between 40 and 60%,[16] elective surgery to prevent further volvulus should always be considered. The choice rests between some kind of fixation procedure and elective resection of the sigmoid loop with primary anastomosis. The procedure which has been most widely accepted is laparotomy with resection, which is now associated with an operative mortality of around 2–3%. The operation may be performed as a laparoscopically assisted procedure[17] but can also be done through a small incision under local anaesthetic in the elderly.[18]

A variety of fixation procedures have been described. These have been associated with high recurrence rates. An exception to this poor outcome has recently been reported.[19] The technique consists of shortening and broadening the sigmoid mesocolon (mesosigmoplasty). Recurrence was seen in only two of 125 patients followed-up for a mean of 8.2 years.

Volvulus of the transverse colon

Volvulus affecting the transverse colon is much less common than sigmoid volvulus, accounting for 2.6% of all cases of colonic volvulus in one series.[20] Predisposing conditions include pregnancy, chronic constipation, distal colonic obstruction and previous gastric surgery. The plain abdominal radiograph usually shows gas-filled loops of large intestine with wide fluid levels. The condition is often mistaken for sigmoid volvulus and the diagnosis is rarely made preoperatively. After operative diagnosis is made and the transverse colon untwisted, evidence of distal obstruction should be sought. The choice of treatment is either an emergency excision of the transverse colon or an extended right hemicolectomy. The rarity of the condition makes definitive statements difficult to support from the published literature but in general a primary anastomosis after resection is probably safe. An alternative method of treatment advocated by Mortensen and Hoffman[21] consists of suturing the right side of the transverse colon to the ascending colon with a similar procedure on the left side, thus shortening the unattached transverse colon. In the presence of gangrenous bowel and significant peritoneal contamination the safest approach is to resect the colon and exteriorise both ends of colon.

Caecal volvulus

Introduction

Volvulus of the caecum is much rarer than volvulus of the sigmoid colon, representing 28% of all cases of colonic volvulus reported over a 10-year period in Edinburgh.[22] It is likely that incomplete rotation of the mid gut leaves the caecum and ascending colon inadequately fixed to the posterior abdominal wall with an excessive length of mesentery. Conditions which alter the normal anatomy may predispose to caecal volvulus. There is an increased risk of caecal volvulus in pregnancy and some patients are found to have adhesions from previous surgery. There is also an association with distal colonic obstruction. Volvulus usually takes place in a clockwise direction around the ileocolic vessels. Although the term caecal volvulus is used, the condition also involves the ascending colon and ileum. As it twists, the caecum comes to occupy a position above and to the left of its original position. A similar condition which is seen very occasionally is 'caecal bascule'. In this condition the caecum folds upwards on itself, producing a sharp kink in the ascending colon.[23]

Clinical features

It is not usually possible to differentiate between caecal volvulus and other forms of proximal large bowel obstruction on clinical grounds. Some patients will have a previous history of episodes of obstruction which subsequently settled on conservative treatment. The main presenting symptoms are colicky abdominal pain and vomiting.

Figure 5.3 *Plain abdominal radiograph demonstrating a caecal volvulus.*

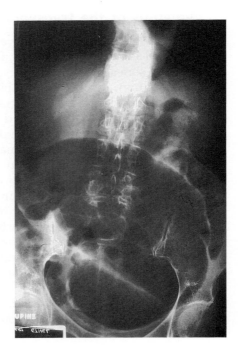

A tympanitic abdominal swelling will usually be present in the mid abdomen.

Radiology

The radiographic features of caecal volvulus have been reviewed by Anderson and Mills.[24] On the supine film a comma-shaped caecal shadow in the mid-abdomen or left upper quadrant with a concavity to the right iliac fossa is diagnostic (Fig. 5.3). There may be small bowel loops lying to the right side of the caecum. A single, long fluid level on the erect film is characteristic. If doubt persists, a contrast enema will show a beaked appearance in the ascending colon at the site of the volvulus.

Treatment

Management of the condition will depend to some extent on the clinical picture. The patient who is unfit for surgical treatment can be considered for colonoscopy since occasional successes have been reported using this method.[25] Laparotomy is necessary in most patients.

If the right colon is gangrenous at operation, the treatment of choice is a right hemicolectomy. The decision about whether a primary anastomosis should be done will be dictated by the circumstances; if there is contamination of the peritoneal cavity resection with exteriorisation of both ends of bowel is the safest option. It should be remembered that there is a markedly increased mortality in patients who have caecal gangrene. A report from the Mayo Clinic demonstrated a mortality rate of 12% in patients with caecal volvulus with a viable caecum whereas the mortality rate increased to 33% if there was colonic gangrene.[2]

There is much more controversy about the procedure of choice in patients who have a viable caecum after reduction of the volvulus. Since derotation alone is associated with high recurrence rate, other forms of treatment have become more widely used. The only definitive approach which prevents recurrence is resection but there is an increased risk of morbidity and mortality. The other two procedures commonly performed for caecal volvulus are caecostomy and caecopexy. Reports on the use of caecostomy demonstrate a wide variation both in terms of recurrence (0–25%) and mortality (0–33%). Some authors express concern over the morbidity of caecostomy and the very occasional serious complications of abdominal wall sepsis and fasciitis are well known in addition to the potential for a persistent fistula. The treatment of caecal volvulus has been reviewed in a large study consisting of 561 published cases.[26] This review showed that caecopexy was associated with a mortality rate of 10% and recurrence rate of 13%. Anderson and Welch[27] described a combined technique of using caecopexy and caecostomy. Using this technique they reported no recurrence after a mean follow-up of 9.8 years. A randomised control trial to resolve the issue of which operative strategy to use in caecal volvulus is unlikely to take place given the number of cases presenting in each institution. If all circumstances are favourable, resection appears to be a justifiable procedure with minimal risk of recurrence, accepting that there may be a small number of patients who will have increased bowel frequency. In other circumstances the minimum procedure compatible with survival becomes the goal. A combination of caecopexy and caecostomy may be the best way of minimising recurrence.

Acute colonic pseudo-obstruction

Acute colonic pseudo-obstruction (ACPO) is the term used to describe the syndrome in which there are symptoms and signs of large bowel obstruction. When these patients are subjected to contrast radiology no mechanical cause for the obstruction can be found. In more than 80% of cases ACPO is associated with other clinical conditions of which at least 50 have been described.[28] The most common of these associated conditions include the puerperium (particularly after Caesarean section), pelvic surgery, trauma and cardiorespiratory disorders. The mortality rate of ACPO is high, partly as a result of underlying disorders. Failure to recognize the condition, leading to inappropriate treatment, is also a contributory factor. The true incidence is hard to ascertain since a number of unrecognised cases are likely to resolve spontaneously. It has been estimated[29] that some 200 deaths per annum in the UK may result from ACPO.

Aetiology

The state of colonic motility at any point in time is determined by a balance of the inhibitory influence of the sympathetic nervous supply and the stimulatory effect of the parasympathetic system. It has been suggested that neuropraxia of the sacral parasympathetic nerves may be a factor in the aetiology of ACPO. This might lead to a failure of propulsion in the left colon and would explain the 'cut-off' between dilated and collapsed bowel which is located on the left side of the large bowel in 82% of cases.[30] It is well recognised that sepsis is a potent stimulus of sympathetic activity and was noted by Jetmore and colleagues in 42% of their patients.[31] Many of the conditions commonly associated with ACPO are likely to result in sympathetic overactivity.

Clinical features

The clinical features may closely mimic those of mechanical large bowel obstruction. Abdominal pain is a feature in over 80% of patients and bowel movements either stop or only small amounts of flatus or liquid faeces are passed.[32] On examination, the abdomen is generally very distended and tympanitic but tenderness is often less than expected. The majority of cases will already have had operative procedures done or have been hospitalised for some time due to some other disorder. Serum electrolytes are often abnormal in this condition.

Radiology

Radiographs of the abdomen in ACPO typically show gross distension of the large bowel with cut-off at the splenic flexure, rectosigmoid junction or less commonly at the hepatic flexure (Fig. 5.4). Gas fluid levels are less commonly seen on the plain radiograph in patients with ACPO when compared to those presenting with mechanical obstruction.[33,34] It has been suggested that a prone lateral view of the rectum may be useful in making the diagnosis since gaseous filling of the rectum will tend to exclude mechanical obstruction.[35] The caecal diameter should be measured since it is believed that the risk of caecal rupture increased greatly when the caecal diameter exceeds 12 cm.[33,34] Sequential abdominal radiographs are valuable in determining progress and guiding therapy. A strong argument may be made for the use of a contrast enema in all cases since the differentiation from mechanical obstruction can be difficult. This is well illustrated in a study reported by Koruth et al.[36] who performed a contrast enema on 91 patients with suspected large bowel obstruction. Of the 79 patients who were thought clinically to have a mechanical obstruction, the diagnosis was confirmed in 50. Of the remaining 29 patients 11 were diagnosed to have other non-obstructing organic causes and 18 patients were shown to have pseudo-obstruction. An interesting

Figure 5.4 *Plain abdominal radiograph of a patient with pseudo-obstruction.*

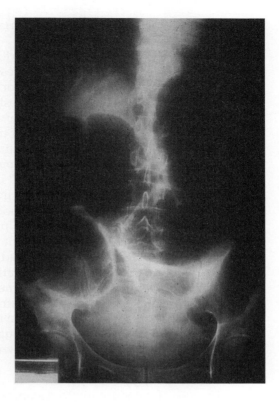

feature of the study were the 12 patients who were thought to have pseudo-obstruction before the water-soluble contrast enema was performed. This examination confirmed the diagnosis of ACPO in 10 but two of the patients were shown to have carcinomas of the colon.

Non-operative management

Many of the patients with ACPO already have fluid and electrolyte imbalance. In most cases central venous pressure monitoring will be necessary and urinary catheterisation be required to monitor hourly urine volumes. The contribution of any medication should be carefully considered and narcotics should be discontinued if at all possible and any other medication which might interfere with peristaltic activity also stopped. A nasogastric tube is routinely inserted to prevent swallowed air from entering the intestines. The use of enemas and flatus tubes is said to be of value in the treatment of early colonic pseudo-obstruction and in a number of patients the water-soluble contrast enema itself may have a useful therapeutic effect. In some patients the condition will resolve without intervention. Bachulis and Smith[33] found that it took an average of 6.5 days for complete resolution to take place in a group of 26 patients treated medically.

Progress should be checked by serial examination of the abdomen and abdominal radiographs.

It is only when the risk of perforation increases substantially that more active intervention is necessary. It has been suggested that decompression should be performed when the caecal diameter approaches 12 cm. Epidural anaesthesia blocks sympathetic outflow and improvement has been observed in a number of patients with ACPO who have had this form of treatment.[37] There has been a recent report on treatment of this condition using guanethidine (an adrenergic blocker) and neostigmine (a parasympathomimetic).[38] The regime used by Hutchinson and Griffiths[38] consisted of giving 20 mg guanethidine in 100 ml of normal saline infused intravenously over 40 min. During this time recordings of blood pressure and pulse were made every 10 min and then 2.5 mg of neostigmine given over 1 min after the guanethidine infusion. In eight of 11 cases the pseudo-obstruction resolved rapidly. Two patients had a problem which may have been attributed to the treatment. One patient had postural hypotension after getting up shortly after the treatment and another patient had excessive salivation. This form of treatment may be worth considering if expectant management fails. There is a risk of bradycardia with cholinergic agonists and it has been suggested that patients with cardiac instability should not be treated with neostigmine.

Colonoscopy

The use of colonoscopy to decompress the colon in ACPO has become well established since it was first suggested by Kukora and Dent,[39] and is successful in 73–90% of cases.[40–42] The procedure can be difficult and tedious, requiring a skilled colonoscopist. Air insufflation must be kept to a minimum. Frequent small volume irrigation is required to ensure good visibility in the colon and maintain colonoscope suction channel patency.

A further advantage of colonoscopy is that necrotic patches can be identified on the colonic mucosa, allowing pre-emptive surgical treatment before perforation supervenes.[43] The risk of perforation of the colon during colonoscopy for this condition has been estimated at around 2%[42] and other complications are very unusual. Is should be emphasised that radiographs taken after successful clinical response often fail to show complete resolution of caecal distension (Fig. 5.5).

One disadvantage of colonoscopic treatment is the tendency for further caecal distension to recur. The overall rate of recurrence following initial colonoscopic decompression varies from 15 to 29%.[31,39,41] There is some difference of opinion about the best method of management of recurrent ACPO but the safety and efficacy of repeat colonic decompression has now been reported.[28,31,41] A potential means of avoiding recurrence is intubation of the caecum with a long intestinal tube passed alongside the colonoscope.[44]

Figure 5.5 *Plain abdominal radiograph of a patient with pseudo-obstruction after colonoscopic decompression.*

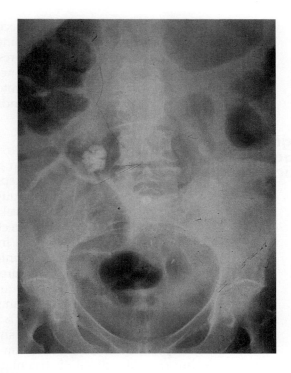

Operative management

In general if colonoscopy is unsuccessful it is probably safest to fashion a tube caecostomy, especially if the caecum is tightly distended. If there are no signs of generalised peritonitis the caecostomy can be fashioned through a small muscle-splitting incision in the right iliac fossa, if necessary under local anaesthetic. An alternative technique is to create a 'blow-hole' caecostomy.[45] This involves suturing the distended caecum to the incised external or internal oblique muscles and once the peritoneal cavity is sealed off, the caecum is opened. Only when perforation of the caecum is suspected should a full laparotomy be performed. If a perforation of the caecum is encountered and the hole is small, tube caecostomy can be performed through the perforation site whereas if multiple perforations are found or extensive necrosis is noted, a right hemicolectomy is the treatment of choice. When resection of the right colon is required, primary anastomosis may be feasible if contamination of the peritoneal cavity is not a feature. Otherwise it is probably safest to bring out an ileostomy and mucous fistula and re-anastomose the two ends of bowel at a later date.

Conclusion

In conclusion, some patients with ACPO can be managed entirely conservatively, employing regular review and frequent plain radiographs of the abdomen to check caecal diameter. As caecal diameter increases in excess of 12 cm, decompression will be required. In selected cases a trial of guanethidine and neostigmine may be worthwhile. The colon can be decompressed with the colonoscope in the majority of cases but failure will necessitate caecostomy. Only if perforation is suspected is a full laparotomy necessary when the approach is determined by the operative findings.

Malignant large bowel obstruction

Introduction

Malignant large bowel obstruction generally occurs in the elderly. Of 168 patients with this condition reported by Gerber et al.[46] 63% were more than 70 years of age. Although carcinoma of the colon is the most common cause of large bowel obstruction in Europe and North America, only one-tenth of colorectal cancers present in this way.[47] Most of these tumours are found in the left side of the colon particularly the sigmoid colon and splenic flexure. The next most common site is the ascending colon. It is rare to find an obstructing carcinoma in the rectum. Both obstruction and perforation occur together in approximately 1% of all colon cancers but in patients who have an obstruction due to cancer 12–19% will have a perforation.[48,49] The perforation may either be at the site of the tumour itself or alternatively a perforation of the caecum occasionally occurs due to back pressure from the distal obstructing lesion.

The influence of obstruction on prognosis of a carcinoma is controversial. Some studies suggest that the apparent adverse effect of obstruction on prognosis is due to the stage of disease rather than obstruction itself. It is suggested that patients who present with obstruction have more advanced disease than those who present with colorectal carcinoma without obstruction.[50] Other reports suggest that obstruction is an independent predictor of poor prognosis.[51,52]

Presentation

The symptoms experienced by patients with large bowel obstruction to some extent depend on the site of obstruction. In right-sided obstruction, particularly at the ileo-caecal valve, the onset of colicky, central abdominal pain may be quite sudden and vomiting is a relatively early feature. If, on the other hand the obstruction is at the recto-sigmoid junction there may be a history of constipation with the patient requiring to use laxatives on an intermittent basis. This clinical picture may give way to increasing constipation and eventual symptoms of complete obstruction. In these circumstances, vomiting is rare.

On examination abdominal distension is the most notable feature; distribution of distension will depend on the level of obstruction. A tympanitic swelling, particularly noted in the right lower quadrant usually signifies caecal distension. Occasionally a mass can be felt but the degree of distension often precludes palpation of the tumour mass.

Figure 5.6
Gastrografin enema demonstrating complete obstruction in the proximal sigmoid colon.

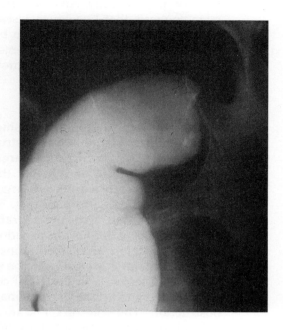

Figure 5.7
Technique of intra-operative colonic irrigation showing extensive colonic mobilisation and exteriorisation.

*Reproduced with permission from J. R. Coll. Surg. Edinb., 1995; **40**: 171–172.*

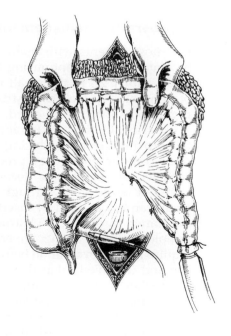

Signs of peritoneal irritation suggests that perforation is either imminent or may already have occurred. Palpation of an irregular liver edge suggests that liver metastases may be present. A palpable mass on rectal examination is likely to be either due to a carcinoma of the rectum or, on occasions, involvement of the anterior rectal wall by a sigmoid carcinoma prolapsing into the pelvis.

Investigative techniques

Plain abdominal radiography using both erect and supine films will usually indicate large bowel obstruction. The pattern of gas distribution in both the small and the large bowel will depend on the site of obstruction but also on whether the ileocaecal valve is competent or not. In all cases of suspected large bowel obstruction a gastrografin enema should be performed (Fig. 5.6) because plain film radiography can be misleading.[36] The gastrografin enema will exclude other conditions such as volvulus or pseudo-obstruction and in addition will cleanse the colon distal to the obstructing lesion. Flexible sigmoidoscopy or colonoscopy may also be useful, particularly if the suspected obstructing lesion is in the distal colon. This investigation is essential to exclude synchronous carcinomas or adenomas below the level of obstruction. The role of CT scan is more controversial but may be helpful in defining the aetiology of colonic obstruction in some cases. In our own practice, CT scan is not routinely done for patients with large bowel obstruction.

Preoperative management

For most patients with malignant large bowel obstruction there will be ample time for optimising the patient's condition before operation (see Chapter 2). In the small number of patients who have evidence of peritonitis as well as obstruction at the time of presentation, more urgent operation is indicated.

Occasionally the gastrografin enema will result in decompression of the proximal colon, reducing the urgency of operation. The goal of converting an emergency procedure into an elective one can also be achieved by endoscopic decompression using laser or diathermy to 'core-out' an opening through an obstructing carcinoma.[53,54] A similar result can be obtained by inserting a metal expandable stent to enlarge the lumen through the obstructing lesion.[55] This may either be done radiologically or using an endoscopic technique. These techniques require further evaluation before they can be recommended for general use and it is likely that they will be of more value in cases of distal obstruction rather than those with proximal carcinomas. It is important to indicate to the patient prior to operation that a stoma may be necessary and if time permits, counselling by the stoma therapist is also worthwhile. The ideal stoma position should be marked on the abdominal wall.

Operative management

Position on the operating table

Patients with right-sided obstruction should be positioned flat on the operating table. Patients with left-sided large bowel obstruction are placed in the lithotomy-Trendelenberg position to allow access to the anus during the procedure for purposes of irrigation of the rectal stump or anal insertion of a surgical stapling instrument. It also allows the surgical assistant to stand between the patient's legs; occasionally the operator can accomplish splenic flexure mobilisation more easily from the same position.

Operative strategy

The abdomen is opened through a generous mid-line incision. If the bowel is tense, it is important to decompress it (a) so that good visualisation of the rest of the abdomen can be accomplished and (b) to prevent spillage of faecal content. In cases of right-sided large bowel obstruction with an incompetent ileocaecal valve the small bowel may well be very distended. The best way of achieving decompression is to milk the contents back into the stomach and aspirate through a large-bore nasogastric tube. If the large bowel is very tense it can often be partly decompressed by inserting a 16 gauge intravenous catheter inserted obliquely through the colonic wall (Fig. 5.2); suction is applied to decompress bowel gas. This is often enough to make it possible to handle the large bowel without fear of rupture. After the bowel is decompressed it is easier to formulate a plan of management. A thorough laparotomy is performed. The location of the primary tumour is sought and with the bowel partly decompressed it is easier to detect synchronous tumours. The presence of direct spread to adjacent structures should also be assessed and peritoneal seedlings looked for. The presence of liver secondaries should be noted. Based on these observations a decision can be formulated about whether the operation is potentially curative or palliative.

When there is a prospect of curative resection standard techniques of radical cancer surgery should be employed including wide excision of the lesion en bloc with the appropriate blood vessels and mesentery. If the lesion is adherent to other structures an attempt should be made to resect part or the whole of these structures with the resected specimen where this is feasible. High cure rates are possible with locally advanced tumours if the lymph nodes are negative and there are no distant metastases but this is only achieved if a radical approach to resection is adopted and clear resection margins obtained.

The presence of liver or peritoneal metastases does not preclude resection of the primary carcinoma. When it is deemed that the operation is a palliative one, if at all possible gastrointestinal continuity should be restored and staged procedures avoided, particularly in patients who have a poor prognosis.

Right-sided obstruction

If there is a closed loop obstruction because of competence of the ileocaecal valve, the caecum and right colon may be very tense. Complete decompression can be achieved as a preliminary to resection by making a small enterotomy in the terminal ileum and a Foley catheter is inserted through the ileocaecal valve and suction applied to the Foley catheter. This technique is particularly useful in cases where there is splitting of the taenia on the caecum, indicating impending rupture. The range of operations available for treatment of right-sided tumours causing obstruction include (1) ileotransverse bypass, (2) right hemicolectomy with exteriorisation of both ends of the large bowel, and (3) a right hemicolectomy with primary anastomosis. There is general agreement that a right hemicolectomy with primary anastomosis is the treatment of choice in most cases. However, this procedure is by no means free of complications. One report noted an operative mortality rate of 17% among 195 patients who had emergency right hemicolectomy with primary anastomosis for obstructing colonic carcinoma.[56] In addition, a leak rate of 10% was noted in 179 patients who had a right hemicolectomy and primary anastomosis for obstruction. This compares with a leak rate of 6% of 759 patients with right colon cancer who were not obstructed.[56] Other studies have shown similar mortality rates. Many of the deaths have resulted from anastomotic failure. Instead of subjecting all patients with obstruction to right hemicolectomy with primary anastomosis, it may be wiser to use a policy of selection, subjecting good-risk patients to primary anastomosis whereas if there are risk factors present for anastomotic failure, patients may be managed with resection and exteriorisation of the bowel ends, particularly if there is contamination of the peritoneal cavity by bowel contents or pus.

The anastomotic technique used will depend on the surgeon's preference. If there is gross disparity in size between the two ends of bowel, it is probably better to perform an open sutured anastomosis using an antimesenteric cut-back to increase the circumference of the smaller end of intestine. An alternative is to use a functional end-to-end anastomosis with stapling devices. A side-to-side anastomosis is performed first of all using a linear cutting stapler which anastomoses the antimesenteric border of the ileum to the antimesenteric border of the colon. The common ileal and colonic end is then stapled off using a linear stapling instrument. If the obstructed bowel is very thickened and oedematous, care requires to be taken with the use of stapling instruments since there is a tendency for the instruments to cut through oedematous bowel.

Only on the relatively rare occasion when locally advanced disease is unresectable should the patient be subjected to an ileo-transverse bypass procedure. There is almost no place for caecostomy in the current management of right-sided large bowel obstruction.

Transverse colon obstruction

Most surgeons would perform an extended right hemicolectomy for patients with transverse colon carcinoma. Decompression of the colon may be necessary to facilitate mobilisation. It will usually be necessary to remove the omentum, together with the colon to ensure a radical approach. For the patient who has a large transverse colon obstructing carcinoma, achieving clearance is often difficult because of involvement of the transverse mesocolon. The splenic flexure will require to be mobilised and a primary anastomosis between ileum and upper descending colon will usually be possible.

Left-sided obstruction

Although there is general agreement that the treatment of choice for right-sided colon tumours is right hemicolectomy with an ileocolic anastomosis, there is no such consensus view regarding tumours which obstruct the left side of the colon. Although the surgical management of obstructing carcinoma of the left colon has been controversial for many years, and remains so, the focus of controversy has progressively shifted. An earlier debate consisted of whether primary resection of obstructing carcinoma (Hartmann's operation) or simple decompression using a loop colostomy should be performed at the time of presentation. Subsequently interest has been focused on whether primary anastomosis after resection performed as an emergency operation is as safe as a two-stage procedure. A current focus of interest centres on which single-stage operation is best for these cases.

In this section, each operative approach will be considered in turn.

Three-stage procedures

The three-stage procedure consists of colostomy, usually a transverse colostomy, resection of the tumour at a second stage, the third stage consisting of colostomy closure. For many years this was the standard approach to the treatment of left-sided large bowel obstruction and in some centres is still the preferred option. The proposed advantages of this approach are first, making the transverse colostomy is a much lesser procedure than primary resection in a group of patients who are often frail. The patient's condition can then be improved before resection is undertaken. A further advantage is that the anastomosis fashioned at the second operation is protected by the transverse colostomy which is then closed at least six weeks later. However, in practice there are a number of disadvantages with this approach. First, a transverse colostomy is not an easy stoma for the patient to manage, particularly if it is situated in the right upper quadrant.[57,58] This is a particular problem for the 25% of patients with left-sided obstruction who are not fit enough to have further surgery for their neoplasm and therefore have a permanent transverse colostomy. A second disadvantage is that these patients have a combined hospital stay of 30–55 days.[59] Although mortality rates of 20% were common in the 1970s with this three-stage approach, the combined mortality of reports from the surgical literature in the late 1980s and early 1990s showed an operative mortality rate of 11%[60–63] which is similar to the operative mortality rates of two-stage and single-stage operations. Most reports show a decreased long-term survival in patients who have three-stage procedures compared with primary resection and delayed anastomosis.[64,65] Despite these disadvantages three-stage operation may still be the treatment of choice in a small number of patients who are unfit for primary resection at the time of presentation.

Two-stage procedures

The suggested advantages of a two-stage procedure over the three-stage procedures are (1) that the tumour itself is removed at the first operation, thereby possibly conferring a better prognosis, (2) that two operations instead of three are necessary, thus reducing the time in hospital, and (3) an anastomosis with its attendant risks of failure are avoided. The operation became popular during the 1970s and still remains the procedure of choice for many surgeons.

How does the procedure stand up to further scrutiny? The overall mortality of the two-stage procedure is around 10%.[49,62] The mean hospital stay is shorter than for the three-stage procedure, ranging from 17[66] to 30 days.[60] One of the disadvantages of this approach is that only around 60% of patients will have bowel continuity restored at a later date. This means that 40% of patients who have a Hartmann's procedure will have a permanent stoma and the attendant problems associated with this.

The second stage of the two-stage operation may be difficult due to dense adhesions. If the rectal stump has been divided intraperitoneally, restoration of bowel continuity is not so much of a problem as in cases in which the rectum has had to be divided below the peritoneal reflection. The timing of the second stage is important. In a study of 80 patients[67] undergoing re-anastomosis after Hartmann's procedure, the most important variable was the length of time between the primary operation and the second stage. There was no anastomotic leakage or mortality in the patients who had the second stage performed more than six months after the Hartmann's resection.

The second stage of the two-stage procedure is increasingly being performed using laparoscopic techniques. Early results suggest that hospital stay may be reduced by performing the procedure laparoscopically but it should be remembered that as with conventional surgery, the second stage may be very difficult indeed and conversion to open surgery may be necessary.

Single-stage procedure

Although isolated reports of primary resection with anastomosis in the treatment of left-sided malignant large bowel obstruction have appeared in the surgical literature since the 1950s, this approach has only recently become popular. Increasingly there have been reports published demonstrating the advantages of primary resection and anastomosis. This policy has been advocated on the basis of a possible shorter hospital stay, reduced mortality and morbidity and the avoidance of a stoma. Two procedures have been developed, incorporating resection and primary anastomosis. First, segmental colectomy (left hemicolectomy, sigmoid colectomy or anterior resection of the rectosigmoid) associated with on-table irrigation, followed by primary anastomosis. Good results have been reported with this procedure with operative mortality rates around 10%,[69,70] anastomotic leakage around 4%[71] and hospital stay approximately 20 days. The alternative technique is subtotal colectomy followed by ileosigmoid or ileorectal anastomosis. This single-stage operation has the merit of avoiding the technical difficulties of intraoperative colonic irrigation and has been reported to have a low operative mortality of 3–11%,[59] low morbidity and hospital stay of around 15–20 days.[72–74]

If these techniques are to be used with good results it is important that surgeons experienced in colorectal surgery perform them. In some circumstances one of these procedures may be preferable to the other, e.g. segmental resection is preferable for lesions at the rectosigmoid whereas subtotal colectomy is the procedure of choice if the tumour lies at the splenic flexure; it is also the best operation if there are synchronous tumours in the colon and in patients with caecal perforation secondary to left-sided malignant obstruction.

If subtotal colectomy with ileorectal anastomosis is selected as the operation of choice the whole colon will require to be mobilised in the usual way. The rectum is washed out in the same way as for elective surgery. After resection of the colon an ileorectal or ileosigmoid anastomosis is performed end-to-end using either a sutured or stapled technique.

When performing segmental resection with on-table irrigation it is useful to have both flexures fully mobilised, allowing the colon to be presented on the surface of the abdomen (Fig. 5.7).[75] After radical resection of the tumour and mesentery is performed, a single piece lavage apparatus is inserted into the proximal end of colon and as much of the bowel content as possible is squeezed into the lavage bag.[76] If the bowel is mobilised thoroughly and presented on the abdominal wall surface, this makes emptying of the colon very much easier. Irrigation is then commenced using either a Foley catheter or needle inserted into the caecum. In our experience only 2–3 litres of normal saline, warmed to body temperature is necessary for the lavage. After lavage is completed, a standard anastomosis is performed between the colon and rectum after a rectal washout has been done.

The first randomised trial comparing these two techniques has recently been reported.[77] This study involved 91 eligible patients recruited by 18 consultant surgeons in 12 centres; 47 were randomised to subtotal colectomy and 44 to on-table irrigation and segmental colectomy. Analysis was on an intention to treat basis. There was no significant difference in operative mortality, hospital stay, anastomotic leakage or wound sepsis between the two groups. There was a significantly higher permanent stoma rate in the subtotal colectomy group compared with the segmental colectomy group (7 versus 1). The high permanent stoma rate in the subtotal colectomy group is partly accounted for by four patients who were randomised to subtotal colectomy but given Hartmann's procedure because this was thought clinically more appropriate by the operating surgeon. Two additional patients had the anastomosis taken down at a later date and a stoma formed.

At follow-up four months after the operation there was a significantly greater number of patients who had three or more bowel movements a day after subtotal colectomy compared with segmental resection (14 of 35 versus 4 of 35). In the study, one patient had 12 bowel movements per day after subtotal colectomy. Nearly one-third of patients randomised to subtotal colectomy had night-time bowel movements during the first few months after operation. In contrast, less than 10% of those who had segmental resection had this problem.

The authors concluded that although the results of both techniques were acceptable, segmental resection following intraoperative irrigation was the preferred treatment for left-sided malignant colonic obstruction. Although the study addressed the immediate and early results after these two procedures it did not investigate the long-term results of either procedure. It has been argued that there are advantages in performing a subtotal colectomy rather than segmental resection in that synchronous tumours will be removed along with the obstructing lesion and because the length of colon left is small there should be less risk of developing a metachronous tumour. To avoid the potential problems of synchronous tumours in patients who are having segmental colectomy our practice recently has been to colonoscope all patients who have a segmental resection at the time of operation to ensure that there are no further adenomas or carcinomas in the colon. On-table irrigation makes visibility at colonoscopy very satisfactory intraoperatively.

Conclusions

For most cases of right-sided malignant colonic obstruction, right hemicolectomy with primary anastomosis is the treatment of choice. This operation can be extended to deal with patients with carcinoma of the transverse colon. For patients who have left-sided malignant colonic obstruction the site of the obstructing lesion is important. For patients who have lesions at the splenic flexure, a subtotal colectomy may be the preferred option. Most other patients who have an obstructing carcinoma in the left colon will be best treated by intraoperative irrigation and segmental colectomy. Patients who are thought to be particularly at risk from lengthy emergency operations are best served by either a transverse colostomy or Hartmann's operation. If good results are to be obtained, selection of patients for the appropriate technique is paramount and meticulous attention to technical detail is essential.

Acute colonic bleeding

Introduction

Bleeding from the colon and rectum accounts for about 20% of all cases of acute gastrointestinal haemorrhage. Acute colonic bleeding is rare so that experience of this problem gained by any clinician is limited. The majority of patients are elderly with a mean age of 66 years reported in one series of 153 cases.[78] The site and source of haemorrhage in the lower gastrointestinal tract is considerably less easy to determine than in the upper gastrointestinal tract. Since bleeding in the majority of patients will settle without intervention the cause of bleeding is often never satisfactorily resolved. Even after examination of the surgically resected specimen the final diagnosis may be uncertain. Not surprisingly, investigation and management of these patients is controversial.

Source of bleeding

The introduction of selective angiography and colonoscopy have made an important contribution to defining the source of acute colonic bleeding. Before these investigations were commonplace, reliance on sigmoidoscopy and barium enema led to the perception that diverticular disease was the cause of severe colonic haemorrhage in 70% of cases.[79] In contrast, more recent reports attribute around 50% of cases to diverticular problems.[80]

Angiodysplasia

In the past 30 years malformations of intestinal blood vessels known as vascular ectasia or angiodysplasia have been diagnosed with increasing frequency as a cause of intermittent bleeding from the large bowel. It has been suggested that angiodysplasia may be acquired through repeated partial low-grade obstruction of submucosal veins which in turn leads to the formation of arteriovenous shunts. Although in 80% of patients angiodysplasia affects the terminal ileum, caecum, ascending colon or hepatic flexure,[81] 20% are present in the descending colon and sigmoid.[82] Associations with coagulopathy and cardiac valvular disease are frequently quoted and were noted in 28% and 25% respectively of the cases in one study.[83] Angiodysplasia causes a spectrum of presentation ranging from unexplained iron deficiency anaemia to acute colonic haemorrhage. Dilated tortuous vessels and distinct 'cherry red' areas are features of angiodysplasia on colonoscopy. In the acute setting and without optimum bowel preparation the relatively subtle appearances are easily missed and the diagnosis is often dependent on arteriography. The angiographic features consist of early filling, tortuous arteries; in the capillary phase dilated lakes of contrast are noted in the wall of the bowel and these drain into large veins which fill earlier than usual (Fig. 5.8).

How common is angiodysplasia in patients who are not bleeding? In one study angiodysplasias were an incidental finding in 3–6% of

Figure 5.8
Mesenteric angiography demonstrating angiodysplasia in the area of the caecum.

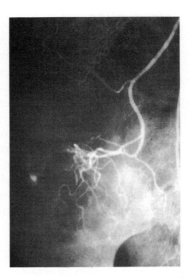

all colonoscopies but in up to 25% of the elderly.[84,85] Despite the fact that bleeding may be coming from angiodysplasia, it is notoriously difficult to demonstrate actual bleeding either by angiography or colonoscopy. Associated ulceration is rarely seen on colonoscopy but would suggest that the bleeding was coming from these lesions if present. The findings of angiodysplasia in a patient with a significant bleed but no active bleeding from the site confronts the surgeon with a dilemma regarding its significance.

Diverticulosis

Although most diverticula occur in the sigmoid colon, approximately 60% of patients who have bleeding of diverticular origin are bleeding from the right colon.[85] Diverticula develop at the site of penetration of nutrient vessels in the colon and bleeding occurs as a result of arterial rupture into the diverticulum. It has been suggested that the tendency for right-sided diverticula to bleed results from the wider necks and domes of these diverticula compared with those on the left side of the colon, leading to thinning of the mucosa overlying the vasa recta.[86] Bleeding tends to be continuous rather than the intermittent bleeding of vascular ectasia; diverticular bleeding remains in many reports the most frequently diagnosed source of acute colonic haemorrhage and also the most common reason for requiring operative intervention.

Other causes

Although vascular ectasia and diverticulosis are important causes of colonic bleeding in the elderly, other causes are occasionally seen. Carcinomas of the left colon cause acute haemorrhage. Patients with inflammatory bowel disease occasionally have a severe lower gastro-intestinal bleed which necessitates surgery. Ischaemic colitis is also a well recognised cause of rectal bleeding.

Presentation

It is very important to take a detailed history from patients with acute colonic bleeding. The nature of bleeding may give clues as to the site of bleeding. Melaena usually signifies bleeding from the upper gastro-intestinal tract (see Chapter 4) but can occasionally occur from small bowel (see Chapter 6) and the proximal colon. If it comes from the proximal colon it is usually small volume bleeding. Large volume fresh bleeding usually indicates a colonic cause but occasionally can also indicate upper gastrointestinal bleeding. A history of previous aortic surgery with insertion of a graft increases the possibility of an aorto-enteric fistula. Abdominal pain may be associated with ischaemic colitis, or inflammatory bowel disease. Bloody diarrhoea suggests inflammatory bowel disease or an infective colitis whereas anal pain is often associated with fissures or haemorrhoids. Abdominal exami-nation is important and digital examination of the rectum should be routine.

Management

Two main patterns are seen in massive colonic haemorrhage. One group, after a significant bleeding episode initially settle down, allowing investigation to proceed in a more leisurely fashion. A second group show evidence of continued haemorrhage or re-bleeding after initial cessation and require urgent investigation. The majority of cases will ultimately stop spontaneously.

Patients require thorough assessment of their haemodynamic status on admission. The overtly shocked patient clearly requires prompt resuscitation but it is important to recognise the symptoms and signs of hypovolaemia before this stage. In a younger, fit patient hypo-tension will be a late event, only apparent after some 30% loss of blood volume. Tachycardia, tachypnoea and narrowing of pulse pressure are all features of significant blood loss requiring prompt action. The elderly and those with underlying systemic disorders will tolerate considerably lesser degrees of blood loss. After establishing good venous access, a full blood count and coagulation study should be done. In cases of acute colonic haemorrhage monitoring of urine output will generally be required and insertion of a central venous catheter will aid in assessing intravascular volume replacement requirements. Nasogastric intubation and lavage of the stomach may be helpful if grossly positive in highlighting the possibility of upper gastrointestinal haemorrhage but a negative lavage occurs in up to 16% of patients with significant upper gastrointestinal bleeding. Upper gastrointestinal endoscopy is the most direct way of excluding bleeding from the upper gastrointestinal tract (see Chapter 4).

Investigative techniques

The aim of investigation is to localise the site of haemorrhage. The methods in common usage are colonoscopy, arteriography and radionuclide scanning. A few centres have built up a large experience of this problem and claim that use of investigative techniques has increased the accuracy of localisation of the bleeding site to around 90%.[87] The majority of patients are looked after by clinicians who have much less experience of the condition and have less access to investigative expertise. Localisation of the bleeding site is often elusive, making the management of these patients demanding and at times perplexing.

Colonoscopy

Colonoscopy was initially thought by most clinicians to have little place in the management of patients with acute colorectal bleeding because of difficulty of visualisation of the colon due to faeces and blood clot. Provided there is an endoscopist of sufficient skill and experience, colonoscopy now forms a part of all protocols for the management of acute bleeding from the large bowel. It can be used immediately after resuscitation in patients who have severe haemorrhage, since the blood acts as a cathartic and if examination is performed when bleeding is active the diagnostic yield may be as high as 76%.[88] An oral purgative or bowel lavage may be given to get rid of blood clot.

There are difficulties with colonoscopy, however. Colonoscopy is technically much more difficult than upper gastrointestinal endoscopy. Interference with vision by blood and faecal material is frequent and even when pathology is identified, establishing the presence of stigmata of recent haemorrhage is more difficult than in the upper gastrointestinal tract. Inconclusive or technically unsatisfactory results are more frequent. There is a variation in the willingness of the colonoscopist to attribute the source of bleeding to observed lesions such as diverticulosis and angiodysplasia and this is reflected in the large variations in the reported incidence of sources of bleeding. Failure to achieve a firm diagnosis may reflect stricter diagnostic criteria rather than inferior diagnostic skill.

As in elective colonoscopy the patient should be closely monitored and receive oxygen therapy. Sedation should be carefully titrated to maintain a cooperative patient. A colonoscope with a wide-bore suction channel is required and excessive insufflation should be avoided since colonic wall distension can exacerbate haemorrhage. It may be useful to perform rigid sigmoidoscopy beforehand to remove large clots from the rectal ampulla. Therapeutic manoeuvres including coagulation by laser, diathermy or heater probe to areas of angiodysplasia and polyp sites are possible.

Angiography

Angiography is extremely helpful when it demonstrates extravasation of contrast into the bowel lumen. This requires that the patient is actively bleeding at a rate of 1–1.5 ml min. Elective angiography of the superior mesenteric artery is performed first since the source of bleeding lies most commonly in the distribution of this vessel. If no bleeding point is seen, an inferior mesenteric angiogram should then be done and more than one contrast injection in each artery may be required to examine the entire territory. If a bleeding point is not visualised and if angiodysplasia is noted on an arteriogram it should not necessarily be assumed that this is the site of bleeding. The site of bleeding has been correctly identified in 58–86% of cases using angiography.[80]

One of the arguments used to support routine use of angiography is its therapeutic potential. Intra-arterial vasopressin therapy can arrest haemorrhage and in a proportion prevent the need for surgery. The technique involves leaving the angiography catheter in the main arterial trunk and commencing infusion at 0.2 units min. Reduction of splanchnic arterial pressure to facilitate the haemostatic plug formation is the goal of this method and appears to work best in diverticular bleeding. In one series of 22 patients, control of haemorrhage was obtained in 20 using vasopressin and although 50% re-bled at varying times afterwards, it was felt that this allowed surgery to be performed electively in 57% of the cases.[80] Vasopressin is contraindicated in patients with significant cardiovascular disease. Complications of diagnostic arteriography occur in up to 9% of patients and include arterial thrombosis, embolisation and renal failure due to the contrast material.

Radionuclide scanning

The introduction of technetium 99m sulphur colloid and technetium 99m-labelled red cell scintigraphy to the investigation of gastrointestinal haemorrhage was particularly important because these are relatively non-invasive investigations. Because of rapid clearance from the blood and high background activity in the liver and spleen, 99m technetium sulphur colloid has largely been replaced by technetium 99m-labelled red cell scanning. This allows the patient to be monitored for up to 24 h after a single injection and may be of value in patients who have intermittent bleeding. Although the technique can be sensitive, rapid movement of extravasated blood along the bowel lumen contributes to inaccuracy in localisation in intermittent imaging. Intestinal irritation from blood in the lumen probably contributes to the marked retrograde as well as an antegrade movement. Because some scans show bleeding but cannot localise it and no confirmatory evidence is found in other patients whose bleeding settles, the results of scintigraphy overall are difficult to quantify. Data from six reports which included 641 patients showed that confirmation of scintigraphic diagnosis ranged from 42% to 97%, the correct localisation from 40% to 97% and incorrect localisation from 3% to 59%.[89]

A widely held view is that scintigraphic imaging is useful as a screening test for patients who have acute lower gastrointestinal bleeding. A major disadvantage of technetium 99m red cell scintigraphy is that it only localises the bleeding to an area of the abdomen. The test is useful in helping to decide which patients require angiography and also is of some help in deciding which vessel should be catheterised for selective angiographic studies.

Overall diagnostic approach

The methods chosen for investigation of patients with acute colonic bleeding will be determined first by the severity of bleeding and second by the expertise of investigation facilities which are available locally. Our own approach is to decide first of all whether the patient may have upper gastrointestinal bleeding. If this seems a possibility then performing upper gastrointestinal endoscopy is important to exclude bleeding from this area of the gastrointestinal tract. In around 80% of patients who present with acute colonic bleeding the haemorrhage will cease spontaneously and in these patients investigation can proceed electively. If bleeding continues, colonoscopy is attempted. This can be preceded by colonic lavage in an attempt to get rid of blood clot. If a source of bleeding is not found on colonoscopy or the view obtained was unsatisfactory, a technetium 99m red cell scan should be arranged, provided the patient remains haemodynamically stable. If the scan is positive, it may act as a useful guide for angiography. Patients who continue to bleed profusely in whom colonoscopy is unsuccessful require surgical intervention.

Treatment

Since colonoscopy is our first-line investigation some patients can also be treated using colonoscopic methods. Hot biopsy forceps are sometimes used to diathermy areas of angiodysplasia. There is a small risk of perforation.[90] The heater probe has been used to treat bleeding diverticula[91] but we have no experience of this method.

Although vasopressin can be infused at angiography and is effective in stopping bleeding in up to 90% of patients with either angiodysplasia or diverticula, there are limitations to the method. Re-bleeding commonly occurs. Most of these patients will require surgical management. For patients who are not fit for surgery, selective arterial embolisation is worth considering.[92]

The rate of blood loss from the colon will determine the urgency of the need for operation. If the bleeding source has been identified, either by angiography or colonoscopy and haemorrhage has not been controlled, laparotomy and segmental excision can be performed with a low operative mortality and risk of recurrent haemorrhage.[80] There is controversy about what to do if a vascular malformation is demonstrated in the right colon while diverticula are noted in the remaining colon but no active bleeding site is demonstrated. Some would advocate segmental right colectomy whereas others would perform subtotal colectomy.

The use of on-table irrigation and intraoperative colonoscopy allows a further opportunity to localise the bleeding site as well as prepare the colon for primary anastomosis in the patient who has vigorous colonic bleeding. Indeed laparotomy, high flow antegrade irrigation and intraoperative colonoscopy has been advocated as the method of management of choice in patients who continue to bleed after resuscitation. Using this approach the bleeding site was identified in seven out of nine cases.[93]

Intraoperative angiography merits mentions as another potential technique in difficult cases. Methylene blue can be injected into an appropriate artery while the surgeon has the colon exposed.

Despite all manoeuvres, localisation of the bleeding point will not be possible in a small percentage of cases and in these cases a subtotal colectomy should be performed. Prior to this, careful exclusion of the cause of bleeding in the small bowel and rectum is mandatory. Intraoperative enteroscopy is the best method of excluding a small bowel cause. The colonoscope can be passed for purposes of enteroscopy either retrogradely from the terminal ileum at the time of laparotomy or antegradely through the mouth, manipulated onwards through the stomach, duodenum and small bowel by the operating surgeon.

Acute colonic diverticulitis

Diverticula are found in the colon more commonly with increasing age. It has been estimated that one-third of the population will have colonic diverticula by the age of 50 whereas two-thirds of people over 80 years will have diverticulosis.[94,95] The vast majority of individuals with colonic diverticula are asymptomatic. However, most patients who require surgical care do so because of an inflammatory complication. Acute diverticulitis can affect any part of the colon. In Western Europe and North America the left side of the colon is more commonly affected whereas in Japan and China right-sided diverticulitis is more commonly seen.[95,96] Diverticulitis is thought to result from inspissation of stool in the neck of a diverticulum with consequent inflammation and possible microperforation. This results in local bacterial proliferation, leading to inflammation in the surrounding colonic wall and mesentery (acute phlegmonous diverticulitis). A collection of pus may form either in the mesentery of the colon or adjacent to the colonic wall. As the collection of pus enlarges it becomes walled-off by loops of small bowel or the peritoneum of the pelvis. Occasionally free perforation into the peritoneal cavity occurs with consequent purulent peritonitis or faecal peritonitis. A grading system has been proposed[97] and has been fairly widely accepted (Table 5.1).

From time to time other complications also arise. A fistula sometimes develops between bowel and another adjacent organ (e.g.

Table 5.1 *Severity grading for acute diverticulitis*

Stage 1 Diverticulitis with pericolic abscess

Stage 2 Diverticulitis with pelvic abscess or localised abscess

Stage 3 Diverticulitis with purulent peritonitis

Stage 4 Diverticulitis with faecal peritonitis

---

bladder). Diverticular disease is responsible for around 10% of all cases of left-sided large bowel obstruction[98] and is frequently difficult to differentiate from malignant left-sided large bowel obstruction on clinical grounds. In addition bleeding is a rare complication of diverticulitis (this problem has been dealt with in the previous section on acute colonic bleeding).

There is evidence that episodes of diverticulitis pursue a more serious course in younger patients and in the very elderly and surgical intervention is more frequently necessary.

Acute diverticulitis of the left colon

Localised disease
A typical patient with localised diverticulitis will complain of pain in the left iliac fossa and is febrile. Examination reveals tenderness and sometimes a mass is palpable. Pelvic examination should be performed in the female patient bearing in mind the possibility of gynaecological pathology. Rectal examination may also give useful information. If sigmoidoscopy is performed it should be done very gently without insufflation of air.

Investigation
Initial assessment includes plain abdominal radiography but there is debate about the nature and timing of additional investigations. Some clinicians believe that initial evaluation will allow cases to be staged and predict the need for surgical intervention. Others believe that evaluation can usefully be deferred until conservative management has failed and a complication requires to be delineated and treated.

In North America CT scanning is the favoured modality. Its advantages include the accurate assessment of the extent of pericolonic involvement and the diagnosis of abscess formation.[99] It is also useful in the therapeutic percutaneous drainage of abscesses. When CT is compared with barium enema there is general agreement that CT provides better definition of the extent and severity of the inflammatory process[100] whereas barium provides better definition of the mucosa of the colon[101] (see also Chapter 1).

Although ultrasonography has not been as widely used as CT scanning in the diagnosis of patients with localised diverticulitis, a recent study showed ultrasound to have a sensitivity of 85% and specificity of 80% compared with the final clinical diagnosis assessed by contrast study or surgical exploration.[102] Ultrasound is also a useful therapeutic modality in abscess drainage. The main disadvantage of ultrasonography is that it is very operator-dependent.

An alternative investigation favoured by many hospitals in the UK is water-soluble contrast enema using gastrografin especially in patients with acute symptoms. No air contrast is used during the examination. The appearances of acute diverticulitis on water-soluble contrast enema are:[103]

1. Diverticulosis with or without spasm
2. Peridiverticulitis
3. Extravasation of contrast

If there are no diverticula present the diagnosis requires to be reviewed. The examination has been shown to be of importance in predicting the need for surgery. Only three of 30 patients who had diverticulosis with or without spasm on gastrografin enema required surgery whereas in 13 of 16 patients with extravasation or peridiverticulitis operation was necessary.[104]

Management

In the absence of generalised peritonitis a conservative policy is adopted. Antibiotic therapy directed at Gram-negative and anaerobic bacteria should be commenced; most clinicians advocate bowel rest initially with fluids and antibiotics given by the intravenous route. If the pain and fever settle within a few days the patient can go home and have a barium enema and sigmoidoscopy performed as an outpatient within a few weeks. It is also our policy to perform colonoscopy if there is any doubt at all on the barium enema examination about the possibility of malignancy.

If the patient continues to be pyrexial and the pain does not settle or the lower abdominal mass is enlarging an ultrasound scan should be requested. A water-soluble contrast enema may also provide useful information at this stage. If there is an abscess visible on ultrasound examination and it continues to enlarge it may be drained percutaneously using ultrasound control although in our experience this is rarely necessary. In the event of localised abdominal signs becoming more generalised or if there is a failure of the infective process to settle despite adequate conservative therapy, operation is indicated. In the small number of patients who require operation for localised diverticulitis a policy of primary resection, on-table irrigation and primary anastomosis is becoming more popular.[105]

Generalised peritonitis

Introduction

Pain from perforated sigmoid diverticulitis usually commences in the lower abdomen mostly on the left side and gradually spreads.

In 25% of cases, however, signs and symptoms are predominantly right-sided.[106] On examination there are signs of generalised peritonitis including tenderness, guarding and rebound tenderness. About a quarter of all patients will have free gas under the diaphragm on plain radiography. Purulent peritonitis is more common than faecal peritonitis. In a report of 93 consecutive patients with perforated diverticulitis and diffuse peritonitis 18 had faecal peritonitis and 75 had purulent peritonitis.[106]

The majority of patients presenting in this way will clearly require operation and there is no merit in pursuing further specific investigations such as gastrografin enema or ultrasound of the abdomen. The main priority at this stage is to resuscitate the shocked patient and since many of them are elderly with poor myocardial reserve, it is best to avoid miscalculations of fluid requirement by central venous pressure measurement. It is a mistake to rush such patients to theatre immediately. A few hours spent on resuscitation in a high dependency area will pay dividends in terms of patient survival. The goals are to restore depleted intravascular and extracellular fluid volume, to re-establish urine flow and maximise myocardial and respiratory function. Antibiotic therapy should be commenced to cover both anaerobic organisms and Gram-negative bacteria. Our practice is to give a combination of cefotaxime and metronidazole intravenously.

Operative management

The patient is operated on in the lithotomy-Trendelenberg position. Good access is best obtained by using a long mid-line incision. Pus and faecal material should be removed from the peritoneal cavity and specimens sent immediately for microscopy and aerobic and anaerobic culture. There is some disagreement about the extent to which the peritoneal cavity should be debrided. The place of intraoperative irrigation of the peritoneal cavity is a further area of controversy. Killingback[107] suggested that the use of 6–10 litres of warm saline solution was of value. The addition of topical antibiotics, although logical, remains to be generally accepted. Using tetracycline lavage (1 g tetracycline in 1 litre 0.9% saline) as the method of treating intraperitoneal infection Koruth et al.[108] reported 82 consecutive emergency colon resections with a 2% residual intraperitoneal sepsis rate. The wound sepsis rate in the same study was 7.3%. This has been our main method of treating intraperitoneal infection and we also have found it to be effective.

Choice of operation

In addition to treating the peritonitis, the main aim of surgical treatment is to minimise the risk of continued contamination of the peritoneal cavity. Until relatively recently it was felt that resection of the colon was too major an undertaking for the acutely ill patient.

In fact the converse appears to apply in that mortality associated with failure to remove the diseased colon is very high. Krukowski and Matheson[109] have shown from an analysis of 57 reports on the treatment of acute diverticular disease that the operative mortality rates of procedures which involve primary resection is less than half the mortality rate of operations which do not include excision of the diseased segment of colon. The mortality rate for 295 patients with generalised purulent or faecal peritonitis due to diverticular disease who were subjected to primary excision was 10% whereas mortality rose to 25% for 813 patients treated using a three-stage procedure.

A further reason for advocating primary resection is the difficulty which is experienced at the time of operation in deciding whether the lesion is a perforating carcinoma or an area of diverticulitis; at laparotomy the appearance of both lesions may be similar when the colon is inflamed and oedematous. It has been estimated that with a pre-operative diagnosis of perforated diverticulitis as many as 25% of patients may be found to have a perforated carcinoma. If there is reasonable suspicion of carcinoma a radical resection of the lesion, together with the colonic mesentery, needs to be performed. Examination of the resected specimen at the earliest opportunity is recommended to aid further decision-making.

Failure to take the resection far enough distally to beyond the sigmoid colon risks recurrence of diverticular disease. Therefore, Hartmann's resection with complete excision of the sigmoid and closure of the rectum with formation of a left iliac fossa colostomy is the procedure advocated by most surgeons. If, however, the operation is exceptionally difficult owing to the colon being very adherent to surrounding structures making safe mobilisation impossible, it may be reasonable to create a proximal stoma, drain the area and transfer the patient to a specialist centre.

Primary anastomosis

There is increasing interest in using primary anastomosis in selected patients who have operations for diverticulitis. The main reasons for increased interest in single-staged operations are first that patients require one operation rather than two. Second, after a Hartmann's operation many patients are left with a permanent stoma either because of unwillingness or unfitness to have further surgery. In addition reversal operations after Hartmann's resection can be very difficult.

Gregg in 1955 was the first to report a resection and primary anastomosis in several patients with perforated diverticulitis without mortality or anastomotic leakage.[110] In their review of the surgical literature Krukowski and Matheson[109] collected 100 cases of resection with primary anastomosis. The operative mortality rate was 9% compared to 12.2% for resection without anastomosis. However, they pointed out that the reported cases are likely to be highly selected and the good results may reflect the enthusiasm and skill of the surgeon performing these procedures rather than the intrinsic merit of the procedure itself. Primary anastomosis is increasingly being recommended in patients with generalised peritonitis without faecal contamination when all other circumstances are favourable. On-table colonic irrigation may further improve the circumstances in which such an operation can be performed. Despite an increasing trend to perform primary anastomosis in patients who have perforated diverticulitis the proportion of patients who are suitable for such a procedure will be small. Only patients with minimal degrees of contamination of the peritoneal cavity should be selected.

Summary

Patients who present with acute conditions of the large bowel require careful assessment and resuscitation. The decision to operate may be difficult and even at laparotomy the choice of procedure can be confusing. If the morbidity and mortality in this difficult area of emergency general surgery are to be kept to a minimum, senior surgical staff must be involved at all stages of patient management. In some instances, advice from, or even transfer to, a specialist colorectal unit may need to be considered after initial resuscitation and assessment.

Acknowledgement

The authors are grateful to Dr D Nicholls, Consultant Radiologist, Raigmore Hospital, Inverness for kindly providing the radiographs shown in Figures 5.1, 5.3 and 5.8.

References

1. Anderson JR, Lee D. The management of acute sigmoid volvulus. Br J Surg 1981; 68: 117–20.
2. Ballantyne GH, Brandner MD, Beart RW, Ilstrup DM. Volvulus of the colon. Ann Surg 1985; 202: 83–92.
3. Schagen Van Leeuwen, JH. Sigmoid volvulus in a West African population. Dis Colon Rectum 1985; 28: 712–16.
4. Sonnenberg A, Tsou VT, Muller AD. The 'institutional colon': a frequent colonic dysmotility in psychiatric and neurologic disease. Am J Gastroenterol 1994; 89: 62–6.
5. Shepherd JJ. Treatment of volvulus of sigmoid colon: A review of 425 cases. Br Med J 1968; 1: 280–3.
6. Sutcliffe MML. Volvulus of the sigmoid colon. Br J Surg 1968; 55: 903–10.
7. Andersen DA. Volvulus in Western India. Br J Surg 1956; 44: 132–43.

8. Rigler LG, Lipschultz O. Roentgenologic findings in acute obstruction of the colon. Radiology 1940: 35: 534–43.
9. Bruusgaard C. Volvulus of the sigmoid colon and its treatment. Surgery 1947; 22: 466–78.
10. Mangiarte EC, Croce MA, Fabian TC et al. Sigmoid volvulus, a four decade experience. Am Surg 1989; 55: 41–44.
11. Hinshaw DB, Carter R. Surgical management of acute volvulus of the sigmoid colon. Ann Surg 1957; 146: 52–60.
12. Knight J, Bokey EL, Chapuis PH, Pheils MT. Sigmoidoscopic reduction of sigmoid volvulus. Med J Aust 1980; 2: 627–8.
13. Starling JR. Initial treatment of sigmoid volvulus by colonoscopy. Ann Surg 1979; 190: 36–9.
14. Arigbabu AO, Badejo OA, Akinola DO. Colonoscopy in the emergency treatment of

colonic volvulus in Nigeria. Dis Colon Rectum 1985; 28: 795–8.

15. Naeeder SB, Archampong EQ. One-stage resection of acute sigmoid volvulus. Br J Surg 1995; 82: 1635–6.

16. Gibney EJ. Volvulus of the sigmoid colon. Surg Gynecol Obstet 1991; 173: 243–55.

17. Leach SD, Ballantyne GH. Laparoscopic management of sigmoid volvulus: modern management of an ancient disease. Semin Colon Rectal Surg 1993; 4: 249–56.

18. Sharon N, Efrat Y, Charuzi I. A new operative approach to volvulus of the sigmoid colon. Surg Gynecol Obstet 1985; 161: 483–4.

19. Subrahmanyam M. Mesosigmoplasty as a definitive operation for sigmoid volvulus. Br J Surg 1992; 79: 683–4.

20. Anderson JR, Lee D, Taylor TV, Ross AH. Volvulus of the transverse colon. Br J Surg 1981; 7: 12–18.

21. Mortensen NJ McC, Hoffman G. Volvulus of the transverse colon. Postgrad Med J 1979; 55: 54–7.

22. Anderson JR, Lee D. Acute caecal volvulus. Br J Surg 1980; 67: 39–41.

23. Weinstein M. Volvulus of the cecum and ascending colon. Ann Surg 1938; 107: 248–59.

24. Anderson JR, Mills JOM. Caecal volvulus: a frequently missed diagnosis. Clin Radiol 1984; 35: 65.

25. Anderson MJ, Okike N, Spencer RJ. The colonoscope in cecal volvulus; report of 3 cases. Dis Colon Rectum 1978; 21: 71–4.

26. Rabanovici R, Simansky DA, Kaplan O, Mavor E, Manny J. Cecal volvulus. Dis Colon Rectum 1990; 33: 765–9.

27. Anderson JR, Welch GH. Acute volvulus of the right colon: an analysis of 69 patients. World J Surg 1986; 10: 336–42.

28. Dorudi S, Berry AR, Kettlewell MGW. Acute colonic pseudo-obstruction. Br J Surg 1992; 79: 99–103.

29. Datta SN, Stephenson BM, Havard TJ, Salaman JR. Acute colonic pseudo-obstruction. Lancet 1993; 341: 690.

30. Vanek VW, Al-Salti M. Acute pseudo-obstruction of the colon (Ogilvie's syndrome): an analysis of 400 cases. Dis Colon Rectum 1986; 29: 203–10.

31. Jetmore AB, Timmcke AE, Gathright JB, Hicks TC, Ray JE, Baker JW. Ogilvie's syndrome: colonoscopic decompression and analysis of predisposing factors. Dis Colon Rectum 1992; 35: 1135–42.

32. Dudley HAF, Paterson-Brown S. Pseudo-obstruction. Br Med J 1986; 292: 1157–8.

33. Bachulis BL, Smith PE. Pseudo-obstruction of the colon. Am J Surg 1978; 136: 66–72.

34. Wanebo H, Mathewson C, Conolly B. Pseudo-obstruction in the colon. Surg Gynecol Obstet 1971; 133: 44–8.

35. Low VH. Colonic pseudo-obstruction: value of prone lateral view of the rectum. Abdominal Imaging 1995; 20: 531–3.

36. Koruth NM, Koruth A, Matheson NA. The place of contrast enema in the management of large bowel obstruction. J R Coll Surg Edinb 1985; 30: 258–60.

37. Lee JT, Taylor BM, Singleton BC. Epidural anaesthesia for acute pseudo-obstruction of the colon. Dis Colon Rectum 1988; 31: 686–91.

38. Hutchinson R, Griffiths C. Acute colonic pseudo-obstruction: a pharmacological approach. Ann R Coll Surg Engl 1992; 74: 364–7.

39. Kukora JS, Dent TL. Colonoscopic decompression of massive nonobstructive cecal dilation. Arch Surg 1977; 112: 512–17.

40. Nivatvongs SN, Vermeulen FD, Fang DT. Colonoscopic decompression of acute pseudo-obstruction of the colon. Ann Surg 1982; 196: 98–100.

41. Strodel WE, Brothers T. Colonoscopic decompression of pseudo-obstruction and volvulus. Surg Clin North Am 1989; 69: 1327–35.

42. Strodel WE, Norstrant TT, Eckhauser FE, Dent TL. Therapeutic and diagnostic colonoscopy in nonobstructive colonic dilatation. Ann Surg 1983; 197: 416–21.

43. Bernton E, Myers R, Reyna T. Pseudo-obstruction of the colon: case report including a new endoscopic treatment. Gastrointest Endosc 1982; 28: 90–2.

44. Stephenson KR, Rodriguez-Bigas MA. Decompression of the large intestine in Ogilvie's syndrome by a colonoscopically placed long intestinal tube. Surg Endosc 1994; 8: 116–17.

45. Gierson ED, Storm FK, Shaw W, Coyne SK. Caecal rupture due to colonic ileus. Br J Surg 1975; 62: 383–6.

46. Gerber A, Thompson RJ, Reiswig OK, Vannix RS. Experiences with primary resection for acute obstruction of the large intestine. Surg Gynecol Obstet 1962; 115: 593–8.

47. Welch JP, Donaldson GA. Management of severe obstruction of the large bowel due to malignant disease. Am J Surg 1974; 127: 492–9.

48. Runkel NS, Schlag P, Schwarz V et al. Outcome after emergency surgery of the large intestine. Br J Surg 1991; 78: 183–8.

49. Umpleby HC, Williamson RC. Survival in acute obstructing colorectal carcinoma. Dis Colon Rectum 1984; 27: 299–304.

50. Korenaga D, Ueo H, Mochida K et al. Prognostic factors in Japanese patients with colorectal cancer: the significance of large bowel obstruction univariate and multivariate analyses. J Surg Oncol 1991; 47: 188-92.

51. Crucitti F, Sofo L, Doglietto GB et al. Prognostic factors in colorectal cancer: current status and new trends. J Surg Oncol 1991; 2 (suppl): 76–82.

52. Serpell JW, McDermott FT, Katrivessis H et al. Obstructing carcinomas of the colon. Br J Surg 1989; 76: 965–9.

53. Bright N, Hale P, Mason R. Poor palliation of colorectal malignancy with neodymium-yttrium-aluminium-garnet laser. Br J Surg 1992; 79: 308–9.

54. Eckhauser ML, Mansour EG. Endoscopic laser therapy for obstruction and/or bleeding colorectal carcinoma. Am Surg 1992; 58: 358–63.

55. Tejero E, Mainar A, Fernandez L, Tobio R, De Gregorio MA. New procedure for the treatment of colorectal new neoplastic obstructions. Dis Colon Rectum 1994; 37: 1158–9.

56. Dudley H, Phillips R. Intraoperative techniques in large bowel obstruction: methods of management with bowel resection. In: LP Fielding, J Welch (eds) Intestinal obstruction, Edinburgh: Churchill Livingstone, 1987, pp. 139–52.

57. Gutman M, Kaplan O, Skornick Y, Greif F, Kahn P, Rozin RR. Proximal colostomy: still an effective emergency measure in obstructing carcinoma of the large bowel. J Surg Oncol 1989; 41: 210–12.

58. Malafosse M, Goujard F, Gallot D, Sezeur A. Traitement des occlusions aigues par cancer du colon gauche. Chirurgie 1989; 115 (Suppl 2): 123–5.

59. Deans GT, Krukowski ZH, Irwin ST. Malignant obstruction of the left colon. Br J Surg 1994; 81: 1270–6.

60. Ambrosetti P, Borst F, Robert J, Meyer P, Rohner A. L'excrese anastomose en un temps dans les occlusions coliques gauche operees en urgence. Chirurgie 1989; 115: (Suppl 2) IVII.

61. De Almeida AM, Gracias CW, dos Santos NM, Aldeia FJ. Surgical management of acute malignant obstruction of the left colon with colostomy. Acta Med Port 1991; 4: 257–62.

62. Gandrup P, Lund L, Balslev I. Surgical treatment of acute malignant large bowel obstruction. Eur J Surg 1992; 158: 427–30.

63. Sjodahl R, Franzen T, Nystrom PO. Primary versus staged resection for acute obstructing colorectal carcinoma. Br J Surg 1992; 79: 685–8.

64. Irvin TT, Greaney MG. The treatment of colonic cancer presenting with intestinal obstruction. Br J Surg 1977; 64: 741–4.

65. Carson SN, Poticha SM, Shields TW. Carcinoma obstructing the left side of the colon. Arch Surg 1977; 112: 523–6.

66. Dixon AR, Holmes JT. Hartmann's procedure for carcinoma of rectum and distal sigmoid colon. J R Coll Surg Edinb 1990; 35: 166–8.

67. Pearce NW, Scott SD, Karran SJ. Timing and method of reversal of Hartmann's procedure. Br J Surg 1992; 79: 839–41.

68. Dudley HAF, Radcliffe AG, McGeehan D. Intraoperative irrigation of the colon to permit primary anastomosis. Br J Surg 1980; 67: 80–1.

69. Murray JJ, Schoetz DJ, Coller JA, Roberts PL, Veidenheimer MC. Intra-operative colonic lavage and primary anastomosis in non-elective colon resection. Dis Colon Rectum 1991; 34: 527–31.

70. Koruth NM, Krukowski ZH, Youngson GG et al. Intra-operative colonic irrigation in the management of left sided large bowel emergencies. Br J Surg 1985; 72: 708–11.

71. Konishi F, Muto T, Kanazawa K, Morioka Y. Intraoperative irrigation and primary resec-

tion for obstructing lesions of the left colon. Int J Colorectal Dis 1988; 3: 204–6.

72. Dorudi S, Wilson NM, Heddle RM. Primary restorative colectomy in malignant left-sided large bowel obstruction. Ann R Coll Surg 1990; 72: 393–5.

73. Stephenson BM, Shandall AA, Farouk R, Griffith G. Malignant left-sided large bowel obstruction managed by subtotal/total colectomy. Br J Surg 1990; 77: 1098–102.

74. Alle JL, Azagra JS, Elcheroth J, Cavenaile JC, Buchin R. La colectomie subtotale en un temps dans le traitement en urgence des neoplasies coliques gauches occlusives. Acta Chir Belg 1990; 90: 86–8.

75. Munro A, Sulaiman MN, Borgstein E, Bachoo P, Bradbury AW. Total colonic mobilisation and exteriorisation facilitates intra-operative colonic irrigation. J R Coll Surg Edinb 1995; 40: 171–2.

76. Munro A, Steele RJC, Logie JR. Technique for intra-operative colonic irrigation. Br J Surg 1987; 74: 1039–40.

77. The SCOTIA Study Group. Single stage treatment for malignant left sided colonic obstruction: a prospective randomized clinical trial comparing subtotal colectomy with segmental resection following intra-operative irrigation. Br J Surg 1995; 82: 1622–7.

78. Dusold R, Burke K, Carpentier W, Dyck WP. The accuracy of Technetium-99m-labeled red cell scintography in localizing gastro-intestinal bleeding. Am J Gastroenterol 1994; 89: 345–8.

79. Noer PF, Hamilton JE, Williams DJ, Broughton DS. Rectal hemorrhage: moderate and severe. Ann Surg 1962; 155: 794–805.

80. Browder W, Cerise EJ, Litwin MS. Impact of emergency angiography in massive lower gastrointestinal bleeding. Ann Surg 1986; 204: 530–6.

81. Cavett CM, Selby H, Hamilton L, Williamson W. Arteriovenous malformation in chronic gastrointestinal bleeding. Ann Surg 1977; 185: 116–21.

82. Santos JCM, Aprilli F, Guimaraes AS, Rocha JJR. Angiodysplasia of the colon: endoscopic diagnosis and treatment. Br J Surg 1988; 75: 256–8.

83. Gupta N, Longo WE, Vernava AM. Angiodysplasia of the lower gastrointestinal tract: an entity readily diagnosed by colonoscopy and primarily managed non-operatively. Dis Colon Rectum 1995; 38: 979–82.

84. Boley SJ, Sammartano R, Adams A et al. On the nature and etiology of vascular ectasias of the colon. Gastroenterology 1977; 72: 650–60.

85. Demarkles MP, Murphy JR. Acute lower gastrointestinal bleeding. Med Clin North Am 1993; 77: 1085–100.

86. Lichtiger S, Kornbluth A, Salomon P et al. Lower gastrointestinal bleeding. In: Taylor MB, Gollan JL, Peppercorn MA (eds) Gastro-intestinal emergencies, 1st edn. Baltimore: Williams and Wilkins, 1992, p. 358.

87. Wright HK. Massive colonic hemorrhage. Surg Clin North Am 1980; 60: 1297–304.

88. Rossini FP, Ferrari A, Spandre M et al. Emergency colonoscopy. World J Surg 1989; 13: 190.

89. Zuckerman DA, Bocchini TP, Birnbaym EH. Massive hemorrhage in the lower gastro-intestinal tract in adults: diagnostic imaging and intervention. Am J Roentgenol 1993; 161: 703–11.

90. Wadas DD, Sanowski RA. Complications of the hot biopsy forceps technique. Gastrointest Endosc 1988; 34: 32.

91. Johnston J, Sones J. Endoscopic heater probe coagulation of the bleeding colonic diver-ticulum. Gastrointest Endosc 1986; 32: 160.

92. Gomes AS, Lois JF, McCoy RD. Angio-graphic treatment of the gastrointestinal hemorrhage: comparison of vasopressin infusion and embolization. Am J Roentgenol 1986; 146: 1031–7.

93. Cussons PD, Berry AR. Comparison of the value of emergency mesenteric angiography and intraoperative colonoscopy with ante-grade colonic irrigation in massive rectal haemorrhage. J R Coll Surg Edinb 1989; 34: 91–3.

94. Mendeloff AL. Thoughts on the epidemi-ology of diverticular disease. Clin Gastro-enterol 1986; 15: 855–77.

95. Kirson SM. Diverticulitis: management patterns in a community hospital. South Med J 1988; 81: 972–7.

96. Sugihara K, Muto T, Morioka Y et al. Diverticular disease of the colon in Japan. Dis Colon Rectum 1984; 27: 531–7.

97. Hinchey EJ, Schaal PG, Richards GK. Treatment of perforated diverticular disease of the colon. Adv Surg 1978; 12: 85–109.

98. Greenlee HB, Pienkos FJ, Vanderbilt PC *et al.* Proceedings: acute large bowel obstruction. Comparison of county, veterans administration and community hospital publications. Arch Surg 1974; 470–6.

99. Lieberman JM, Haaga JR. Computed tomography of diverticulitis. J Comput Assist Tomogr 1983; 7: 431–3.

100. Hulnick DM, Megibow AJ, Balthazar EJ, Naidich DP, Bosniak MA. Computed tomography in the evaluation of diverticulitis. Radiology 1984; 152: 491–5.

101. Smith TR, Cho KC, Morehouse HT, Kratfa PS. Comparison of computed tomography and contrast enema evaluation of diverticulitis. Dis Colon Rectum 1990; 33: 1–6.

102. Verbanck J, Lambrecht S, Rutgeerts L *et al.* Can sonography diagnose acute colonic diverticulitis in patients with acute colonic inflammation? A prospective study. J Clin Ultrasound 1989; 17: 661–6.

103. Kourtesis GJ, Williams RA, Wilson SE. Acute diverticulitis; safety and value of contrast studies in predicting need for operation. Aust NZ J Surg 1988; 58: 801–4.

104. Kourtesis GJ, Williams RA, Wilson SE. Surgical options in acute diverticulitis. Value of sigmoid resection in dealing with the septic focus. Aust NZ J Surg 1988; 58: 955–9.

105. Rothenberger DA, Wiltz O. Surgery for complicated diverticulitis. Surg Clin North Am 1993; 73: 975–92.

106. Dawson JL, Hanon I, Roxburgh RA. Diverticulitis coli complicated by diffuse peritonitis. Br J Surg 1965; 52: 354.

107. Killingback M. Management of perforative diverticulitis. Surg Clin North Am 1983; 63: 97–115.

108. Koruth NM, Hunter DC, Krukowski ZH, Matheson NA. Immediate resection in emergency large bowel surgery: a 7 year audit. Br J Surg 1985; 72: 703–7.

109. Krukowski ZH, Matheson NA. Emergency surgery for diverticular disease complicated by generalised and faecal peritonitis: a review. Br J Surg 1984; 71: 921–7.

110. Gregg RO. The place of emergency resection in the management of obstructing and perforating lesions of the colon. Surgery 1955; 27: 754–61.

6 Acute conditions of the small bowel and appendix (including perforated peptic ulcer)

Ian Bailey
Jeremy J. T. Tate

Introduction

Acute disease of the small bowel, from which appendicitis is differentiated, contributes substantially to the workload of the general surgeon and many patients will present as emergencies. There are many causes of small bowel disease and due to the mobility and position of the bowel within the abdominal cavity, disease in any intra-abdominal organ or any part of the investing layers of the abdominal cavity may involve the small bowel secondarily. The pattern of acute small bowel disease varies with the age of the patient – some conditions are more common in young people, others in an older population. The incidence of acute surgical small bowel pathology is difficult to estimate overall but is probably second to appendicitis as the site of disease requiring urgent surgical intervention.

Small bowel disease manifests itself in one of four main ways:

1. Intestinal obstruction
2. Localised peritonitis
3. Generalised peritonitis
4. Intestinal haemorrhage

These categories are not mutually exclusive and more than one type of pathological process may exist in each clinical episode. Usually one category predominates but the clinical picture may change if the presentation or treatment is delayed.

Treatment of small bowel disease may be operative or conservative and the timing of any surgical intervention requires as much consideration as the causes and specific treatment of small bowel disease.

Table 6.1 *Causes of small bowel obstruction*

Within the lumen

Gall stone
Food bolus
Bezoars
Parasites (e.g. ascaris)
Enterolith
Foreign body

Within the wall

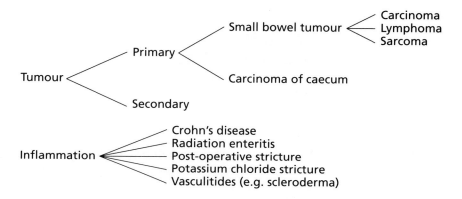

Outside the wall

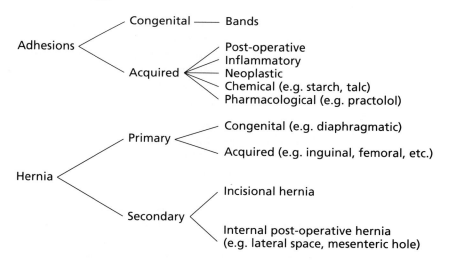

Intussusception

Volvulus

Small bowel obstruction

Aetiology

Table 6.1 gives a broad classification for the many causes of small bowel obstruction. The commonest cause in the USA and Europe is adhesions secondary to previous surgery whereas in the third world countries it is hernia. In order to avoid unnecessary surgery, and to ensure the correct surgical approach is employed, an attempt should be made to diagnose the cause of the obstruction preoperatively where possible or, at least, to eliminate conditions which might require special treatment. In practice, the cause of the obstruction is often diagnosed at operation.

Mechanisms

The small bowel will respond to obstruction by the onset of vigorous peristalsis. This produces colicky abdominal pain usually in the central abdomen as the small bowel is largely of mid-gut embryological origin. As the obstruction develops, the proximal intestine dilates and fills with fluid producing systemic hypovolaemia. Further fluid is lost through vomiting which occurs early in most cases of small bowel obstruction.

As the process continues, the risk of complications increases with eventual infarction and perforation. At this point peristalsis will cease and the abdomen becomes silent. The aim of management should be to intervene before such complications develop.

If there is a volvulus of a loop of intestine around a point of adhesion there is a 'closed-loop' obstruction. Gangrene may occur rapidly in this situation whereas radiological appearances may be less impressive.

Presentation

The typical clinical presentation of small bowel obstruction is central abdominal colicky pain, vomiting, which is often bile stained, abdominal distension and a reduction or absence of flatus. Vomiting may be less of a feature and a greater degree of abdominal distension observed if the blockage is in the distal ileum. Bowel sounds increase and may be audible to the patient. Localised peritonitic pain and tenderness may develop. In some patients there may be an obvious causative feature such as an irreducible hernia. The presence of surgical scars is important as is any history of previous intra-abdominal pathology.

Although small bowel obstruction can occur without development of abdominal pain, the absence of this symptom should be viewed with caution. This is particularly the case in postoperative patients where small bowel obstruction and intestinal ileus can be difficult to differentiate.

The history and examination of the patient should be sufficiently detailed to allow a diagnosis of small bowel obstruction and to determine possible causes. Complicated small bowel obstruction, with ischaemia or perforation, should be readily detectable by marked abdominal tenderness. It is essential to assess the patient's general state, particularly the degree of dehydration and its effect on the patient so that adequate resuscitation is undertaken prior to any planned surgical treatment.

Investigation

Investigative techniques will vary with the different clinical presentations. Investigations are required to assess:

1. The general state of the patient
2. To confirm the diagnosis of small bowel obstruction
3. To establish the cause of small bowel obstruction

Blood tests

Routine blood tests are needed to detect possible electrolyte disturbance, pre-existing renal failure and anaemia. A leucocytosis is common but might indicate an infective process whereas a neutrophil count greater than $20\,000 \times 10^9\,l^{-1}$ is a feature suggesting possible intestinal ischaemia. Arterial blood gases may be helpful in particularly ill patients. Other blood tests to detect possible ischaemic bowel are discussed in Chapter 1, as is the role of both plain and contrast radiology.

Plain abdominal X-ray will confirm a diagnosis of small bowel obstruction by demonstration of diluted small bowel loops. Sparse colonic gas and a dilated stomach containing a large air-bubble may also be present. An erect abdominal radiograph may be helpful to the non-expert because fluid levels are easily seen whereas there may be uncertainty regarding the presence of bowel loops on the supine film. Additionally, the distribution of the dilated bowel on an erect film may help to distinguish small bowel obstruction from large bowel obstruction when it is not clear from other features. Occasionally specific diagnostic features can be helpful, such as the presence of a calcified gallstone and gas in the biliary tree in gallstone ileus.

Ultrasound examination of the abdomen has generally been thought unhelpful in small bowel obstruction as the gas-filled loops greatly reduce the sensitivity of the investigation. A recent study, however, has questioned this view, suggesting ultrasonography can identify fluid-filled loops of obstructed proximal bowel and collapsed distal bowel.[1] Ultrasound can demonstrate peristalsis and may help to distinguish mechanical obstruction from ileus.

CT scan is not limited by bowel gas and can be useful in assessing patients with a previous history of intra-abdominal malignancy.

Management

General management

The first step is resuscitation of the patient with intravenous fluids and administration of supplemental oxygen. This may need to be aggressive and both colloids and crystalloids should be used. Urinary catheterisation and central venous pressure management can be helpful, particularly in elderly patients or those with co-existing morbidity. Adequate fluid replacement must be given rapidly if surgical intervention is planned.

Decompression of the stomach with a nasogastric tube will reduce vomiting in most patients, decompress the bowel and reduce the risk of airway contamination by aspiration. Fluid lost via the nasogastric tube should be replaced with additional intravenous crystalloids and potassium.

Analgesia should be given early and in adequate doses. The analgesia requirement needs to be reviewed regularly in the early stages of management and opiates are generally required, intravenously if necessary (e.g. hypovolaemic patient). These will not mask signs of localised or generalised peritonitis and there is no justification to withhold adequate analgesia while waiting for further clinical assessment.

Prophylaxis against thrombo-embolic problems should be considered, particularly in elderly patients or those with malignancy. Subcutaneous heparin is most suitable as it is short acting (see Chapter 2).

Expectant management

Intravenous fluids and nasogastric aspiration are the two components of the 'drip and suck' regimen which is the first-line treatment for most patients with obstruction. Spontaneous resolution will occur in up to 70% of patients with obstruction secondary to adhesions. Signs suggestive of infarction (continuing abdominal pain and failure of clinical improvement over 24–36 hours) are indications for surgery (see also Chapter 1).

Surgical management

The particular circumstances of any given case determine the relative need for surgical intervention. Some of the commonest features in decision making are listed in Table 6.2.

Operative principles

Once a decision to operate has been made, patients should be fully resuscitated, treatment of co-morbidity optimised and the stomach emptied with a nasogastric tube. The wide range of possible surgical procedures should be explained to the patient. Prophylactic antibiotics are generally indicated. Deep vein thrombosis prophylaxis may be given also but may exclude use of epidural anaesthesia and should be discussed with the anaesthetist.

Table 6.2 *Small bowel obstruction: indications for surgery*

Absolute indication (surgery as soon as patient resuscitated)	Relative indication (surgery within 24 h)	Trial of conservatism (wait and see and/or investigate)
Generalised peritonitis	Palpable mass lesion	Incomplete obstruction
Visceral perforation	'Virgin' abdomen	Previous surgery
Irreducible hernia	Failure to improve (continuing pain, high n-g aspirates)	Advances malignancy
Localised peritonitis		Diagnostic doubt (possible ileus)

Generally, a mid-line incision is the most flexible when the diagnosis is unknown. If the patient has a previous midline incision, this should be used but it may be helpful to extend it cranially or caudally so that the peritoneal cavity can be entered through a virgin area rather than directly through the back of the scar. In particular, loops of small bowel may be densely adherent to the back of the old scar and it can be difficult to recognize a change in tissue plane before the lumen of the bowel is entered. Although this is not a major problem if the small bowel is normal, it is clearly best avoided. If the bowel wall is diseased, the surgeon may be forced to create an ileostomy if there is iatrogenic injury to the dilated intestine; previously irradiated bowel is one example.

Having entered the abdominal cavity, the first step is to identify the point at which the dilated bowel proximal to the obstruction point changes to collapsed distal bowel. It is important to demonstrate that such a change is present as this confirms the diagnosis of mechanical obstruction and identifies the obstructing point. The presence of uniformly dilated small bowel, or no definite point of change in diameter of the bowel, suggests that the clinical diagnosis of mechanical obstruction may be incorrect.

Dilated proximal bowel can be decompressed, usually by milking the contents proximally and aspirating via the nasogastric tube which should be of a large size. Alternatively, a suction catheter may be inserted through a small enterotomy. Decompression is particularly useful in a distal obstruction as a large number of dilated loops can be difficult to handle. The large amount of fluid within the bowel makes it heavy and if it is removed from the abdominal cavity, it should be supported so that the mesentery is not stretched or damaged. The large surface area of dilated loops results in considerable insensible fluid loss. If it is anticipated that the viscera will lie outside the abdominal cavity for a significant length of time, it should be placed in a waterproof 'bowel' bag or wrapped in moist swabs. The dilated bowel may be friable and should be handled with care.

Having identified the point of obstruction, the cause is dealt with. If it is due to adhesions, they should be divided as completely as possible. It is not necessary or helpful, however, to divide every adhesion within the abdomen as these will inevitably reform. Only the adhesions necessary to identify the point of obstruction and those causing the obstruction, should be divided. It is essential to recognise the patient in which the clinical diagnosis of mechanical small bowel obstruction is incorrect and the presence of adhesions does not, in itself, confirm the diagnosis.

The small bowel should be resected if it is clearly ischaemic or there is disease in the bowel at the point of obstruction. Anastomosis may be carried out if both ends of the bowel are healthy. Proximal decompression above the anastomosis is rarely necessary. Exteriorisation of the bowel is indicated, however, if there is a generalised disease of the bowel with obstruction at one point as anastamotic dehiscence is more likely. An ileostomy may be indicated in patients with Crohn's disease as part of their long-term management, and the possibility of such a step should be recognised, considered and discussed with the patient prior to undertaking the exploratory laparotomy.

Special conditions

Radiation enteritis

Patients can present with an acute abdomen during radiotherapy due to radiation enteritis. This can present considerable diagnostic difficulties as the patients are often neutropenic or suffering other side effects of their treatment yet have marked abdominal signs. The possibility of a primary pathology, such as acute appendicitis arising during the course of radiotherapy, must be borne in mind but these patients should be managed expectantly if possible.

A more common acute presentation is with adhesions due to previous radiotherapy and these patients normally have obstructive symptoms. Again, a conservative management policy is the best course as the laparotomy is fraught with difficulty. The adhesions are often dense and, if the small bowel is inadvertently injured during mobilisation, it is very likely that it will not heal where it is repaired or anastomosed. If it is necessary to resect the small bowel in such a situation, the proximal end should invariably be brought out as an ileostomy.

Malignant obstruction

Primary tumours of the small bowel are rare but can be the cause of acute small bowel obstruction. A diagnosis, is such situations, is rarely made pre-operatively and surgical management at laparotomy will depend on the exact nature of the disease.

A more common problem is the patient with advanced intra-abdominal malignancy, with or without a past history of surgical treatment of intra-abdominal malignancy who presents with bowel obstruction. These patients usually respond to initial conservative management and thus emergency laparotomy is less likely to be carried out. If the obstruction fails to settle, or rapidly recurs, there is usually time to carry out appropriate investigations to determine the extent of the disease. Ascites can be a confusing clinical factor in such a patient. When surgery is necessary, the exact procedure will depend on the operative findings. The choice usually lies between a resection and bypass procedure.

Not all patients have obstruction due to their malignant process. One study of patients who present with obstruction following previous treatment of intra-abdominal malignancy, either by surgery or radiotherapy suggested that, in around one third of such patients, the obstruction is due to a cause other than secondary malignancy.[2]

A recent study from Japan showed that of 85 patients who had previously undergone surgery for gastric cancer and were subsequently readmitted to hospital with intestinal obstruction, the cause was benign adhesions in 20%.[3]

The results of bypass entero-enterostomy, for malignant adhesions, are generally poor with short periods of patient survival. For this reason there is growing expertise in the medical management of intestinal obstruction by palliative care physicians.[4] The principles involve the use of fluid diet, steroids and Octreotide. The results of such management are variable but it does offer the opportunity to spare a patient in the terminal phase of their disease the morbidity of laparotomy.

A third option of surgical management, which is appropriate in a small minority of patients, is placement of percutaneous gastrostomy and feeding jejunostomy to decompress the bowel proximal to an obstructing point and maintain nutrition. The jejunostomy may have to be placed at laparotomy but feeding gastrostomies are highly effective at decompressing an obstructed stomach and are more acceptable than use of a long-term nasogastric tube. Total parenteral nutrition (TPN) may be required in place of a jejunostomy. Advanced malignancy is a common indication for TPN in America but is less popular in the UK unless facilities exist to manage the patient at home.

Groin hernia

Any hernia can present with intestinal obstruction. If presentation is delayed, gangrene may have occurred and a bowel resection may be necessary. A Richter's hernia involves part of the circumference of the bowel wall and the lumen is not obstructed. Infarction of the trapped bowel wall segment will still occur but there will be exquisite localised tenderness over a potential hernia site and the indication for surgical intervention is usually clinically apparent.

A patient with acute symptoms of a hernia which is irreducible should have urgent surgery. The hernia should be repaired in the usual way although the risk of complications is increased and a full treatment course of antibiotics should be given. In most cases, direct approach to the hernia is appropriate. The incarcerated tissue may reduce under anaesthesia and it is unlikely, should this occur, that there will have been strangulation. It is debatable, therefore, whether a full laparotomy to inspect spontaneously reduced tissue from the hernia is indicated but the possibility that a gangrenous loop of bowel has dropped back into the abdominal cavity should always be kept in mind. This is usually readily apparent in the early postoperative period.

A final consideration is the patient who has an asymptomatic hernia who develops acute intestinal obstruction and who then may demonstrate signs of an apparently irreducible swelling. The intestinal obstruction raises intra-abdominal pressure and this will, in turn, produce the irreducible hernia. The unwary may find the hernia difficult to reduce and, in their efforts to do so, elicit tenderness. This is likely to occur in patients with ascites and large bowel obstruction due to colorectal cancer. Thus, it is worth obtaining a plain abdominal X-ray in all patients with an irreducible hernia and apparent bowel obstruction. The absence of dilated small bowel loops, or the presence of a dilated colon, should suggest the possibility that the apparently 'incarcerated' hernia is a secondary effect of some other intra-abdominal pathology.

Enterolith obstruction

This is rare. The commonest types are gallstone ileus and bezoars. Gallstone ileus typically occurs in the elderly female and is due to the development of a cholecystoduodenal fistula after an episode of acute cholecystitis. The gallstone may be visible on a plain abdominal radiograph. At surgery the stone should be removed by proximal enterotomy, the intestine proximal to the obstruction should be carefully palpated to exclude the presence of a second large gallstone and the gall bladder should be left alone as cholecystectomy in this situation is difficult and unnecessary.

Bezoars may arise in psychiatric patients, the normal population who have over indulged in particular types of food, e.g. peanuts, and those who have ingested a foreign body. Rarely they can occur with material that is collected within a jejunal diverticulum.

Intussusception

This form of obstruction is rarely diagnosed preoperatively in adults. In children, acute presentation is usually to the paediatric department and the main differential diagnosis is gastrointestinal infection. This is discussed in more detail in Chapter 10. Intussusception in adults is usually caused by benign or malignant tumours of the bowel which should be treated on their merit once detected at laparotomy.

Connective tissue disorders

There are several systemic connective tissue disorders which can affect the gastrointestinal tract and result in a loss of peristaltic power.

These patients generally present with chronic symptoms and the presence of the underlying disorder is established. Occasionally symptoms suggesting acute gastrointestinal obstruction are present and the differentiation between full mechanical obstruction and ileus can be difficult. Expectant management of these patients should be pursued whenever possible. The obstructed episode may progress to perforation of the bowel and the patient can present with free gas visible on plain abdominal films. Surgical intervention should be based on the clinical condition of the patient and a laparotomy is not always necessary. If peritonitis is present, the perforated bowel should be resected and consideration given to bringing the proximal bowel out as an ileostomy. If an anastomosis is performed, there may be difficulties with the healing so that anastomotic dehiscence is relatively common. In addition, postoperative ileus is common and the differentiation of a further episode of mechanical obstruction, or continuing ileus, presents a major diagnostic challenge.

Intestinal obstruction in the early postoperative period

Gastrointestinal ileus can occur after any intra-abdominal operation. The surgeon may also be asked to see patients who have undergone orthopaedic or gynaecological procedures who have apparent bowel obstruction. Each case must be judged on its merits but the differentiation between true mechanical obstruction and paralytic ileus can be difficult. In patients who genuinely have a mechanical obstruction, appropriate surgical intervention is frequently delayed as a result of this diagnostic dilemma. The use of dilute barium or water-soluble contrast small bowel studies in these patients may be helpful.[5] Ultrasound is also useful as it may demonstrate lack of peristalsis which would support the diagnosis of an ileus.

Laparoscopy

Following the introduction and development of laparoscopic surgery there have been a few reports regarding the use of laparoscopy and laparoscopic surgery in the treatment of small bowel obstruction and the division of band adhesions.[6] It must be pointed out, however, that this is a risky procedure due to the distended loops of small bowel and laparoscopy must be performed with great care and using an 'open technique'. It is probably most appropriate when the cause of the adhesive obstruction is likely to be a single band such as might occur in a patient who has previously had an appendicectomy, but no other major abdominal surgery. Unless the surgeon has extensive experience in laparoscopic surgery conventional open surgery should be the choice for the treatment of intestinal obstruction which requires operation.

Peritonitis Small bowel pathology may present as an acute abdomen with localised and generalised peritonitis. This may represent the end-stage of any condition causing obstruction but this section considers those conditions which present with primarily inflammatory signs.

Crohn's disease

Crohn's disease is a chronic relapsing inflammatory disease which can affect any part of the gastrointestinal tract. A common presentation is inflammation of the terminal ileum and this occasionally presents as an acute abdomen. The small bowel alone is affected in approximately 30% of cases and the small bowel and colon together in 50%. The incidence of Crohn's disease is highest in the United States, the United Kingdom and Scandinavia and is rare in Asia and Africa, suggesting that dietary factors are important. Similar to appendicitis, the disease can appear at any age but is most frequent in young adults and there may be a familial tendency.

The disease is probably an immunological disorder although the exact mechanism is unclear. The final pathway is probably a micro-vasculitis in the bowel wall, with the precipitating cause unknown as yet.

Presentation

A typical acute clinical episode presents with abdominal pain, diarrhoea and possible fever. These symptoms can be acute in onset in a patient who has previously been entirely well. An acute presentation is more likely in young adults hence the differential diagnosis of Crohn's disease in patients with suspected appendicitis.

Two other clinical presentations occur although they are less likely to be acute. First, resolving Crohn's disease will produce fibrosis in the ileum which can cause obstructive symptoms. These tend to be subacute or chronic, however, and an acute presentation with small bowel obstruction is rare. Second, entero-enteric or entero-cutaneous fistula occurs in Crohn's disease because of the transmural inflammation that is a characteristic histological finding.

Investigation

A patient who presents with right iliac fossa pain, but in whom the symptoms are more insidious than typical appendicitis, should give rise to clinical suspicion. Non-specific inflammatory markers may be markedly elevated (white cell count, platelet count, alkaline phosphatase and ESR). These markers can, however, be raised in acute appendicitis and will not differentiate Crohn's disease. An ultrasound scan may show thickening of the bowel wall or a mass and if these signs are present further investigation should be undertaken. A positive white cell scan or small bowel enema can suggest the diagnosis.

Mesenteric ischaemia

Mesenteric ischaemia may be acute or chronic. Chronic mesenteric ischaemia can also be termed mesenteric claudication and is usually caused by a stenosis in the proximal part of the superior mesenteric artery. Patients develop cramp-like abdominal pains after eating, due to the increased oxygen requirements to the small intestine which cannot be met by failure to increase blood flow due to the stenosis. The disease is usually associated with atherosclerosis and the investigation of choice is mesenteric angiography. Further management should be taken over by a specialist vascular surgeon and will not be discussed further here.

Acute mesenteric ischaemia can affect anywhere in the gastrointestinal tract, but is most common in the small bowel and colon. Acute ischaemia to the small bowel will usually produce infarction, whereas ischaemia to the large bowel may present less dramatically with bloody diarrhoea and abdominal pain which often settles over the course of a few days and is termed ischaemic colitis. Delayed strictures may occur.

Acute small bowel ischaemia

Acute small bowel ischaemia is caused by either thrombosis or embolus. Thrombosis may occur in the superior mesenteric artery or its branches usually associated with underlying atherosclerosis. Embolus is often associated with atrial fibrillation when the patient may have mural thrombosis in the atrium which dislodges and impacts itself somewhere in the superior mesenteric artery distribution. Venous thrombosis in the distribution of the superior mesenteric vein is a less common cause of acute small bowel ischaemia, but may be related to increased blood coagulability, portal vein thrombosis, dehydration, infection, compression and vasoconstricting drugs.

Early detection of acute mesenteric ischaemia is difficult and failure to detect this condition early continues to be one of the major causes of morbidity and mortality. The diagnosis is usually more common in an elderly patient who gives a history of vague abdominal pain getting worse, often colicky in nature. There may be a background history of atherosclerosis, but not invariably so. Examination findings are often unremarkable, lulling the clinician into a false sense of security. Detection of atrial fibrillation or decreased peripheral pulses should alert the clinician to an underlying vascular problem, but even then early diagnosis remains the exception rather than the rule. The investigations for possible mesenteric ischaemia have been discussed in detail in Chapter 1 and will not be repeated. Angiography may be useful if the diagnosis is suspected, but by this stage a more appropriate investigation is likely to be laparoscopy or laparotomy. Patients in whom a diagnosis is suspected should be resuscitated and prepared for abdominal surgery. Once the diagnosis has been confirmed a decision needs to be made as to whether the ischaemic bowel is infarcted or salvageable by vascular reconstruction. If the underlying cause is thrombosis then resection should be performed, but if an embolus is present then exploration of the superior mesenteric artery with removal of the embolus may save an extended small bowel resection. This procedure is difficult and may require associated vascular reconstruction and advice should be sought from a specialist vascular surgeon.

If surgical resection is carried out, primary anastomosis may be performed providing the blood supply to both proximal and distal margins is adequate. If embolectomy and reconstruction have been performed then both distal and proximal ends should be brought out as stomas with repeat laparotomy performed in 48 hours. There is a tendency among some vascular surgeons to staple off the proximal and distal ends of bowel, forcing the surgeon to re-explore the patient in 48 hours rather than performing an anastomosis and basing further management on clinical condition. Following straightforward thrombosis it is safe to perform primary anastomosis providing good pulses are evident in both proximal and distal resection margins. Attention must still be given in the postoperative period to the general condition of the patient in order that any possible secondary ischaemic event can be detected early.

Unfortunately the majority of patients with mesenteric ischaemia only have the diagnosis made at laparotomy and the small intestine is invariably infarcted and requires resection. If the whole of the superior mesenteric artery has been affected the majority of small bowel and part of the proximal colon will often be involved and no resection should be performed. The patient should receive intravenous opiates, and be kept well sedated as death will occur shortly afterwards.

Meckel's diverticulum

Meckel's diverticulum is a remnant of the omphalomesenteric or vitelline duct. It arises from the anti-mesenteric border of the distal ileum approximately two feet from the iliocaecal valve. It may contain ectopic tissue, usually gastric, and is estimated to be found in approximately 2% of patients. Meckel's diverticulum may remain completely asymptomatic throughout life, particularly if it has a broad base and does not contain ectopic gastric mucosa. Occasionally a band may exist between the Meckel's diverticulum and the umbilicus which can cause small bowel obstruction. This should be treated as for a congenital band adhesion although resection of the diverticulum should accompany the division of the band. Occasionally the diverticulum may intussuscept also causing obstruction. Again this will require reduction and excision. The other two common complications of Meckel's diverticulum are inflammation, when the patient presents with signs and symptoms similar to acute appendicitis, and haemorrhage. Acute inflammation is rarely suspected before surgery and the patient is usually diagnosed on the operating table once a normal appendix has been found through a right iliac fossa incision. In the presence of inflammation the Meckel's diverticulum should be excised and the small bowel repaired. Occult gastrointestinal bleeding may occur from a Meckel's diverticulum which contains ectopic gastric mucosa and the diagnosis is usually established by a red cell scan. The treatment is surgical resection.

Haemorrhage

Disease of the small intestine is an occasional cause of acute gastro-intestinal haemorrhage. There are no specific clinical features which distinguish the small bowel as the source rather than the colon, but it is important to exclude bleeding from a gastroduodenal source at an early stage by upper gastrointestinal endoscopy (see Chapter 4). The most commonly encountered causes are vascular malformation, peptic ulceration in a Meckel's diverticulum and small bowel tumour. These are all treated by resection.

One of the major problems at operation is that a vascular abnormality may produce no external signs. The mobility and variable anatomical layout of the small bowel means that it can be difficult to identify a bleeding point which has been demonstrated by red cell scan or angiography. In the latter case a catheter should be passed by the radiologist into the mesenteric branches as close as possible to the bleeding point to aid surgical localisation. If this has not been possible, interoperative enteroscopy may be helpful. Occasionally the only option is to place segmental soft bowel clamps throughout the small intestine resecting the segment which fills up with blood after a period of waiting. Blind resection is, however, often unrewarding and the risks of rebleeding are high.

Acute appendicitis

Acute appendicitis is the most common intra-abdominal surgical emergency and has an incidence of 7–12% in the population of USA and Europe. Although frequently described as a childhood illness, the peak incidence is towards 30 years of age. It is slightly more common in males (1.3–1.6 × the incidence in females) but the operation of appendicectomy is more common in women.

Pathology

The aetiology of acute appendicitis is bacterial infection secondary to blockage of the lumen but the predisposing factors are unknown. There is little seasonal variation although there may be familial tendency. The incidence has been falling since the 1930s and this is assumed to be secondary to improved living standards and general hygiene. Changes in dietary habits with an increase in dietary fibre may also be a factor as appendicitis is less common in those countries with a high roughage diet (e.g. Central Africa).

Blockage of the appendiceal lumen is assumed to be the mechanism in many cases of appendicitis. A blockage has been observed to be caused by faecoliths, parasitic worms, tumours of caecum or the appendix itself and enlargement of lymphoid aggregates within the appendix wall. In many cases, however, the cause of the obstruction is unknown. Barium contrast studies typically fail to demonstrate an appendiceal lumen in patients with acute appendicitis.

The pathology of acute appendicitis is classically described as suppurative, gangrenous or perforated. Typically there is a full thickness inflammation of the appendix wall and, as the disease progresses, adjacent tissues, particularly the omentum, may also become inflamed. Haemorrhagic ulceration and necrosis in the wall indicate gangrenous appendicitis and subsequent perforation may be associated with localised peri-appendiceal abscess or generalised peritonitis.

Clinical features

The presentation of acute appendicitis may be widely variable but the classical history is of central abdominal pain over 12–24 h shifting to the right iliac fossa. Nausea and vomiting are common but diarrhoea less so. On examination, the patient usually exhibits a low grade pyrexia and localised peritonism in the right lower quadrant. Rebound tenderness may be effectively demonstrated by percussion of the abdominal wall rather than the crude method of deep palpation and sudden release.

Appendicitis can occur at any age and, although the main peak is young adults, there is a second peak around the seventh decade. The condition is most difficult to diagnose at the extremes of age; in the very young due to the lack of history and frequent late presentation and in the elderly because of a wider list of differential diagnoses and often less impressive physical signs. Acute appendicitis should be considered in the differential diagnosis of virtually any patient with an acute abdomen.

A further factor which may produce atypical signs is the variation in the position of the appendix. A retrocaecal appendix can give rise to tenderness in the right upper quadrant whereas a pelvic appendix may be associated with central abdominal discomfort. Rectal examination tends to be of little value in the diagnosis of acute appendicitis even when the organ lies in the pelvis. It is not always necessary to routinely carry out a rectal examination in patients where a diagnosis of appendicitis has been established from abdominal examination.[7] Equally, studies in children have failed to support the theory that pelvic abscess can be detected by a rectal examination with any degree of reliability although, clearly, it is indicated if this diagnosis is suspected.

Acute appendicitis is one of a relatively dwindling number of conditions in which a decision to operate may be based solely on clinical findings. In this context, the description of classic history and/or the presence of localised peritonism are highly predictive of acute appendicitis. Features such as high fever, non-localising abdominal tenderness or prolonged history tend to make the diagnosis less likely. The risk of morbidity and mortality is significantly increased if the appendix perforates and, thus, to err on the side of overdiagnosing acute appendicitis remains accepted best surgical practice. As discussed in Chapter 1, if in doubt, laparoscopy offers an alternative to, what may turn out to be, an unnecessary laparotomy.

Atypical presentation

Appendix mass

The natural history of acute appendicitis left untreated is that it will either resolve or become gangrenous and perforation will occur. An alternative outcome is that the appendix becomes surrounded by a mass of omentum which walls off the inflammatory process and prevents inflammation spreading to the abdominal cavity yet resolution of the condition is delayed. Such a patient usually presents with a longer history (a week or more) of right lower quadrant abdominal pain, appears systemically well and has a tender palpable mass in the right iliac fossa. This condition is best managed conservatively as the risk of perforation has passed and removal of the appendix at this late stage can be difficult. In older patients, a diagnosis of carcinoma of the caecum, which has obstructed the appendix, must be considered and excluded by barium enema or colonoscopy.

Appendix abscess

If the appendix becomes walled off by omentum but has perforated, an abscess will develop localised to the peri-appendiceal region. This may be in the right paracolic gutter, the subcaecal area or the pelvis. There may be a mass but, unlike an appendix mass, the patient is systemically unwell with significant abdominal tenderness. This condition is best treated by surgical intervention through a standard right iliac fossa incision. A residual necrotic appendix is usually found and can be resected. Tissues and organs adjacent to the abscess will be friable and should be handled with care. The abscess cavity is drained.

Chronic appendicitis

In the past, there has been an assumption that a patient who is thought to have appendicitis, but presents late and does not undergo immediate surgery, should have a delayed appendicectomy. More recently, however, there has been some evidence that the incidence of appendicitis in patients managed conservatively is no greater than in the normal population and interval appendicectomy is unnecessary. Patients with true relapsing or chronic appendicitis are rare and often difficult to diagnose as the symptoms may be atypical and short lived. In genuine cases, the macroscopic appearance of the appendix is abnormal and, thus, the diagnosis is best established by laparoscopy, following which the appendix can be removed.

Investigations

Baseline investigations

The majority of these investigations have been discussed at length in Chapter 1.

Urinalysis is helpful; although pus cells and microscopic haematuria can occur in appendicitis, their absence may be useful in excluding urinary tract diseases from a differential diagnosis.

Plain abdominal radiograph is of virtually no help in the diagnosis of acute appendicitis and is not routinely indicated. Barium enema can be carried out on an urgent basis without bowel preparation. Its value lies in the ability to exclude appendicitis rather than to confirm the diagnosis as complete filling of the appendiceal lumen rarely occurs in acute appendicitis but failure to fill the lumen is less predictive. This limitation, together with the practicalities of arranging an urgent barium enema, the lack of bowel preparation and its relatively invasive nature, particularly for young patients, limit its practical application.

Differential diagnosis

Just as appendicitis should be considered in any patient with abdominal pain, virtually every other abdominal emergency can be considered in the differential diagnosis of suspected appendicitis. Some of the more common conditions which present in a similar fashion include gastroenteritis and mesenteric lymphadenitis, gynaecological diseases, right-sided urinary tract disease and disease of the distal small bowel. Gynaecological disorders are probably the most important group because the removal of a normal appendix is highest in young women. Acute salpingitis, Mittelschmerz pain and complicated ovarian cyst may all be difficult to differentiate. Torsion of an ovarian cyst usually presents with a notable acute onset of pain and may sometimes be distinguished on clinical grounds. It is important to recognise ruptured ectopic pregnancy and females of childbearing age should routinely have a pregnancy test (although appendicitis is not uncommon in the first trimester of pregnancy).

Diagnostic dilemmas

The continuing development of ultrasound techniques and laparoscopic surgery have both prompted the view that the proportion of normal appendices removed (typically up to 20% of patients operated on) is unacceptably high. Although it is clearly advantageous to spare patients unnecessary surgery, the morbidity and mortality of failing to diagnose appendicitis until perforation has occurred is greater than that associated with removal of a normal appendix. If the diagnostic tools discussed in Chapter 1 are not readily available, the best policy remains early surgery when there is clinical suspicion of acute appendicitis.

Management

A positive diagnosis of acute appendicitis requires urgent surgery as any further delay will result in a higher proportion of perforation.[8] Where the diagnosis is in doubt, patients who are systemically well and/or have mild signs, can be managed conservatively for 12–24 h[9] with regular review or investigations as described in Chapter 1. All patients should be resuscitated with intravenous fluids and adequate analgesia. Studies support the view that treatment with narcotic analgesia does not adversely affect the ability to diagnose appendicitis on clinical grounds and, indeed, may assist diagnosis by relieving the patient's anxiety.[10] Analgesia should therefore *not* be withheld pending clinical review.

Intravenous antibiotics may be given once a decision has been made to operate. A recent study has demonstrated that simple appendicitis may be treated with antibiotics only, but there is a risk of recurrent attacks.[11]

Conventional appendicectomy

A classical appendicectomy incision is made over the point of maximum tenderness and this usually lies on a line between the anterior superior iliac spine and umbilicus in the right iliac fossa. The skin incision should be horizontal and placed in a skin crease if possible to achieve a satisfactory cosmetic result. The abdominal wall muscles may be separated in the traditional 'muscle splitting' fashion or the abdominal cavity may be entered at the lateral margin of the rectus muscle, with retraction of the muscle fibres medially. This lateral rectal approach may be associated with less postoperative discomfort. A right-sided Pfannensteil incision is used by some surgeons in female patients because it allows ready access to the pelvis for the diagnosis and treatment of gynaecological conditions should these be present. This incision is inconvenient, however, if the caecum lies outside the pelvis or the appendix is retrocaecal. The need for such an approach has been replaced by the wider availability of diagnostic laparoscopy and this incision is no longer recommended.

Once the abdominal cavity has been entered the appendix should be located by gentle palpation and it may be most easily mobilised from the inflammatory adhesions by finger dissection. If it is obviously inflamed, it should be removed and no further laparotomy carried out. If the appendix is macroscopically normal, examination of the terminal ileum, small bowel mesentery and pelvis, both by palpation and direct visualisation with retraction of the abdominal wall, should be undertaken. Any free peritoneal fluid should be examined and cultured. The presence of bile staining indicates bowel perforation at some point, such as perforated peptic ulcer, and a full laparotomy is indicated.

It used to be traditional to bury the appendix stump but there is now general recognition that simple ligation of the stump is adequate,[12] but if the appendix is perforated at the base formal oversew of the caecal pole is advised. Leaving an excessively long stump should be avoided as this will inevitably become ischaemic and can produce symptoms postoperatively. Peritoneal lavage and surgical drains are unnecessary unless there is an established abscess cavity.

All patients should receive prophylactic antibiotics against the risk of wound infection which is the commonest complication of appendicectomy. Regimens vary but the two most common are metronidazole alone or in combination with a broad-spectrum cephalosporin or penicillin. A single dose is as effective as three doses for wound prophylaxis. In perforated appendicitis, however, a full treatment course over five days is recommended. Prophylaxis against deep venous thrombosis is usually omitted in young patients as the risk is low and early postoperative mobilisation is possible. It should be routinely employed in older patients.

Laparoscopic appendicectomy

The value of laparoscopic appendicectomy is currently a major topic of controversy in the management of acute appendicitis. Discussion of diagnostic laparoscopy has been presented in Chapter 1 and if it has been undertaken, and the appendix is well visualised and relatively mobile, it is relatively simple to remove the appendix by laparoscopic techniques. The basic principles of laparoscopic appendicectomy mirror those of conventional open surgery. The appendix mesentery is usually divided first and may be cauterised with bi-polar diathermy, tied in continuity with ligatures or controlled by application of haemostatic clips. The appendix itself is usually ligated with a preformed loop ligature. An alternative, highly effective and rapid technique, is to apply an endoscopic stapling device to the appendix which is divided as the first step. The vascular pedicle is then tied with a loop ligature before division. Unfortunately, the stapling device is expensive.

The inflamed appendix should be removed through an endoscopic port or, if it is excessively swollen, placed in a bag for retrieval as it is essential to remove the appendix through the abdominal wall without contaminating the soft tissues. This minimises the risk of wound infection which appears to be significantly lower than after conventional surgery.[13,14]

There have been various descriptions of operative technique for laparoscopic appendicectomy and different positions for port placement are used. If ports are placed low in the abdominal wall, the cosmetic result may be improved but some surgeons prefer to place one port in the right upper quadrant and one in the lower abdomen to allow the classical positioning of the long axis of laparoscopic instruments at right angles to each other. There is no evidence to suggest that one approach is better than another. The main technical problem during laparoscopic appendicectomy is freeing adhesions in an advanced case, particularly if the appendix is gangrenous as it can disintegrate with repeated instrumentation. If a 'difficult' appendix is encountered, the laparoscope can be used to transluminate the abdominal wall, allowing accurate placement of a conventional surgical incision and it may be possible to keep this to a smaller size than would otherwise have been used.

A technique of laparoscopic assisted appendicectomy has been described[15] whereby the appendix is approached through a small incision in the right iliac fossa. Under laparoscopic view the appendix and caecal pole are delivered onto the abdominal wall after release of the pneumoperitoneum and appendicectomy carried out. Once the stump has been closed the caecum is returned to the peritoneal cavity, the abdominal incision closed and laparoscopic inspection then carried out after re-producing the pneumoperitoneum.

One of the reported complications of laparoscopic appendicectomy is leaving too long a stump and risking recurrent symptoms.[16] Care must be taken to ensure that the entire appendix has been fully mobilised to avoid this complication. There have now been many reports comparing open and laparoscopic appendicectomy. Some have suggested an advantage associated with the laparoscopic approach,[13,17] whereas others have shown no difference between the two techniques.[18,19]

The normal appendix

If a standard incision is made, conventional teaching suggests that a normal appendix should be removed to prevent confusion in the future should right iliac fossa pain recur. This hypothesis has never been fully tested and one would imagine that most patients are capable of understanding whether their appendix had been removed or not provided they are given this information. On the other hand, removal of a normal appendix is associated with minimal morbidity although the wound infection rate is the same for removal of a normal appendix as for a non-perforated inflamed appendix. In practice, a normal appendix should probably be left behind only in exceptional circumstances, such as Crohn's disease affecting the caecum at the base of the appendix, and even then some surgeons would still advocate removal to prevent future diagnostic dilemma.

Removal of a normal appendix at diagnostic laparoscopy is not mandatory and should not be undertaken if a definitive diagnosis for the patient's symptoms, such as pelvic inflammatory disease, is established. If no cause for symptoms is discovered, there are two arguments in favour of removing the appendix. First, there is a small incidence of appendicitis on histological examination of a macroscopically normal appendix.[20] Second, the removal of the appendix prevents the development of a diagnostic dilemma in a patient who continues to get abdominal symptoms and signs following laparoscopy. It could also be argued that a major advantage of laparoscopy in suspected appendicitis is the ability to remove a normal appendix easily and with very low morbidity.

The counterargument suggests that all operative interventions or procedures are associated with some form of risk and if the appendix is normal at laparoscopy there needs to be good reason to remove it. Each surgeon will no doubt determine their own thoughts on this matter and decisions may vary between patients and the clinical presentation.

Postoperative complications and outcome

Hospital stay

The duration of hospital stay depends on local resources, policies, the patient's general condition and any co-existing disease. It is not clear whether laparoscopic surgery reduces hospital stay; this has been shown in some randomised studies[13,14,17] but not in others.[18,19] Much may depend on local factors. Reports of routine early discharge (24–48 h) after conventional appendicectomy[21] suggest that a full diet and early mobilisation are well tolerated by the majority of patients.

Wound infection

This is the commonest postoperative complication, occurring in 15% of patients on average following a conventional right iliac fossa incision. In most cases there is superficial cellulitis and this responds to antibiotics. In a smaller number of cases there will be dehiscence of the wound and purulent discharge. Occasionally, surgical intervention may be required to drain a collection in the abdominal wall. The current practice of early discharge results in many wound infections developing once the patient is at home and the possibility of this complication should always be discussed with the patient.

There is no clear evidence that injection of local anaesthetic into the wound is associated with any alteration in the incidence of wound infection but there is also minimal benefit in reducing postoperative wound pain.[22,23] The skin may be closed with interrupted stitches or a continuous suture and this does not appear to affect wound infection rates or subsequent management. Some surgeons prefer to leave the skin incision open if there has been gross contamination of the wound in perforated appendicitis. The subsequent cosmetic result of such a scar is usually entirely satisfactory but healing takes several weeks.

Other septic complications

Pericaecal fluid collections are relatively common and are usually indicated by the presence of abdominal discomfort and a low grade pyrexia. This can be diagnosed by ultrasound and treated by aspiration; drainage is rarely necessary. Pelvic abscess is a rare complication which presents with low abdominal discomfort and swinging pyrexia. The symptoms may be delayed by ten days or more and a soft tender mass may be palpable on rectal examination but this is not always the case. Again, ultrasound diagnosis is required and, if pus is aspirated, a percutaneous drain should be placed if possible. Occasionally, a pelvic abscess may be difficult to drain percutaneously. The options are to treat the patients with antibiotics, try and drain the abscess into the rectum or to proceed to surgical drainage through the abdomen. The decision is influenced by the local circumstances and general condition of the patient. Prolonged use of antibiotics should be avoided and further attempts made at drainage if the collection is not resolving on repeated ultrasound examinations.

In patients who have undergone laparoscopic appendicectomy for a perforated appendicitis, signs of generalised peritonitis can develop in the first 48 hours. This may be due to dissemination of infected fluid through the abdominal cavity, possibly by circulation of the carbon dioxide used to create the pneumoperitoneum. The main differential diagnosis in this situation is iatrogenic injury to the intestine and, if in doubt, re-laparoscopy is indicated.

Prognosis

The mortality of appendicitis is associated with the age of the patient and delayed diagnosis (perforated appendix). Recent data have revealed a mortality of 0.24% and morbidity of 7.7% in 6596 patients undergoing open appendicectomy between 1990 and 1992.[24]

A further prognostic consideration is the incidence of subsequent tubal infertility after appendicectomy. Again, studies suggest that whereas surgery may be associated with adhesions, subsequent fertility is only adversely affected in patients with perforated appendicitis.[25]

Perforated peptic ulcer

Incidence

Current data suggests the incidence of perforated peptic ulcer over the last 15 years is on the decline although it has risen in elderly females.[26] As discussed in Chapter 1 perforated peptic ulcer is an important differential diagnosis to consider in patients who are admitted with acute abdominal pain, but only represents approximately 3% of this group of patients. Despite improvements in resuscitation techniques, antibiotic therapy and anaesthesia, the mortality associated with perforated peptic ulcer has not changed over the last two decades remaining around 25%.[27] This is almost certainly due to the fact that the age-mix of the disease has changed during this time with more elderly (female) patients presenting with perforated peptic ulcers many of whom have serious concomitant medical illnesses.

Initial assessment and diagnosis

In the initial assessment of a patient with a suspected perforated ulcer it is important to elucidate drug history (particularly steroid therapy and treatment with non-steroidal anti-inflammatory drugs), a previous history of duodenal ulcer disease and, in particular, whether *Helicobacter pylori* has been identified or treated. Other important factors include the patient on intensive care following major trauma, burns or sepsis who develops acute abdominal pain due to an acute perforated 'stress' peptic ulcer. The general assessment and investigation of patients with suspected perforated peptic ulcers have been described in detail in Chapter 1.

Management

As all emergency surgeons will attest, in the majority of patients who undergo surgery for a perforated peptic ulcer the greater omentum has become firmly adherent to the perforation and all that is required is a simple peritoneal toilet. In these cases the surgeon will usually remove the omental plug to inspect the perforation before performing a patch repair using the same piece of omentum. This persuaded surgeons to evaluate non-operative treatment for perforated peptic ulcers with some success.[28] This form of treatment should only be advocated, however, in the fit patient in whom there is no generalised peritonitis and in whom a contrast meal has demonstrated no leak of contrast from the duodenum. Sick elderly patients are best treated by surgery following full resuscitation as there is a higher incidence of intra-abdominal sepsis following non-operative treatment which is less well tolerated by many elderly patients. Non-operative treatment involves nasogastric suction, intravenous fluids and broad spectrum antibiotics with regular reassessment to confirm that generalised peritonitis does not occur. The important message provided by the studies of non-operative treatment for perforated peptic ulcers is that immediate surgery is unnecessary and there is plenty of time to adequately resuscitate the patient before embarking on surgical treatment.

However, most patients with perforated peptic ulcers will undergo surgery. This can be performed using a standard laparotomy or by laparoscopy.

Open surgical repair of perforated peptic ulcer

A standard upper midline abdominal incision is usually used although a small transverse right upper quadrant incision provides good access to the first part of duodenum and is particularly appropriate in elderly ill patients, especially if the operation has to be performed under local anaesthesia due to concomitant medical illness. The principle of the operation is to perform a thorough peritoneal toilet with large quantities of normal saline lavage fluid with an antibiotic such as tetracycline. A piece of omentum is then brought up and sutured over the perforation of the duodenum without any direct attempt made to close the perforation itself. Perforated pre-pyloric ulcers should be treated similarly, but more proximal gastric ulcers are best resected where possible and if this is likely to lead to significant stenosis then a patch repair can be performed, but a biopsy should be taken from the ulcer edge to exclude malignancy. On some occasions it may be best to proceed with partial gastrectomy. The majority of perforated peptic ulcers are caused by *Helicobacter pylori*,[29] so definitive surgery is not required. However, for perforated chronic duodenal ulcers, previously shown to be *H. pylori* negative, it is reasonable to perform definitive anti-ulcer surgery.[30]

Laparoscopic repair of perforated peptic ulcer

There have now been many reports in the surgical literature confirming the possibility of closing perforated peptic ulcers using the laparoscopic approach.[31] Thorough peritoneal lavage can be carried out through a wide-bore suction probe inserted down a laparoscopic port and in those cases where the omentum is firmly adherent to the duodenum no further procedure is required. If a perforation is evident then a patch repair can be carried out using intracorporeal or extracorporeal laparoscopic knot tying or alternatively a plug of gelatin can be inserted into the perforation and fixed with fibrin glue.[32] In a prospective study of 100 consecutive patients with perforated duodenal ulcers treated by laparotomy or laparoscopy there was no difference in hospital stay, but the operation took longer laparoscopically.[33] One might therefore conclude at the present time that there are inadequate data to support routine use of laparoscopy in the repair of perforated peptic ulcers. However, the study quoted[33] was not randomised and further data are awaited from randomised controlled trials.

Following repair of perforated peptic ulcer in the early postoperative period it is reasonable to treat all patients for *H. pylori* infection unless there is good evidence that the ulcer is caused by non-steroidal anti-inflammatory drugs. Repeat endoscopy should be considered at six weeks to confirm ulcer healing and, at the same time, a biopsy can be taken from the gastric antrum to determine *H. pylori* status. Persistent ulceration will then require further treatment, either by another course of *H. pylori* eradication therapy or long-term anti-acid treatment. Some surgeons prefer to investigate patients depending on persistence of clinical symptoms, but the policy described above allows those patients whose ulcers have healed to stop long-term therapy and at the same time identifies those patients who may develop recurrent complications so that they can be treated before these complications occur.

References

1. Ogata M, Mateer JR, Condon RE. Prospective evaluation of abdominal sonography for the diagnosis of bowel obstruction. Ann Surg 1996; 223: 237–41.
2. Walsh HPJ, Schofield PE. Is laparotomy for small bowel obstruction justified in patients with previously treated malignancy? Br J Surg 1984; 71: 933–5.
3. Nakane Y, Okumura S, Akehira K et al. Management of intestinal obstruction after gastrectomy for carcinoma. Br J Surg 1996; 83: 133.
4. Parker MC, Baines MJ. Intestinal obstruction in patients with advanced malignant disease. Br J Surg 1996; 83: 1–2.
5. Zer M, Kaznelson D, Feigenberg Z, Dintsman M. The value of gastrografin in the differential diagnosis of paralytic ileus versus mechanical intestinal obstruction. Dis Colon Rectum 1977; 20: 573–9.
6. Paterson-Brown S. Emergency laparoscopic surgery. Br J Surg 1993; 80: 279–83.
7. Dixon JM, Elton RA, Rainey JB, Macleod DAD. Rectal examination in patients with pain in the right lower quadrant of the abdomen. Br Med J 1991; 302: 386–8.
8. Moss JG, Barrie JL, Gun AA. Delay in surgery for acute appendicitis. J R Coll Surg Edinb 1985; 30: 290–3.
9. McLean AD, Stonebridge PA, Bradbury AW, Rainey JB, McLeod DAD. Time of presentation, time of operation, and unnecessary appendicectomy. Br Med J 1993; 306: 307.
10. Attard AR, Corlett MJ, Kidner NJ, Leslie AP, Fraser IA. Safety of early pain relief for acute abdominal pain. Br Med J 1992; 305: 554–6.
11. Eriksson S, Granström L. Randomized controlled trial of appendicectomy versus antibiotic therapy for acute appendicitis. Br J Surg 1995; 82: 166–9.
12. Engstrom L, Fenyo G. Appendicectomy: assessment of stump invagination: a prospective, randomized trial. Br J Surg 1985; 72: 971–2.
13. Kum CK, Ngoi SS, Goh PMY, Tekant Y, Isaac JR. Randomized controlled comparing laparoscopic and open appendicectomy. Br J Surg 1993; 80: 1599–600.
14. McAnena OJ, Austin O, O'Connell PR, Hederman WP, Gorey TF, Fitzpatrick J. Laparoscopic versus open appendicectomy; a prospective evaluation. Br J Surg 1992; 79: 818–20.
15. Byrne DS, Bell G, Morrice JJ, Orr G. Technique for laparoscopic appendicectomy. Br J Surg 1992; 79: 574–5.
16. Milne AA, Bradbury AW. 'Residual' appendicitis following incomplete laparoscopic appendicectomy. Br J Surg 1996; 83: 217.
17. Cox MR, McCall JL, Toouli J et al. Prospective randomized comparison of open versus laparoscopic appendectomy in men. World J Surg 1996; 20: 263–6.
18. Tate JJT, Dawson JW, Chung SCS, Lau WY, Li AKC. Laparoscopic versus open appendicectomy; prospective randomised trial. Lancet 1993; 342: 633–7.
19. Martin LC, Puente I, Sosa JL et al. Open versus laparoscopic appendectomy. Ann Surg 1995; 222: 256–62.
20. Lee W-Y, Fan S-T, Yiu T-F, Chu K-W, Suen H-C, Wong K-K. The clinical significance of routine histopathologic study of the resected appendix and safety of appendiceal inversion. Surg Gynecol Obstet 1986; 162: 256–8.
21. Salam IMA, Fallouji MA, El Ashaal YI et al. Early patient discharge following appendicectomy: safety and feasibility. J R Coll Surg Edinb 1995; 40: 300–2.
22. Dahl JB, Moiniche S, Kehle H. Wound infiltration with local anaesthetics for post operative pain relief. Acta Anaesthesiol Scand 1994; 38: 7–14.
23. Turner GA, Chalkiadis G. Comparison of preoperative with postoperative lignocaine infiltration on postoperative analgesic requirements. Br J Anaesth 1994; 72: 541–3.
24. Baigrie RJ, Dehn TCB, Fowler SM, Dunn DC. Analysis of 8651 appendicectomies in England and Wales during 1992. Br J Surg 1995; 82: 933.
25. Mueller BA, Daling JR, Moore DE et al. Appendectomy and the risk of tubal infertility. N Engl J Med 1986; 315: 1506–7.
26. Jibril JA, Redpath A, Macintyre IMC. Changing pattern of admission and operation for duodenal ulcer in Scotland. Br J Surg 1994; 81: 87–9.

27. Irvin TT. Mortality and perforated peptic ulcer: a case for risk stratification in elderly patients. Br J Surg 1989; 76: 215–18.

28. Crofts TJ, Park KGM, Steele RJC, Chung SSC, Li AKC. A randomized trial of non-operative treatment for perforated peptic ulcer. N Engl J Med 1989; 320: 970–1.

29. Sebastian M, Prem Chandran VP, Elashaal YIM, Sim AJW. *Helicobacter pylori* infection in perforated peptic ulcer disease. Br J Surg 1995; 82: 360–2.

30. Donovan AJ, Vinson TL, Maulsby GO, Gewin JR. Selective treatment of duodenal ulcer perforation. Ann Surg 1979; 189: 627–36.

31. Sunderland GT, Chisholm EM, Lau WY, Chung SCS, Li AKC. Laparoscopic repair of perforated peptic ulcer. Br J Surg 1992; 79: 785.

32. Tate JJT, Dawson JW, Lau WY, Li AKC. Sutureless laparoscopic treatment of perforated duodenal ulcer. Br J Surg 1993; 80: 235.

33. Lau WY, Leung KL, Zhu XL, Lam YH, Chung SCS, Li AKC. Laparoscopic repair of perforated peptic ulcer. Br J Surg 1995; 82: 814–16.

7 Pancreaticobiliary emergencies

Jeremy N. Thompson

Introduction

This chapter describes the management of acute conditions of the pancreas, bile ducts and gall bladder. The non-emergency treatment of pancreaticobiliary disease, the management of late complications of acute disease and pancreaticobiliary trauma are not considered in detail as these are dealt with elsewhere in this series. See Hepatobiliary and Pancreatic Surgery (James Garden, ed).

The topics discussed in this chapter include acute gall bladder disease, acute cholangitis, acute pancreatitis, iatrogenic injury to the bile duct, haemorrhage from the biliary tract or pancreas and gall-stone ileus. Jaundice caused by obstruction to the bile ducts requires urgent investigation and treatment but is not a true emergency unless complicated by cholangitis.

Acute gall bladder disease

Disease spectrum and aetiology

Most (95%) acute gall bladder disease is related to stones which produce a spectrum of symptoms. At one end there is a short-lived episode of acute abdominal pain lasting less than 1–2 h, at the other prolonged abdominal pain associated with evidence of a systemic inflammatory response culminating in either empyema of the gall bladder, of gall bladder necrosis with perforation and localised abscess formation or biliary peritonitis. Such severe complications of gall bladder stone disease are uncommon, indeed most patients with gall bladder stones are asymptomatic. Recurrent short-lived episodes of abdominal pain, so-called biliary colic, is the commonest presentation. A more protracted episode of inflammation occurs in 10–20% of patients with symptomatic gallstones and leads to the clinical syndrome of acute cholecystitis. Both these presentations are usually caused by impaction of a stone in the neck of the gall bladder or in the cystic duct. This produces acute obstruction to the gall bladder and prevents emptying. Prolonged obstruction is frequently complicated by bacterial infection, and may lead to empyema, or to gall bladder wall necrosis with perforation and either localised abscess formation around the gall bladder (pericystic abscess) or more rarely generalised biliary peritonitis. Bacteria can be cultured from gall bladder bile in 20% of patients with stones and 50% of patients with acute cholecystitis.[1] Upper gastrointestinal bacteria such as *Escherichia coli*, *Klebsiella* and *Enterococcus* are frequently found. Bacterial infection in acute cholecystitis is usually a secondary event. Obstruction to gall bladder emptying produces a prostaglandin-mediated inflammatory response within the mucosa with the resultant exudation of a protein-rich fluid into the gall bladder lumen. Secondary bacterial infection may lead to suppurative cholecystitis (empyema). Prolonged obstruction without infection leads to formation of a mucocele. Relief of gall bladder obstruction by stone disimpaction leads to resolution of acute cholecystitis, but patients remain at high risk of recurrent attacks. Ischaemia of the gall bladder wall particularly the fundus, occurs in 25% of patients with acute cholecystitis, possibly caused by increased gall bladder pressure (Laplace's law). Ischaemia may lead to necrosis (gangrene) and perforation.

In approximately 5% of patients acute gall bladder disease is not related to gall bladder stones (Table 7.1). Acalculous cholecystitis usually occurs in patients who are severely ill on an intensive care unit.[2] Prolonged absence of enteric feeding, which frequently occurs in critically ill patients, is associated with distension of the gall bladder and sludge formation because of the absence of stimulation to gall bladder contraction. Such a gall bladder may become inflamed leading to systemic illness with localised peritonitis, probably because of a chemical injury to the gall bladder mucosa from concentrated bile acids. Cytomegalovirus (CMV) infection of the gall bladder is seen in patients with AIDS and *Salmonella* cholecystitis also occurs. Emphysematous cholecystitis is a rare condition in which gas is seen in the gall bladder wall or lumen on plain radiograph or ultrasound scanning.[3] A primary bacterial cause is usual and anaerobic bacteria, especially Clostridia, are often present. Some 20% of patients are diabetic.

Rarely the gall bladder is supported by a mesentery from the liver or lies freely within the peritoneal cavity. These gall bladders may undergo torsion and present acutely. Preoperative diagnosis is the exception.

Ischaemic cholecystitis may follow operation if the cystic artery or right hepatic artery are ligated without cholecystectomy, or be a complication of vascular disease such as polyarteritis nodosa or bacterial endocarditis. More frequently it complicates radiological embolisation of the liver. Hepatic artery chemotherapy may also cause acute cholecystitis, but this is normally prevented by prophylactic cholecystectomy.

Clinical features and investigation

The prevalence of gallstones increases with age and is higher in women. About 30% of women and 15% of men in the United

Table 7.1 *Causes of acute gall bladder disease*

Gallstones
Chemical/bile salts injury
Primary infection e.g. Salmonella
                        CMV
                        Clostridia
                        Other
Torsion of gall bladder
Ischaemia
        – iatrogenic, e.g. surgery, embolisation
        – vascular disease

Kingdom will develop gall bladder stones. The majority of patients are untroubled by their stones.

Biliary pain is variable in location, although most commonly localises to the right upper abdomen. Epigastric, retrosternal and left hypochondrial pain may also occur and there is commonly radiation to the right scapular region. Pain lasting more than 1–2 h implies acute cholecystitis which is associated with systemic signs of inflammation and evidence of localised peritonitis. Inspiration produces pain when a hand is pressed in the right subcostal region but not the left (positive Murphy's sign). A gall bladder mass is palpable in 20–25% of patients, usually representing inflamed tissues adherent to a distended gall bladder, particularly the greater omentum.

Laboratory investigations may show evidence of systemic inflammation with a leucocytosis, raised ESR and C-reactive protein. Liver function tests may be deranged and the serum amylase mildly elevated. Hyperbilirubinaemia up to 100 μmol l^{-1} occurs in 25% of patients with acute cholecystitis often in the absence of bile duct stones.[4] More marked jaundice or abnormalities of liver function test which fail to return to normal following resolution of the acute inflammation are suggestive of ductal obstruction by stones. Marked elevation of the serum amylase should suggest the alternative diagnosis of acute pancreatitis (see below). Blood cultures may be positive in patients with suppurative cholecystitis. Blood glucose levels should be checked particularly as diabetic patients have a higher complication rate.

Ultrasound scanning is the investigation of first choice; it not only identifies gall bladder stones with a high accuracy but may also demonstrate evidence of acute inflammation with gall bladder distention, wall thickening and localised pericystic fluid (Fig. 7.1). A positive ultrasound Murphy's sign is often present with acute cholecystitis, the inflamed gall bladder causing pain when impacting against the ultrasound probe on inspiration. The diameter of the common bile duct can also be accurately measured although the detection of ductal

Figure 7.1
An ultrasound scan showing an acutely inflamed gall bladder with wall thickening (arrowed) and luminal stones.

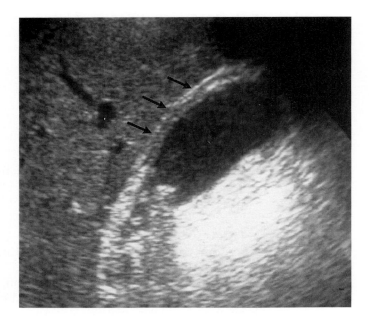

stones is less reliable. Abscess formation within the liver or around the extrahepatic gall bladder may be seen. Small gall bladder stones or crystals (microlithiasis) may be difficult or impossible to detect on ultrasound scanning, which cannot therefore be used to completely exclude gall bladder stones.

Plain abdominal radiograph will show calcified gall bladder stones but these occur in only 15–20% of cases. When ultrasound scanning is difficult or equivocal CT scanning may be necessary to confirm the clinical diagnosis of acute gall bladder disease. Biliary radionucleotide scanning with Tc-99m iminodiacetic acid derivatives is less reliable, non-filling of the gall bladder occurring in fasting conditions in the absence of acute disease. Rarely gas may be seen within the wall of the gall bladder either on ultrasound scanning or plain abdominal radiograph. Air may also be seen within the biliary system in patients who have had a previous biliary-enteric anastomosis, sphincterotomy, or sphincteroplasty, or who have developed a spontaneous fistula from the gall bladder to the gastrointestinal tract, usually the duodenum.

The differential diagnosis of acute cholecystitis includes acute pancreatitis, perforation of a duodenal or gastric ulcer, acute cholangitis, acute appendicitis, perihepatitis (the Curtis–Fitz–Hugh syndrome), ureteric colic, myocardial infarction and hepatic congestion (right-sided cardiac failure or hepatitis). Differentiation is usually straightforward on clinical grounds and urgent investigation, but the diagnosis is occasionally difficult.

Management

Most acute gall bladder disease may be managed non-operatively. Biliary colic usually resolves spontaneously within 1–2 h and requires analgesia and later investigation. Prolonged biliary colic or acute cholecystitis normally requires hospital admission, intravenous fluids, analgesia and systemic antibiotic therapy. Antibiotics active against enteric bacteria should be chosen, a cephalosporin or a broad spectrum penicillin being the usual first choice. A nasogastric tube is not normally required. Most patients improve on such a regimen, but all should be carefully monitored as a few will develop progressive disease despite this treatment. Failure of the systemic disturbance to resolve and increasing evidence of local peritonitis are indications for interventional treatment.

Although most patients with acute cholecystitis can be managed non-operatively initially, those presenting with empyema of the gall bladder and evidence of severe systemic sepsis may need emergency intervention, and patients with biliary peritonitis require urgent laparotomy. Occasionally laparotomy is required because of diagnostic uncertainty, but this is uncommon.

If emergency intervention is necessary the alternatives are either decompression of the gall bladder percutaneously under ultrasound or CT guidance or operation. If operation is undertaken cholecystectomy is preferable but should only be undertaken by surgeons with considerable experience of elective surgery. There will be marked inflammation around the gall bladder and in Calot's triangle. Although cholecystectomy is usually possible when performed by an experienced surgeon either at laparoscopic or open operation, the essential step is one of gall bladder decompression rather than its complete removal. Decompression can be easily accomplished by Foley catheter cholecystostomy.[5] If cholecystectomy is attempted, aspiration of the distended gall bladder helps dissection; the fluid should be cultured. Frequently there is an oedematous plane of cleavage between the acutely inflamed gall bladder and the liver bed which is easily separated. Occasionally the gall bladder wall is densely adherent to the liver bed; this part of the gall bladder wall may be left and the mucosa cauterised with diathermy. If dissection is considered hazardous in the region of Calot's triangle, a subtotal cholecystectomy with stone removal and over-sewing of the neck of the gall bladder provides a satisfactory long-term result. A fundus-first dissection technique may be helpful. Rarely a stone impacted in the neck of the gall bladder may compress or erode into the common hepatic duct, the Mirizzi syndrome[6] (Fig. 7.2). In these patients the bile duct is at risk of injury during cholecystectomy particularly during operation for acute cholecystitis. If suspected, the gall bladder should be opened and the impacted stone removed. Inspection and palpation from within the gall bladder lumen will then be possible. If a Mirizzi syndrome exists, the gall bladder neck can be over-sewn or a Roux

Figure 7.2 *An ERCP showing a Mirizzi syndrome. A large stone is seen eroding into the common hepatic duct (arrowed).*

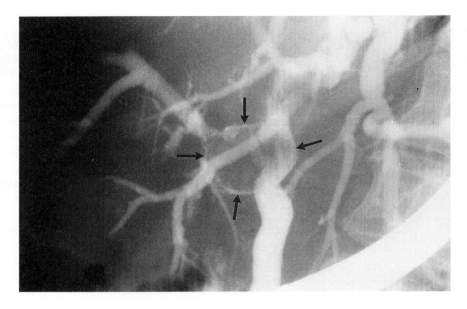

loop of jejunum anastomosed to the gall bladder remnant or the common duct.

Percutaneous catheter drainage of the gall bladder is particularly valuable in patients who are considered to be at high operative risk, for example elderly patients with multiple medical problems or those on an intensive care unit with other serious illness. Good results are reported using percutaneous gall bladder drainage, the catheter is passed trans-hepatically to reduce the risk of intraperitoneal leakage.[7] However, if gall bladder perforation has caused biliary peritonitis emergency cholecystectomy is necessary, and should be combined with evacuation of bile and peritoneal lavage. If tube compression alone is performed, elective cholecystectomy can be undertaken later when the patient's condition has improved.

Cholangiography may be obtained at the time of cholecystectomy or indeed after percutaneous gall bladder drainage. However, unless there is concern about possible co-existent cholangitis (see below) the surgeon should not struggle to perform cholangiography in a seriously ill patient. If indicated, endoscopic cholangiography may be obtained and any incidental ductal stones dealt with following recovery from acute cholecystitis. The results of emergency cholecystectomy demonstrate an increased complication rate and mortality when compared with elective operation.[8] This probably reflects the status of patients undergoing emergency gall bladder surgery, although percutaneous decompression of the gall bladder will now avoid emergency operation in many high risk patients.

Most patients (at least 70%) respond to non-operative management for acute gall bladder disease and they should preferably undergo early cholecystectomy during the same hospital admission. This can

Figure 7.3 *An algorithm for the management of acute gall bladder disease.*

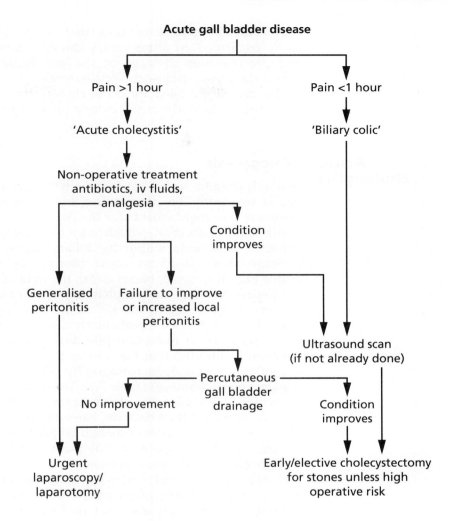

Acute gall bladder disease

Pain >1 hour

Pain <1 hour

'Acute cholecystitis'

'Biliary colic'

Non-operative treatment
antibiotics, iv fluids,
analgesia

Condition
improves

Generalised
peritonitis

Failure to improve
or increased local
peritonitis

Ultrasound scan
(if not already done)

Percutaneous
gall bladder
drainage

No improvement

Condition
improves

Urgent
laparoscopy/
laparotomy

Early/elective cholecystectomy
for stones unless high
operative risk

be performed on the next available elective operating list. Early chole-cystectomy following acute gall bladder disease during the same hospital admission has been shown to be as safe as delayed opera-tion, shortens total hospital stay and avoids the risk of recurrent episodes of acute disease.[9,10] Patients who have undergone operative cholecystostomy or catheter gall bladder drainage may undergo later cholecystectomy when their condition is improved. For patients at high operative risk, who have responded to non-operative therapy or who have been treated by percutaneous gall-bladder decompression, an expectant policy may be adopted although the patient and rela-tives should be warned of the high risk (approximately 50% over one year) of recurrent acute gall bladder disease. An algorithm for the management of acute gall bladder disease is shown in Fig. 7.3.

Patients with acute acalculous and emphysematous cholecystitis have a high complication rate and a 30–50% mortality.[2,3] Diagnosis is often difficult because of associated illness but once suspected is easily confirmed on ultrasound scanning. Treatment is by antibiotics and percutaneous drainage of the gall bladder. Biliary peritonitis occasionally necessitates cholecystectomy.

The overall mortality for acute cholecystitis is less than 5%, death occurring particularly in the elderly and diabetic.

Acute cholangitis

Pathogenesis

Acute cholangitis occurs less frequently than acute gall bladder disease but is frequently life threatening and requires immediate therapy. There are two requirements for the development of acute cholangitis, first biliary obstruction (which may be incomplete) and second the presence of bacteria within the biliary system.[11] Raised intrabiliary pressure above 20–25 cm water (normal 7–14 cm) leads to reflux of bile and, if infected, bacteria into the liver sinusoids and thence to the hepatic venous and lymphatic systems causing bacteraemia and in some cases to septic shock.[12] Acute cholangitis is usually associated with benign disease particularly ductal stones, but is less common in the presence of malignant bile duct obstruction unless iatrogenic infection is introduced at the time of biliary intervention (endoscopic retrograde cholangiopancreatography (ERCP) or percutaneous transhepatic biliary drainage) (Table 7.2). The explanation for this difference in incidence of cholangitis almost certainly relates to the presence or absence of biliary tract bacteria. Bacteria are common in the presence of ductal (75–90%) stones or benign biliary strictures (80–90%) but less common in the presence of malignant obstruction (25–40%) unless there is coincidental stone disease.[13]

E. coli, *Klebsiella* and *Enterococcus* are the most frequent bacterial cultures from the bile of patients with acute cholangitis. However, anaerobic bacteria may also be found in up to 25% of patients. The

Table 7.2 *Causes of acute cholangitis*

Gallstones in bile duct
Biliary stent/tube occlusion
Benign biliary strictures
– papillary stenosis
– post cholecystectomy
– primary sclerosing cholangitis
– chronic pancreatitis
– idiopathic
Biliary-enteric anastomotic stricture
Malignant bile duct obstruction
Radiological/endoscopic cholangiography or biliary therapy
Oriental cholangiohepatitis

route by which these bacteria reach the bile is uncertain, possibilities include ascending infection (particularly after sphincterotomy or biliary-enteric anastomosis), portal venous, hepatic arterial or lymphatic spread. Bacteria may also reach the bile duct indirectly via the gall bladder.

Clinical features and investigation

Patients with acute cholangitis classically present with Charcot's triad of fever with rigors, jaundice and upper abdominal pain.[14] There is a spectrum of clinical disease from a short-lived fever and discomfort which resolves spontaneously to a rapidly fatal condition. In severe cases patients will also have depression of their mental state and evidence of septic shock.[15] Because these patients are often elderly and confused at the time of presentation the history of abdominal pain may not be readily apparent and abdominal signs minimal. The jaundice is often only slight or moderate particularly in the early stages of disease. For these reasons acute cholangitis should be considered in all patients presenting with sepsis for which there is no clear cause. A history of biliary disease should alert the surgeon to the possibility of cholangitis. Mild jaundice (or cholestatic liver function tests) or upper abdominal tenderness in association with evidence of sepsis should lead to a working clinical diagnosis of acute cholangitis. Treatment should not be delayed for investigation which should be used to confirm the clinical diagnosis. Mild jaundice frequently accompanies sepsis from other causes particularly if there is portal pyaemia, but jaundice in the presence of sepsis should *always* lead to consideration of a diagnosis of acute cholangitis.

Liver function tests usually (>90%) show elevation of serum bilirubin and marked elevation of alkaline phosphatase and gamma-glutamyl transferase suggestive of cholestasis. Occasionally occlusion to one or more intrahepatic ducts leads to cholangitis without jaundice because part of the liver is draining normally. Other liver tests may also be deranged including the transaminases and prothrombin time. In addition there will be evidence of a systemic response to infection with leucocytosis, raised ESR and C-reactive protein. Blood cultures, which should be taken in all patients, grow enteric Gram-negative organisms in 50% of cases. The serum amylase is mildly elevated (35% of patients) and occasionally markedly elevated suggesting possible associated acute pancreatitis.

Plain abdominal radiographs are usually unhelpful but may show calcified gallstones or aerobilia. Imaging with ultrasound scanning is the investigation of first choice and this normally shows evidence of bile duct dilatation and gallstone disease. Ductal stones are frequently missed on both ultrasound and CT scanning, but these investigations may show multiple liver abscesses. Cholangiography is always required at some stage in the investigation of patients who have presented with acute cholangitis, but may be delayed until the acute stage of the disease has resolved unless the patient fails to respond to initial treatment (see below). Interventional cholangiography raises biliary pressure and should always be covered by antibiotic treatment because of the risk of recurrent acute cholangitis. Magnetic resonance cholangiography may replace diagnostic percutaneous transhepatic cholangiography (PTC) and ERCP, but most patients who present with acute cholangitis require endoscopic therapy for their biliary obstruction.

The differential diagnosis of acute cholangitis includes acute cholecystitis, acute pancreatitis, pyelonephritis, hepatitis and hepatic abscess. The presence of rigors, marked cholestasis and reduced abdominal signs favours cholangitis rather than cholecystitis.[16] If doubt exists patients should be treated as if they had acute cholangitis.

Management

Immediate therapy for acute cholangitis consists of intravenous fluid replacement and systemic antibiotic therapy. Intensive care treatment is necessary in patients with septic shock. Urinary catheterisation and careful monitoring of urine output is necessary in all seriously ill patients as acute cholangitis is a potent cause of renal failure. Antibiotic therapy is started with a broad spectrum antibiotic such as one of the newer penicillins or a third generation cephalosporin. Aminoglycosides may be used in combination with these or other agents but monitoring of their serum levels is required to avoid nephrotoxicity. Whichever antibiotics are chosen they should cover Gram-negative enteric bacteria, *Enterococcus* and also anaerobes.

Failure of the patient to respond to these measures over a period of 12–24 h is an indication for urgent biliary decompression. This may be achieved by one of three methods: endoscopic, percutaneous transhepatic or operative. ERCP is the procedure of choice in this situation if facilities and expertise are available.[17,18] Biliary decompression must be achieved if at all possible either by ductal stone clearance or by endoscopic placement of a biliary stent or nasobiliary drain. ERCP without biliary decompression is liable to exacerbate the patient's condition. If ERCP fails or is not possible, for example in the presence of previous gastric surgery, then percutaneous transhepatic biliary drainage should be considered. This technique has the advantage of accessing the biliary tree above the site of obstruction and thus rapidly providing decompression of the obstructed ducts. Treatment of the cause of the biliary obstruction can be delayed until the patient has recovered. If both of these techniques are unavailable or fail, recourse has to be taken to operative decompression of the biliary tract. Such operations in patients who have failed to respond to other measures carry a very high mortality (30–50%). Biliary decompression must be obtained, usually by insertion of a T-tube into the common bile duct. Protracted explorations of the bile duct should be avoided and the

Figure 7.4 *An algorithm for the management of acute cholangitis.*

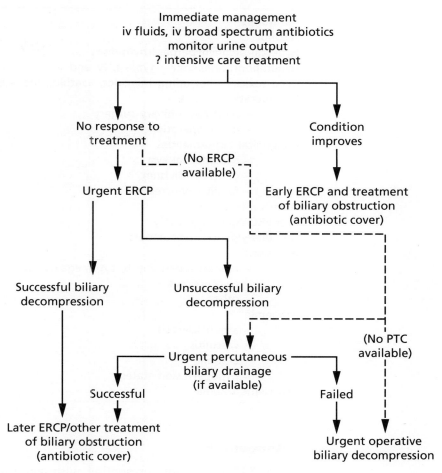

patient's stones or stricture dealt with at a later stage. An algorithm for the management of acute cholangitis is shown in Fig. 7.4. The overall mortality of patients presenting to hospital with acute cholangitis is 15–25%.

Acute pancreatitis

Acute pancreatitis is a life-threatening illness which can occur at any time from childhood to old age. The incidence varies geographically and is related to the prevalence of gallstones and alcohol consumption of the population. Although the condition still carries a 10% overall mortality a number of advances in the diagnosis and management of acute pancreatitis have been made over recent years. This section deals in detail only with the early management of an attack of acute pancreatitis.

Table 7.3 *Causes of acute pancreatitis*

Gallstones
Alcohol
Hypercalcaemia/hyperparathyroidism
Hyperlipoproteinaemia – types I, IV and V
Drug toxicity – including thiazides, azathioprine, steroids
Postoperative
     – pancreaticobiliary surgery
     – other operations
Congenital abnormalities
     – choledochal cyst
     – pancreas divisum
     – familial pancreatitis
Ascaris infestation
Post-ERCP/sphincterotomy
Ampullary/pancreatic tumours
Infections
     – mumps, Coxsackie B, cytomegalovirus
     – cryptococcus
     – other
Ischaemic
     – atherosclerosis
     – vasculitis
     – embolic
     – hypoperfusion states
Pancreatic trauma

Pathogenesis

Up to 80% of patients presenting with acute pancreatitis either have a history of excessive alcohol consumption (greater than 40 units per week) or are found to have gallstone disease. There are a large number of other rarer causes for acute pancreatitis and these are listed in Table 7.3. In children and teenagers congenital causes are most frequent and these include choledochal cyst, familial pancreatitis and pancreas divisum. A history of abdominal trauma should always be excluded as this may produce rupture of the pancreas.

Stones in the biliary system cause acute pancreatitis by impacting at the lower end of the common bile duct. The exact mechanism by which acute pancreatitis is initiated is uncertain although possibilities include obstruction to the pancreatic duct, the reflux of infected bile into the pancreatic ductal system via the common channel at the lower end of the bile and pancreatic ducts, and the reflux of duodenal contents into the pancreatic duct following disruption of the sphincter mechanism by passage of a stone. Almost all patients (90%) with gallstone-related acute pancreatitis will pass at least one gallstone in their

Figure 7.5 *A small stone (arrowed) impacted in the lower bile duct in a patient with acute pancreatitis. Note the wide low-inserted cystic duct.*

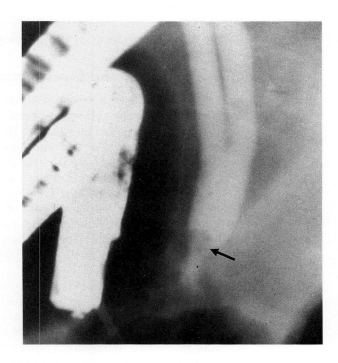

stool within a few days of the attack.[19] The earlier cholangiography is performed in the course of an attack of acute pancreatitis the higher the incidence of ductal stones.[20] Patients with progressive severe pancreatitis may be found to have a gallstone impacted at the lower end of the bile duct (Fig. 7.5). These findings suggest that gallstone impaction rather than its passage is the critical factor in the initiation and continuation of an attack of gallstone-related acute pancreatitis. The stones that cause acute pancreatitis are normally small and are found in patients with wide cystic ducts and long common channels.[21] Most such stones are formed in the gall bladder and are passed through the cystic duct into the common bile duct prior to impaction at the lower common bile duct. Large stones in a gall bladder with a narrow cystic duct will not lead to acute pancreatitis. Very small gall bladder stones (microlithiasis) and cholesterol crystals within the bile may be undetectable by any imaging technique and yet cause acute pancreatitis.

The pathogenesis of alcohol-related acute pancreatitis is uncertain.[22] Attacks often follow an alcohol binge and may be precipitated by the concurrent consumption of a fat-rich meal. Alcohol may have a direct toxic effect on pancreatic cells, lead to the production of protein plugs within small pancreatic ducts, produce pancreatic ischaemia or indirectly lead to pancreatitis by causing hyperlipoproteinaemia. Patients who consume alcohol may also have gallstones or another cause for acute pancreatitis, and moderate alcohol consumption should not lead to the definite diagnosis of alcohol related pancreatitis. Many patients with alcohol-related pancreatitis suffer from recurrent attacks of acute pancreatitis culminating in the development of chronic pancreatitis.

Clinical features and investigation

Patients present with a range of clinical disease, from mild epigastric discomfort to severe abdominal pain with signs of widespread peritonitis and severe systemic illness. The pain is usually located in the central upper abdomen and radiates to the upper lumbar region. Repeated vomiting is common and a useful distinguishing symptom from other causes of severe upper abdominal pain. The pain may be relieved by sitting upright or forward and by flexion of the hips and knees. Examination shows signs of upper abdominal peritonitis. Patients with severe attacks may also be confused and in shock. Bruising around the umbilicus (Cullen's sign) and in the flanks (Grey Turner's sign) are uncommon and usually indicate severe haemorrhagic disease.

The diagnosis is confirmed by a marked rise in serum amylase (greater than 1000 iu l[-1]), lipase, trypsin or elastase. Mild to moderate elevations of serum levels of these enzymes are not diagnostic of acute pancreatitis, and may occur in other causes of acute abdominal pain such as intestinal ischaemia, cholecystitis and gastrointestinal perforation. Hyperlipidaemic serum prevents accurate amylase estimation, although this can be measured after serial dilution. Blood should be taken at the time of admission for liver function tests as these may be useful in identifying the probable cause of acute pancreatitis.[23] Significant elevations of bilirubin, alkaline phosphatase and particularly alanine and aspartate transaminases are highly suggestive of a gallstone cause for pancreatitis. Marked elevation of bilirubin suggests continued bile duct obstruction by a stone and raises the possibility of concurrent acute cholangitis (see above). Full blood count, serum calcium, glucose, C-reactive protein, and arterial blood gases should also be taken as base line measures and for prediction of the severity of the attack, which may be judged by using the Ranson[24] or Glasgow[25] criteria (Table 7.4). These criteria divide patients into those predicted to have a mild or a severe attack. The APACHE-2 scoring system, C-reactive protein (>150 mg l[-1]), interleukin-6, and trypsinogen activation peptide estimations have also been used to assess severity of illness.[26] These predictive measures are useful for comparative studies of different treatment regimens, and may also provide an indication for early intervention for example by ERCP in patients with gallstone disease (see below). They also identify the one-third of patients who are likely to develop severe pancreatitis and who require intensive monitoring and therapy.

Open peritoneal aspiration and lavage has also been used as a method of assessing the severity of attack, and can provide useful information but is not currently widely used, largely because it appears to have no clear therapeutic role.[27,28]

Table 7.4 *Prognostic grading system*

Ranson	Glasgow/Imrie
At admission/diagnosis	**Within 48 hours**
Age > 55 years	Age > 55 years
WBC > 16 000 mm^{-3}	WBC > 15 000 mm^{-3}
Blood glucose > 10 mmol l^{-1}	Blood glucose > 10 mmol l^{-1}
AST > 250 SF units dl^{-1}	(not diabetic)
LDH > 350 IU l^{-1}	Serum albumin < 32 g l^{-1}
	Blood urea > 16 mmol l^{-1}
Within 48 hours	(no response to iv fluids)
Haematocrit fall > 10%	LDH > 600 IU l^{-1}
Blood urea nitrogen rise > 5 mg dl^{-1}	Pao_2 < 60 mmHg
Serum calcium < 2.0 mmol l^{-1}	AST/ALT > 100 IU l^{-1}
Pao_2 < 60 mmHg	Serum calcium < 2.0 mmol l^{-1}
Base deficit > 4 mEq l^{-1}	
Estimated fluid sequestrian > 6 l	

Three or more positive criteria in either system predicts a severe attack of acute pancreatitis.

WBC, white blood cells; LDH, lactate dehydrogenase; AST, aspartate aminotransferase; ALT, alanine aminotransferase.

An erect chest radiograph is usually performed to exclude evidence of free gas within the peritoneal cavity. Plain abdominal radiographs often show features suggestive of acute pancreatitis including a dilated loop of small bowel in the left upper abdomen (the 'sentinel loop') and colonic dilatation up to the mid or distal transverse colon ('colon cut-off' sign).

Urgent ultrasound scanning to identify gall bladder stones should be obtained and this may also give information about the extent of pancreatic inflammation although poor images are often obtained because of gaseous bowel distension. CT scanning in the initial stages of an attack of acute pancreatitis is often unnecessary although this investigation is of value in assessing patients with complicated or severe disease in the later stages of their acute illness. CT scans early in the course of acute pancreatitis show diffuse pancreatic enlargement with loss of surrounding fat planes and often peripancreatic fluid collections. A 'normal' CT scan does not exclude acute pancreatitis, but an abnormal scan may be useful to confirm the diagnosis.

Occasionally in patients presenting late after the onset of abdominal pain the diagnosis is uncertain particularly if amylase levels are not markedly elevated. In such patients estimation of the urinary amylase : creatinine clearance ratio (>8% suggests acute pancreatitis) may be valuable, as may estimation of other serum pancreatic enzymes such as trypsin. CT scanning of the pancreas in these patients may also serve to confirm the diagnosis of acute pancreatitis.

ERCP occasionally has a role in the diagnosis of acute pancreatitis, for example in demonstrating evidence of pancreatic duct disruption in patients with traumatic cause, and also has a probable therapeutic role in severe gallstone-related disease (see below).

Management

The early management of patients with acute pancreatitis includes measures to sustain the patient through the insult of this disease and other measures designed to prevent the progression of acute pancreatitis or the development of complications. Initial measures include intravenous fluid replacement including the use of blood products if necessary, analgesia, nasogastric suction (except in mild attacks) and treatment for hypoxia, hyperglycaemia and hypocalcaemia should these occur. Large volumes of intravenous fluid, particularly colloids, may be required to maintain an adequate central venous pressure, blood pressure and urinary output. In severe cases inotropic support and ventilation may be required. Oral feeding should be delayed until the patient is over the acute attack. Prophylaxis against upper gastro-intestinal ulceration with antacids or inhibition of acid secretion is advisable in patients with severe disease. Nutritional support by total parenteral feeding may also be required.

A large number of drugs have been tested both experimentally and clinically in acute pancreatitis in an attempt to reduce pancreatic secretion, inhibit activated pancreatic enzymes, prevent infection of pancreatic and peripancreatic tissues, and reduce the inflammatory response.[29] Few have been shown to be beneficial by randomised clinical trial. Recent studies suggest that early antibiotic therapy reduces the septic complication rate and mortality of severe acute pancreatitis and such treatment is recommended.[30] Preliminary clinical studies also suggest that Lexifant which is a platelet-activating factor antagonist may reduce the severity of an attack of acute pancreatitis if started during the early stages of the disease.[31]

There has been much recent interest in the role of early ERCP and endoscopic sphincterotomy for patients with gallstone-related acute pancreatitis. At least three randomised controlled trials of early ERCP have been reported.[32-34] Although the results have been variable at least two of these trials suggest benefit in terms of reduced complication rates and possibly also mortality. This benefit appears to be confined to those patients with gallstone-related disease who are predicted to have a severe attack. ERCP and sphincterotomy may benefit patients with acute gallstone-related pancreatitis in two ways, first by removing a stone impacted at the lower end which is acting as a continuing source of pancreatic inflammation and, secondly, by relieving biliary tract obstruction with possible associated acute cholangitis. ERCP and endoscopic sphincterotomy are both occasional inducers of acute pancreatitis, but in expert hands at least, the fear that ERCP would exacerbate an existing attack of acute pancreatitis appears to be unfounded. For those patients with a predicted severe attack of acute pancreatitis in whom gallstones are suspected early expert ERCP and sphincterotomy is recommended.

Emergency surgery has little role in the early stages of acute pancreatitis. Urgent biliary surgery for acute gallstone pancreatitis has been advocated but a randomised clinical trial showed no benefit.[35] A diagnostic laparotomy or laparoscopy may be appropriate if there is diagnostic doubt, particularly when pancreatic enzyme markers are only modestly elevated. If such an operation is performed and evidence of acute pancreatitis found at laparotomy then it is reasonable to proceed with cholecystectomy and T-tube drainage of the bile duct if gallstones are identified or are thought to be the likely cause of pancreatitis. Peritoneal lavage and insertion of large drains in the region of the pancreas may also be of value, although there is evidence that abdominal drains may cause infection of pancreatic and peripancreatic necrosis.

Most patients (80%) improve over 2–3 days after initial treatment. The others fail to respond rapidly and may deteriorate. For these patients debridement of necrotic peripancreatic and pancreatic tissue may be required particularly if there is evidence of bacterial infection within this necrotic tissue. The indications for such surgery and the techniques used are beyond the remit of this chapter.

Following recovery from an attack of gallstone-related acute pancreatitis cholecystectomy should normally be undertaken during the same hospital admission to prevent further episodes of acute pancreatitis. If the cause is uncertain further investigation to exclude gallstones or other treatable causes of acute pancreatitis should be undertaken, including repeat ultrasound scan and ERCP. Advice on alcohol avoidance should be given to those who have recovered from alcohol-related acute pancreatitis. Such advice is often ignored and many patients are destined to recurrent bouts of acute pancreatitis, although these episodes are frequently less severe.

Haemorrhage from the biliary tract or pancreas

Bleeding into the biliary tract (haemobilia) or pancreatic ductal system (Wirsungorrhagia) is a rare occurrence. Patients present with upper gastrointestinal bleeding which may be severe. Haematemesis, rectal bleeding and melaena may all occur and the cause of bleeding is usually not identified on initial investigation. Blood may be seen coming from the ampulla of Vater in the second part of the duodenum on upper gastrointestinal endoscopy but often no site of bleeding is identified.

Haemobilia usually follows trauma to the liver which is often iatrogenic.[36] A small amount of haemobilia following percutaneous liver biopsy is not infrequent although severe bleeding is uncommon. Haemobilia also occurs after other percutaneous or operative procedures on the liver, or more rarely the biliary tract. Blunt or penetrating trauma to the liver, gall bladder or bile ducts may also be complicated by significant haemobilia. Patients usually complain of upper abdominal pain (biliary colic) and often have a mild obstructive jaundice. Bleeding into the pancreatic duct is usually seen in patients with established chronic pancreatitis but may cause acute pancreatitis. Pancreatic inflammatory cysts may erode into peripancreatic blood vessels, and if these communicate with the pancreatic ductal system result in gastrointestinal bleeding.

Visceral angiography is the investigation of choice. In the majority of cases an arterial abnormality will be identified, and this can often be successfully treated by radiological embolisation. It is important to occlude the artery both proximal and distal to the site of haemorrhage as the liver and pancreas have many collateral blood vessels which open up rapidly following arterial occlusion to fill vessels retrogradely. For this reason surgical ligation of a main pancreatic or hepatic artery is usually unsuccessful in controlling bleeding in these patients, and has the additional disadvantage of preventing subsequent radiological access to the site of bleeding.

Gallstone ileus

Gallstone migration into the small bowel through a fistula between the gall bladder and the duodenum may lead to small intestinal obstruction if the stone is unable to pass through the distal ileum. The management of intestinal obstruction is described in more detail in Chapter 6 and will not be discussed in detail here. Gallstone ileus may be diagnosed on plain abdominal radiograph, when, in addition to the signs of small bowel obstruction, air may be seen within the biliary tract (aerobilia) and more rarely a calcified gallstone identified in the lower right abdomen.

Laparotomy is required and if possible the stone should be gently massaged through the ileocaecal valve into the caecum, otherwise it must be removed through an enterotomy. The proximal small bowel should be carefully checked for further stones as these may lead to recurrent small bowel obstruction if not removed. For most patients no treatment is required for the cholecyst-duodenal fistula which may be safely left intact.

Bile duct injury at cholecystectomy

Bile duct injury may occur at laparoscopic or open cholecystectomy. Sometimes there are dense inflammatory adhesions in Calot's triangle, but many injuries occur in 'straightforward' cholecystectomies. Often injury is not recognised until after operation when bile is noticed in the abdominal drain (if present), the patient becomes jaundiced or develops signs of biliary peritonitis.

If the bile duct injury is recognised during cholecystectomy an attempt at bile duct repair should be undertaken. The most experienced biliary surgeon available should be called and a laparoscopic procedure converted to open operation. Small incisions into the bile duct may be repaired directly. Transection of the bile duct is often associated with loss of some bile duct tissue, but if the two ends of the bile duct can be approximated easily without tension a direct repair over a T-tube is acceptable. The alternative, and possibly better, procedure is reconstruction in the form of an hepaticojejunostomy Roux en Y. Suturing the blind end of the Roux loop to the anterior abdominal wall and marking its location with clips or metal suture material may be useful for later percutaneous anastomotic dilatation. A transanastomotic tube drain is recommended and this can be brought out through the abdominal wall from the blind end of the Roux loop.

If the injury is not recognised until after cholecystectomy the requirement for urgent surgery varies with the presentation. Jaundice requires urgent investigation with ultrasound scanning and usually ERCP to confirm the presence of biliary obstruction and identify the cause. If the bile duct is completely occluded by a clip or suture material ERCP will only show the distal bile duct and percutaneous transhepatic cholangiography will be required to define the upper extent of the biliary stricture. Patients presenting with postoperative jaundice are usually fit enough to be transferred to an expert biliary surgical centre for definitive repair.

Patients presenting with a biliary leak through their abdominal wound drain require urgent ERCP to identify the site of the leak, which frequently is coming from either the cystic duct stump or a small bile duct which was draining directly into the gall bladder through the gall bladder bed (duct of Luschka). If these are identified endoscopic biliary stenting will reduce intraductal biliary pressure and allow closure of the site of leakage. The stent can then be removed approximately 4–6 weeks later. If leakage is seen from the bile duct itself it may also in some cases be possible to pass an endoscopic stent across the site of leakage into the upper bile duct and to treat the patient non-operatively. Often, however, this is not possible particularly if complete transection of the bile duct has occurred. Under these circumstances, if the patient's condition is stable and there is no evidence on ultrasound scanning of extensive intra-abdominal bile leakage, a period of external biliary drainage may be accepted whilst the patient is stabilised and transferred.

If the patient presents with biliary peritonitis then urgent laparotomy is required. The abdominal bile should be evacuated and a peritoneal lavage performed. If the site of bile leakage can be identified and closed without difficulty this should be attempted, if not wide bore drains should be inserted in the region of the leak and an external biliary fistula accepted at this stage. No attempt at complex biliary repair should be undertaken. Postoperatively the patient's condition should be stabilised prior to transfer for definitive repair at a later date.

Note to reader This chapter has dealt with the early management of straightforward biliary and pancreatic emergencies. The reader should refer to Hepatobiliary and Pancreatic Surgery (James Garden, ed) of this series for more detailed information regarding some of the more complex problems.

References

1. Claesson BEB, Holmund DEW, Martzsch TW. Microflora of the gallbladder related to duration of acute cholecystitis. Surg Gynecol Obstet 1986; 162: 531–5.
2. Cornwell EE, Rodriguez A, Mirvis SE, Shorr RM. Acute acalculous cholecystitis in critically injured patients. Ann Surg 1989; 210: 52–5.
3. Mentzer RM Jr, Golden GT, Chandler JG. A comparative appraisal of emphysematous cholecystitis. Am J Surg 1975; 129: 10–15.
4. Dumont AE. Significance of hyperbilirubinaemia in acute cholecystitis. Surg Gynecol Obstet 1976; 142: 855–7.
5. Kaufman M, Weissberg D, Schwartz I, Moses Y. Cholecystostomy as a definitive operation. Surg Gynecol Obstet 1990; 170: 533–7.
6. Mirizzi PL. Sindrome del conducto hepatico. J Int Chir 1948; 8: 731–2.
7. Van Steenbergen W, Ponette E, Marchal G et al. Percutaneous transhepatic cholecystostomy for acute complicated cholecystitis in elderly patients. Am J Gastroenterol 1990; 85: 1363–8.
8. McSherry CK. Cholecystectomy, the gold standard. Am J Surg 1989; 158: 174–8.
9. Jarvinen JH, Hastabacka J. Early cholecystectomy for acute cholecystitis. A prospective randomised study. Ann Surg 1980; 191: 502–5.
10. Norrby S, Herlin P, Holmin T, Sjodahl R, Tagesson C. Early or delayed cholecystectomy in acute cholecystitis? A clinical trial. Br J Surg 1983; 70: 163–5.
11. Lipsett PA, Pitt HA. Cholangitis: non-toxic and toxic. In: Blumgart LH (ed.) Surgery of the liver and biliary tract, 2nd edn. Edinburgh: Churchill Livingstone, 1994; pp. 1081–9.
12. Huang T, Bass JA, Williams RD. The significance of biliary pressures in cholangitis. Arch Surg 1969; 98: 629–35.
13. Lipsett PA, Pitt HA. Acute cholangitis. Surg Clin North Am 1990; 70: 1297.
14. Charcot JM. Lecons sur les maladies du fore des voies biliares et des veins. Paris, Faculte de Medicine de Paris. Recueillies et Publices par Bourneville et Sevestre 1877.
15. Reynolds BM, Dargan EL. Acute obstructive cholangitis: a distinct clinical syndrome. Ann Surg 1959; 150: 299.
16. Pitt HA, Cameron JL. Acute cholangitis. In: Way LW, Pelligrini CA (eds) Surgery of the gallbladder and bile ducts. Philadelphia: W B Saunders, 1987, pp. 295–313.
17. Lai ECS, Mok, FPT, Tan ESY et al. Endoscopic biliary drainage for severe acute cholangitis. N Engl J Med 1991; 326: 1582.
18. Gogel HK, Runyon BA, Volpicellia NA et al. Acute suppurative cholangitis due to stones: treatment by urgent endoscopic sphincterotomy. Gastrointest Endosc 1987; 33: 210.
19. Acosta JM, Ledesma CL. Gallstone migration as a cause of acute pancreatitis. N Engl J Med 1974; 290: 484–7.
20. Neoptolemos JP, Carr-Locke DL, London NJ et al. ERCP findings and the role of endoscopic sphincterotomy in acute gallstone pancreatitis. Br J Surg 1988; 75: 954–60.
21. Armstrong CP, Taylor TV, Jeacock J, Lucas S. The biliary tract in patients with acute gallstone pancreatitis. Br J Surg 1985; 72: 551–5.
22. Singh M, Simsek, H. Ethanol and the pancreas. Gastroenterology 1990; 98: 1051–62.
23. Neoptolemos JP, Hall AW, Finlay DF, Berry JM, Carr-Locke DL, Fossard DP. The urgent diagnosis of gallstones in acute pancreatitis: a prospective study of three methods. Br J Surg 1984; 71: 230–3.
24. Ranson JHC, Rifkind KM, Roses DF, Fink SD, Eng K, Spencer FC. Prognostic signs and the role of operative management in acute pancreatitis. Surg Gynecol Obstet 1974; 139: 69–81.
25. Osborne DH, Imrie CW, Carter DC. Biliary surgery in the same admission for gallstone-associated acute pancreatitis. Br J Surg 1981; 68: 758–61.
26. Imrie CW. Biliary acute pancreatitis. In: Blumgart LH (ed.) Surgery of the liver and

biliary tract, 2nd edn. Edinburgh: Churchill Livingstone, 1994: 613–22.

27. Mayer AD, McMahon MJ, Corfield AP *et al*. Controlled clinical trial of peritoneal lavage for the treatment of severe acute pancreatitis. N Engl J Med 1985; 312: 399–404.

28. McMahon MJ, Playforth MJ, Pickford IR. A comparative study of methods for the prediction of severity of attacks of acute pancreatitis. Br J Surg 1980; 67: 22–5.

29. Ranson JHC. Acute pancreatitis. In: Braasch JW, Tompkins RK (eds) Surgical disease of the biliary tract and pancreas – multidisciplinary management. St Louis: Mosby, 1994; pp. 432–72.

30. Johnson CD. Antibiotic prophylaxis in severe acute pancreatitis. Br J Surg 1996; 83: 883–4.

31. Kingsnorth AN, Galloway SW, Formela LJ. Randomized, double-blind phase II trial of Lexipafant, a platelet activating factor antagonist, in human acute pancreatitis. Br J Surg 1995; 82: 1414–20.

32. Neoptolemos JP, Carr-Locke DL, London NJ, Bailey IA, James D, Fossard DP. Controlled trial of urgent endoscopic retrograde cholangiopancreatography and endoscopic sphincterotomy versus conservative treatment for acute pancreatitis due to gallstones. Lancet 1988; ii: 979–83.

33. Nowak A, Blaszczyska M, Nowakowska-Dulawa E, Marek T. Endoscopic sphincterotomy in therapy of acute biliary pancreatitis. In: Proceedings of the 2nd United European Gastroenterology Meeting, 1993.

34. Fan S-T, Lai ECS, Mok FPT, Lo C-M, Zheng S-S, Wong J. Early treatment of acute biliary pancreatitis by endoscopic papillotomy. N Engl J Med 1993; 4: 228–32.

35. Kelly TR, Wagner DS. Gallstone pancreatitis: a prospective randomised trial of the timing of surgery. Surgery 1988; 104: 600–5.

36. Sandblom PH. Haemobilia. In: Blumgart LH (ed.) Surgery of the liver and biliary tract, 2nd edn. Edinburgh: Churchill Livingstone, 1994, pp. 1259–74.

8 Anorectal sepsis

Roger Grace

Anorectal sepsis is a common surgical emergency; approximately 13 000 patients present to hospital each year in England and Wales. Sepsis is commoner in men than women and can occur at any age group but is commonest in the third and fourth decade. Anorectal sepsis occurs in children but it is not common.[1]

Although regarded as a minor problem by many surgeons the associated pain, the need for surgery, the loss of time from work and the incidence of recurrent sepsis are certainly not regarded as minor by the patients and overenthusiastic surgery can result in significant long-term problems with continence. The diagnosis and management of any fistula in association with acute anorectal sepsis lies in the province of an experienced colorectal surgeon.

Aetiology

A knowledge of the surgical anatomy of the anal canal and the microbiology of the abscess are crucial to the understanding of the aetiology of anorectal sepsis and at the same time it should be remembered that the incidence, the management and the success of the management of an acute abscess may be influenced by concurrent disease.

Surgical anatomy

The anal canal should be regarded as a 3–4 cm muscular tube lined by epithelium. This muscular tube has two components; the internal sphincter which is a thickening of the circular muscle extending down from the rectum and the external sphincter which is somatic in origin and surrounds the anal canal with its uppermost fibres running into the puborectalis element of levator ani. The dentate line in the mid anal canal marks the site of the embryonic proctodeal membrane. The anal glands lie between these two muscle groups in the so-called intersphincteric, or intermuscular, space and their ducts pass through the internal sphincter to open into the anal canal at the dentate line. The fibres of the longitudinal muscle extending down from the rectum also lie in this space. The epithelium above the dentate line is columnar in origin whereas that below is squamous with an intermediate area

Table 8.1 *Classification of abscesses in patients with anorectal abscess and fistulae*

Location	Number	%
Perianal	437	42.7
Ischiorectal	233	22.8
Intersphincteric	219	21.4
Supralevator	75	7.3
Submucous (high intermuscular)	59	5.8

Ramanujam PS, Prasad M, Abcarian H, Tan AB. Perianal abscesses and fistulas: a study of 1023 patients. Reproduced with permission, Dis Colon Rectum 1984; 27: 593–7.

between them called the transitional zone. The ischiorectal fossa lies outside the external sphincter and is a 'space' containing fat. The cryptoglandular[2–6] theory suggests that the majority of abscesses begin as an infection within the anal glands that is as an intersphincteric, or intermuscular abscess and the anatomical definition of any abscess is dependent on the direction in which the abscess tracks; the direction of the track defines the anatomy of the associated fistula. The incidence of different types of abscess is shown in Table 8.1.

Perianal abscess
The intersphincteric abscess drains downwards between the internal and external sphincters to present at skin level as a perianal abscess (intersphincteric fistula).

Ischiorectal abscess
The intersphincteric abscess drains laterally through the external sphincter into the ischiorectal fossa to present at skin level as an ischiorectal abscess (transphincteric fistula).

Intersphincteric abscess/submucous abscess
The intersphincteric abscess may remain localised within the intersphincteric space, presenting as such, but it may also track medially to present as a submucous abscess below the mucosa of the anal canal (intersphincteric fistula).

It would seem reasonable to suggest that a patient presenting with an intersphincteric abscess has an abscess which has presented clinically before beginning to track medially, laterally or downwards and there are certainly no data to explain why any one anorectal abscess should track in one direction rather than another.

Supralevator abscess or pelvic abscess
There are two exceptions to the above anatomical definitions. The first is a perianal abscess which does not relate to an intersphincteric origin (see microbiology) and the second is the supra levator abscess, or

pelvic abscess which begins above the levator plate and is associated with inflammatory disease within the pelvis; it tracks through the levator plate into the ischiorectal fossa normally presenting laterally to the anal canal (extrasphincteric fistula).

Perianal abscesses are commoner than ischiorectal abscesses but not surprisingly in recurrent sepsis ischiorectal sepsis is commoner than perianal. This is a reflection of the fact that not all perianal abscesses are associated with a fistula (see microbiology) and the fact that the intersphincteric (or low) fistula associated with perianal sepsis is much easier to define and treat in the primary phase than is the transphincteric fistula associated with an ischiorectal abscess.

Microbiology

The microbiology of the pus holds the second key to the aetiology of anorectal sepsis for not all abscesses are associated with a fistula in ano. The literature in relation to microbiology and ano-rectal sepsis, however, is small and until 1982[7] the relation between abscess, fistula and microbiology had not been recognised. There was, however, some evidence before this to suggest a relationship. In 1964 Wilson[8] reported the two year results of anorectal sepsis treated by incision, curettage and primary suture under antibiotic cover. An organism was cultured in 69/100 patients; only 3/45 (6.7%) patients developed recurrent sepsis following staphylococcal sepsis whereas 12/24 (50%) occurred after coliform sepsis. In 1971 Mazier[9] related the staphylococcus to the sepsis of hydradenitis suppurativa. In 1973[10] a retrospective study noted the high incidence (16.9%) of *Staphylococcus aureus* in those patients whose pus had been sent for culture and in 1977 Page and Freeman[11] reported an incidence of *Staph. aureus* of 23.6% in acute anorectal sepsis.

This incidence of staphylococcal sepsis belied the thought that all anorectal sepsis was secondary to intersphincteric sepsis for *Staphylococcus aureus* is a skin organism that does not have access to the anal glands. This apparent anomaly became clear in 1982;[7] in a simple prospective study all anorectal abscesses were drained by a single surgeon and the pus was sent for culture; a fistula, if found, was laid open. A second examination under anaesthesia was performed 7–10 days later without knowledge of the microbiology and if a fistula was found at this stage it was laid open. Of the 114 patients who grew bowel organisms 62 (54.4%) were found to have a fistula; no patient out of 34 with skin derived organisms had a fistula ($P<0.0005$).

In the same year, in contradistinction, however, Whitehead et al.[12] in a retrospective study, with the surgery being performed by surgeons in training, suggested that 9 (28%) of 32 patients with skin-derived organisms apparently had a fistula in association with the anorectal sepsis; he did, however, emphasise the positive incidence of gut specific *Bacteroides* in association with anorectal sepsis.

The two senior authors then reported the results of a joint study in 1986[13] in which the surgery was performed in Wolverhampton and the pus was posted to Doctor Ekyn at St Thomas' Hospital. The surgical protocol was as in 1982[7] but the microbiology was much more sophisticated. In a population of 80 patients 53 had a fistula and of these 45 (84.9%) grew *Escherichia coli* and 47 (88.7%) grew gut-specific *Bacteroides*; only one patient with a fistula grew *Staph. aureus* and this was in a patient who also grew gut-specific organisms. Of the 27 patients who had no fistula eight (29.6%) grew *Staphylococcus aureus* and 17 (63%) grew anaerobes that were not gut specific ($P < 0.0001$).

Subsequently evidence from Henrichsen and Christiansen[14] supported these findings with five fistulas found in 21 patients with bowel-derived organisms and no fistula in seven patients with skin-derived organisms. Fielding and Berry[15] showed that 88% of patients whose abscess was associated with a fistula, and 75% of those with recurrent sepsis, grew bowel-derived organisms; these high yields were identified in spite of a pus swab being sent to the laboratory for culture rather than encouraging their surgeons to send pus in a bottle.

Nicholls *et al.*[16] had raised the problem associated with sophisticated microbiology required to differentiate between bowel and skin-derived *Bacteroides* in a routine NHS laboratory and came to the rather negative conclusion that this inability to differentiate negated the requirement to send pus for routine microbiology. Their own figures, however, showed that 78% of the abscess with a fistula grew coliforms compared to 29% in the no-fistula group; their yield of *Staph. aureus* (two out of 46 patients), was much lower than most series.

Further indirect evidence was obtained by Seow-Choen *et al.*[17] who looked at the microbiology of chronic anal fistulae in 25 patients; 69 isolates representing 17 species were obtained; all organisms were gut derived. They commented that the majority of the growths were obtained only from enrichment and they suggested that the chronic inflammation in anal fistulae does not seem to be maintained by either excessive numbers of organisms or by organisms of an unusual type. The gut-derived organism basis for the aetiology of intersphincteric sepsis would have been difficult to uphold if they had grown skin-derived organisms.

There have been no subsequent data published to contradict the conclusion that intersphincteric sepsis is associated with the presence of gut derived organisms whereas skin-derived sepsis is merely a boil which happens to originate alongside the anal canal.

Anorectal sepsis in children

Anorectal sepsis is not common in children. Over a five-year period in a District General Hospital serving a population of 300 000 only 16 patients presented to the Department of Surgery[1] and the largest reported study, devoted merely to abscesses, relates to only 29 patients over eight years.[18] Within the context of this low incidence the incidence below the age of two would appear to be higher than that between two and twelve, and below two years sepsis mainly occurs in boys. The incidence of an associated fistula in ano is much higher in boys than in girls.[19]

Four authors have looked at the microbiology of anorectal sepsis in children; Brook and Martin[20] grew a total of 87 isolates from 28 patients; 66 of these were gut derived and 13 were skin derived; eight, as reported, were indeterminate. They did not, however, relate their findings to the anatomy, the abscess or the presence of a fistula; they particularly commented on the low incidence of *Staph. aureus*. Enberg *et al.*,[18] however, isolated *Staph. aureus* in 35% of 29 children and said it was their commonest isolate; they claimed there was no correlation between the finding of a fistula (7/29 patients) and the microbiology. Abercrombie[1] found gut organisms in 10/12 children, with skin organisms in only one patient and no growth in the other, but unfortunately did not relate the microbiology to the six children who had a fistula. Al-Salem[21] found gut organisms in 9/11 boys but only in 1/7 girls presenting with a perianal abscess; one boy and one girl grew both *E. coli* and *Staph. aureus*. Five girls and one boy grew *Staph. aureus* alone. Five boys, but no girls, were subsequently found to have a fistula in ano; microbiology was not related to the finding of a fistula.

Anorectal sepsis in special situations

Diabetes

There is a definite incidence of diabetes in patients with anorectal sepsis; in the very large series from Cook County Hospital[22] this was 4.7%. Some of the patients were known diabetics but the remainder, presenting with anorectal sepsis, were found to be new diabetics. This figure is very similar to 12/33 (5.1%) in the Birmingham study.[23] Successful surgical management of the abscess requires good management of the diabetes.

Inflammatory bowel disease

Anorectal sepsis is associated with both ulcerative colitis and Crohn's disease but is commoner in Crohn's disease. Anorectal sepsis usually presents in patients with known inflammatory bowel disease but may occasionally be the presenting feature. Of the patients presenting to Cook County Hospital[22] with acute anorectal sepsis 1% had underlying inflammatory bowel disease but no data were given as to the split between Crohn's disease and ulcerative colitis. In Birmingham[23] 9/233 (3.9%) had Crohn's disease and only one had ulcerative colitis. This incidence is mirrored by the two Wolverhampton[7,13] studies where 9/245 (3.7%) had Crohn's disease and only two had ulcerative colitis.

Malignant disease

Anorectal carcinoma,[23,24] lymphoma[25,26] and leukaemia[27] have all been reported as presenting in association with anorectal sepsis. In the experience of the author the prognosis of patients presenting with malignant disease closely involved with this type of sepsis is very poor. Avill[24] reported three cases of carcinoma of the rectum presenting in 1 year whereas in Birmingham[23] over a 2-year period 4/233 patients had an underlying carcinoma of the rectum.

Hydradenitis suppurativa

Hydradenitis suppurativa is a chronic low-grade sepsis of skin probably associated with an abnormality of the apocrine glands. The microbiology has been extensively studied and it is suggested that the organisms most frequently cultured are the anaerobic Gram positive cocci and the asaccharolytic group of bacteroides.[28]

Fulminating anorectal sepsis: Fournier's gangrene

Under this heading it is best to group those patients with gas-forming infections which may not be clostridial in origin but are associated with a synergistic action of aerobe and anaerobe microorganisms. Abcarian and Eftaiha[29] introduced the phrase 'free-floating anus' and described 24 cases of fulminating anorectal sepsis with massive tissue necrosis; their most commonly cultured organisms were *E. coli*, *Bacteroides* species and *Peptostreptococcus*. The term Fournier's gangrene has been used to describe tissue necrosis which extends anteriorly towards the scrotum and penis; it may also arise from a urological origin as well as anorectal sepsis.

Recurrent anorectal sepsis

There is no good prospective study of anorectal sepsis in relation to the incidence of recurrence and most retrospective studies are compromised by inadequate follow-up data; in studies relating to primary anorectal sepsis, however, most authors quote a high incidence of previous sepsis in their reported populations. In three studies (Cardiff,[10] Wolverhampton/STH,[13] Kovalcik et al.[30]) the incidence was around 30% whereas in the first Wolverhampton study it was 41%.[7] In the two Wolverhampton studies,[7,13] 82 and 84% of the recurrent abscesses were at the same site as the previous abscess. Chrabot[31] prospectively studied 100 patients with recurrent abscesses. In 32 patients the primary diagnosis was hydradenitis suppurativa and this high incidence probably reflects the nature of their population under study. In the other 68 patients, however, 53 had an associated fistula. Unfortunately their study gave no details in relation to microbiology. Mortensen[32] reported that all recurrent abscesses from which bacteria were cultured grew bowel-derived organisms.

Presentation of anorectal sepsis

Acute anorectal sepsis may present in four different ways:

1. Patients with a perianal or ischiorectal abscess present with a short history of painful lump by the canal. A number of patients will unfortunately have been given antibiotics by their general practitioner. On examination the painful lump will generally be obvious.
2. Patients with an intersphincteric abscess which has not tracked, or with a submucous abscess will present with acute anal pain of short duration and their pain is often such that they decline the invitation to sit down in the consulting room; on immediate examination there is nothing to see and the diagnosis is only confirmed on examination under anaesthetic.
3. Some patients will present with a history of painful lump, which may or may not have been treated with antibiotics, but they will also give a story of relief of pain following the discharge of pus.
4. Some patients will present with a history of recurrent episodes of a painful lump which has discharged spontaneously only to recur at a later date; these patients may also give a story of being treated by the general practitioner with antibiotics and some may give a story of having undergone a previous surgical procedure. It is likely that all the patients who present with recurrent sepsis have an associated fistula in ano.

Fulminating sepsis or Fournier's gangrene

Patients with fulminating anorectal sepsis present with a short history of pain with massive cellulitis and necrosis extending forward to involve the perineum and, in the male, the scrotum and penis; it may also spread forwards on to the anterior abdominal wall. The patient is toxic and ill. The patients are often diabetic. This is a form of the so-called necrotising fasciitis.[33]

Investigation

Endoanal ultrasound

There is no place for endoanal ultrasound in the management of anorectal sepsis unless the investigation is undertaken under anaesthetic; the acute discomfort associated with anorectal sepsis prevents this investigation being undertaken while the patient is awake.

Optimistic titles in the literature such as: 'Anal endosonography in the evaluation of perianal sepsis and fistulae in ano,[34] 'Intra-rectal ultrasound in the evaluation of perirectal abscesses',[35] and 'Ultrasound of perianal and perirectal fistula and/or abscess in Crohn's disease',[36] might make one think otherwise. However, Law's[34] data relate to chronic sepsis/fistula and Cataldo et al.[35] although suggesting in their summary that they were studying 24 cases of perianal abscess and fistula, do not identify the anatomical site of the abscess in the 19 patients in whom it was demonstrated both on ultrasound and surgery. However, they do discuss fistula and internal openings. In the study by Tio et al.[36] all patients had Crohn's disease; their first group of 17 patients complained of severe pain during and after defecation and all underwent ultrasound under anaesthetic. Their second group comprised 15 patients who did not require surgery.

All three studies suggested that abscess cavities could be demonstrated by ultrasonography along with fistula tracks but Law[34] admitted that the identification of an internal opening was not wholly successful.

CT scanning and MRI

Although there may be a place for CT scanning or MRI of the anal canal in the subsequent investigation of a patient with a fistula following anorectal sepsis there is no place for either of these investigations in the immediate management of acute anorectal sepsis.

Management

Accepted management of acute anorectal sepsis in the United Kingdom has been to perform any surgical procedure, whatever this may be, under general anaesthetic. In the United States, as a result of financial pressures from the insurance companies, many surgeons will now perform the chosen procedure under local anaesthetic, often in the office rather than in hospital. Commendably not all American surgeons agree and from Chicago Abcarian[37] commented that, in view of the recurrence rate, formal examination under general anaesthetic at the time of the initial anorectal abscess is not only clinically effective, but also cost effective.

The objectives of surgery for acute anorectal sepsis are:

1. To relieve the symptoms.
2. To reduce the hospital stay and time off work to a minimum.
3. To prevent recurrent sepsis.

Surgical procedures

1. Simple linear drainage of the abscess will relieve the symptoms and will be associated with a minimal hospital stay and time off work but will do nothing to prevent recurrent sepsis if this sepsis is associated with a fistula.
2. Drainage using a cruciate incision, that is a de-roofing procedure, will relieve the symptoms but the wound is large and the stay in hospital and time off work will be longer; it will also do nothing to reduce the incidence of recurrent anorectal sepsis.
3. Incision and primary suture with[8] or without[38] antibiotic cover will relieve the symptoms, will be associated with a minimal hospital stay and time off work but, it does nothing to reduce the incidence of recurrent anorectal sepsis; the use of local gentamycin in a biologically absorbable collagen along with systemic clindamycin does not improve the results when compared to clindamycin alone.[32]

There can be no disagreement that relief of symptoms is the first and immediately the most important objective of surgery. The patient, not unreasonably, and for many reasons, wishes to limit the time spent in hospital and the time lost from work to a minimum but with the incidence of recurrent sepsis being as high as it is when any underlying fistula has not been treated, there is a very good argument for placing the third objective, that is the reduction in the incidence of recurrent sepsis, before the more immediate objective relating to the time in hospital and time off work.

Best practice in acute anorectal sepsis should therefore be as follows.

1. Examination under anaesthetic (EUA) will define the anatomical limit to the abscess. Normally this means establishing whether or not the ischiorectal fossa is involved, and at the same time looking into the anal canal for evidence of pus discharging through an internal opening. This will define the diagnosis of an associated fistula. If a fistula is demonstrated it is important to remember that any induration associated with the sepsis may make it difficult to be certain as to the relationship of the fistula track to the sphincter complex.
2. Sigmoidoscopy to ensure there is no underlining disease.
3. Linear drainage of the abscess to relieve the symptoms and then pus (in a bottle) is sent for microbiological analysis.
4. When the surgeon is confident as to his diagnosis a low or intersphincteric fistula may be laid open at this stage.
5. A high or transphincteric fistula may be noted with a view to a further EUA at a later date or a seton suture may be placed along the track for drainage and subsequent management as indicated.
6. If no fistula is demonstrated no further surgical procedure is undertaken. The patient is discharged within 24 hours and returns to the next outpatient clinic with further management depending on the microbiology.

Skin-derived sepsis means that the abscess is not associated with a fistula and no further surgical procedure is required; the patient may be discharged.

If bowel-derived sepsis is found, the surgeon may perform a further EUA within two weeks by which time the induration will have settled. The track of any predetermined fistula, or any fistula demonstrated at this examination may be treated as indicated, that is, laid open or managed with a seton suture.

If no fistula is found the patient is discharged for follow-up in the clinic.

The subsequent natural history of such an abscess will be as follows.

1. The patient will present with a recurrent abscess.
2. The patient will present with a fistula.
3. The patient may have no further trouble but with time the incidence of further trouble does increase.

Scenarios 1. and 2. will require treatment as indicated. In a patient with a recurrent abscess at the same site as the previous sepsis the evidence is very strong that there is an underlying fistula and it is in this situation that endoanal ultrasound[34] or MRI[39] may be valuable to identify the track of the fistula if it is not clinically obvious.

Surgical damage to the anal canal

In the acute phase the anatomy of the anal canal may not be easy to assess and unnecessary damage to the sphincter mechanism is unacceptable surgical practice. Inexperienced surgeons should merely drain the abscess and allow the acute symptoms to settle before referring the patient to an experienced colorectal surgeon for further treatment; an experienced surgeon, however, may proceed as previously indicated. In 1987 Schouten et al.[40] produced excellent results in relation to recurrence rate from a primary partial internal sphincterectomy in the treatment of anorectal sepsis but they did admit to imperfect control of flatus (22.3%) and soiling in 13.4% of the patients they studied. A later study[41] compared the results of incision, drainage and fistulectomy with primary partial internal sphincterectomy (36 patients) with incision and drainage alone (34 patients). The recurrence rate in the two groups was 2.9% and 44.6% ($P < 0.0003$), respectively, but there was an incidence of anal function disturbances in 39.4% in the fistulectomy/sphincterectomy group; interestingly it was also 21.6% in the incision and drainage alone group. These authors suggested that because the combined recurrence rate was only 40.6% in the incision and drainage group, and because of the increased anal function disturbances after partial internal sphincterectomy, fistulectomy should be reserved as a second-stage procedure if necessary. Their period of follow-up, however, was only 3 years and it is likely that their 40.6% recurrence rate will rise with time.

Lunniss and Phillips,[42] although admitting that culture of gut organisms was a sensitive method of detecting an underlying fistula, suggested that it was not particularly specific (80%). They suggested that the demonstration of sepsis in the intersphincteric space in association with an anorectal abscess was 100% sensitive and 100% specific for detection of an underlying fistula and that the demonstration was facilitated by a radially placed incision. They then went on to say that this procedure was simple, accurate and well within the skills of a surgical trainee. This was a dangerous statement for the trainee involved had a particular interest and expertise in anorectal disease, and this procedure is not recommended for surgeons in training.

Role of antibiotics

There is no place in the management of acute anorectal sepsis for antibiotics except when the surgeon feels that the abscess has progressed to fulminating anorectal sepsis or Fournier's gangrene (see below).

Management of special situations

Inflammatory bowel disease
All acute abscesses should be drained. Low fistulae in both ulcerative colitis and Crohn's disease may probably be safely laid open. High fistulae are best treated with a seton suture for long-term drainage.

Malignant disease
Management requires drainage of the abscess and then standard management of the underlying malignant disease.

Fulminating anorectal sepsis or Fournier's gangrene
Fulminating anorectal sepsis is associated with a significant incidence of both morbidity and mortality. Surgical management requires mandatory wide excision of necrotic tissue back to healthy bleeding tissue at both skin and subcutaneous levels. Surgery is drastic and all involved tissues must be excised. This is the only situation in acute anorectal sepsis when systemic antibiotic therapy is indicated and the use of wide-spectrum antibiotics, adjusted as indicated by the results of culture, will be required.

Hydradenitis suppurativa
The extent of any surgical procedure is determined by the extent and severity of the disease. The oedematous folds of skin may need to be excised but conservative and minimal surgery with preservation of skin produces very good results and healing may be surprisingly impressive. Wide excision and grafting, however, may sometimes be required when the sepsis is widespread. There is no place for antibiotic therapy.

Conclusions

1. An understanding of the anatomy and microbiology of anorectal sepsis is essential for good surgical management.
2. Unnecessary damage to the sphincter complex as a result of surgery is unacceptable surgical practice.
3. Inexperienced surgeons should merely aim to relieve the symptoms by draining the pus.
4. The management of fistula in ano in association with acute anorectal sepsis is the province of surgeons with an interest in colorectal surgery.
5. The only place for antibiotics in the management of acute anorectal sepsis is in association with fulminating sepsis or Fournier's gangrene.

References

1. Abercrombie JF, George BD. Perianal abscesses in children. Ann Roy Coll Surg 1992; 74: 385–6.

2. Nesselrod JP. In: Christopher F (ed.) A textbook of surgery, 5th edn. Philadelphia and London: Saunders, 1949, p. 1092.

3. Eisenhammer S. The internal anal sphincter and the ano-rectal abscess. Surg Gynaecol Obstet 1956; 103: 501–6.

4. Eisenhammer S. A new approach to the ano-rectal fistulous abscess based on the high intermuscular lesion. Surg Gynaecol Obstet 1958; 106: 595–9.

5. Eisenhammer S. The ano-rectal and ano-vulval fistulous abscess. Surg Gynaecol Obstet 1961; 113: 519–20.

6. Parks AG. Pathogenesis and treatment of fistula-in-ano. Br Med J 1961; 1: 463–69.

7. Grace RH, Harper IA, Thompson RG. Anorectal sepsis: microbiology in relation to fistula in ano. Br J Surg 1982; 69: 401–3.

8. Wilson DH. The late result of anorectal abscess treated by incision, curettage and primary suture under antibiotic cover. Br J Surg 1964; 51: 828–831.

9. Mazier WP. The treatment and care of anal fistulas. A study of 1000 patients. Dis Colon Rectum 1971; 14: 134–44.

10. Buchan R, Grace RH. Anorectal suppuration: the result of treatment and the factors affecting the recurrence rate. Br J Surg 1973; 60: 537–40.

11. Page RE, Freeman R. Superficial sepsis: the antibiotic choice for blind treatment. Br J Surg 1977; 64: 281–4.

12. Whitehead SM, Leach RD, Ekyn SJ, Phillips I. The aetiology of perirectal sepsis. Br J Surg 1982; 69: 166–8.

13. Ekyn SJ, Grace RH. The relevance of microbiology in the management of anorectal sepsis. Ann R Coll Surg 1986; 62: 364–72.

14. Henrichsen S, Christiansen J. Incidence of fistula in ano complicating anorectal sepsis: a prospective study. Br J Surg 1986; 73: 371–2.

15. Fielding MA, Berry AR. Management of perianal sepsis in a district general hospital. J R Coll Surg Edinb 1992; 37: 232–4.

16. Nicholls G, Heaton ND, Lewis AM. Use of bacteriology in anorectal sepsis as an indicator of anal fistula: experience in a district general hospital. J R Soc Med 1991; 84: 318–19.

17. Seow-Choen F, Hay AJ, Heard S, Phillips RKS. Bacteriology of anal fistulae. Br J Surg 1992; 79: 27–8.

18. Enberg RN, Cox RH, Burry VF. Perirectal abscess in children. Am J Dis Child 1974; 128: 360–1.

19. Shafer AD, McGlone TP, Flanegan RA. Abnormal crypts of morgagni. The cause of perianal abscess and fistula in ano. J Paediatr Surg 1987; 22: 203–4.

20. Brook I, Martin WJ. Aerobic and anaerobic bacteriology of perirectal abscess in children. Paediatrics 1980; 2: 282–4.

21. Al-Salem AH, Laing W, Talwalker V. Fistula in ano in infancy and childhood. J Paediatr Surg 1994; 29: 436–8.

22. Ramanujam PS, Prasad ML, Abcarian H. Perianal abscess and fistulas: a study of 1023 patients. Dis Colon Rectum 1984; 27: 593–7.

23. Winslett MC, Allan A, Ambrose NS. Anorectal sepsis as a presentation of occult rectal and systemic disease. Dis Colon Rectum 1988; 31: 597–600.

24. Avill R. The management of carcinoma of the rectum presenting as an ischiorectal abscess. Br J Surg 1984; 71: 665.

25. Steele RJC, Eremin O. Krajewski AS, Ritchie GL. Primary lymphoma of the anal canal presenting as perianal suppuration. Brit Med J 1985; 291: 311.

26. Porter AJ, Meagher AP, Sweeney JL. Anal lymphoma presenting as a perianal abscess. Austr NZ J Surg 1994; 64: 279–81.

27. Troiani RT, DuBois JJ. Surgical management of anorectal infection in the leukaemiac patient. Milit Med 1956; 10: 558–61.

28. Finegold SM. Anaerobic bacteria in human disease. New York: Academic Press, 1977.

29. Abcarian H, Eftaiha M. Free floating anus: a complication of massive anorectal infection. Dis Colon Rectum 1983; 26: 516–21.

30. Kovalcik PJ, Peniston RL, Cross GH. Anorectal abscess. Surg Gynaecol Obstet 1979; 190: 884–6.

31. Chrabot CM, Prasad ML, Abcarian H. Recurrent anorectal abscesses. Dis Colon Rectum 1983; 26: 105–8.

32. Mortensen J, Kraglund K, Klaerke M, Jaeger G, Savane S, Bone J. Primary suture of

anorectal abscess: a randomised study comparing treatment with clindamycin versus clindamycin and gentacoll. Dis Colon Rectum 1995; 38: 398–401.

33. Thompson H, Cartwright K. Streptococcal necrotising fasciitis in Gloucestershire. Br J Surg 1995; 82: 1444–5.

34. Law PJ, Talbot RW, Bartram CI. Anal endosonography in the evaluation of perianal sepsis and fistula in ano. Br J Surg 1989; 76: 752–5.

35. Cataldo PA, Senagore A, Luchtefeld MA. Intrarectal ultrasound in the evaluation of perirectal diseases. Dis Colon Rectum 1993; 36: 554–8.

36. Tio TL, Mulder CJJ, Wijers OB, Sars PRA, Tygal GNJ. Endosonography of the perianal and perirectal fistula and/or abscess in Crohn's disease. Gastrointest Endosc 1990; 36: 331–6.

37. Winslett MC, Allan A, Ambrose NS. Anorectal sepsis as a presentation of occult rectal and systemic disease: Editorial comment Abcarian H. Dis Colon Rectum 1988; 31: 597–600.

38. Stewart MPM, Laing MR, Krukowski ZH. Treatment of acute abscesses by incision, curettage and primary suture without antibiotics; a controlled clinical trial. Br J Surg 1985; 72: 66–7.

39. Lunnis PJ, Barker PG, Sultan AH *et al*. Magnetic resonance imaging of fistula in ano. Dis Colon Rectum 1994; 37: 708–18.

40. Schouten WR, Van Vroonhoven Th, Van Berlo CLJ. Primary partial internal sphincterectomy in the treatment of anorectal abscess. Neth J Surg 1987; 392: 43–5.

41. Schouten WR, Van Vroonhoven Th. Treatment of anorectal abscess with or without primary fistulectomy. Dis Colon Rectum 1991; 34: 60–3.

42. Lunnis PJ, Phillips RKS. Surgical assessment of acute anorectal sepsis is a better predictor of fistula than microbiological analysis. Br J Surg 1994; 81: 368–9.

9 Abdominal trauma

Iain D. Anderson

Introduction

Trauma presents a continuing challenge. Accidental injury is the leading cause of death in the young (age <35 years) and some half a million patients require hospital admission for the treatment of injury each year. With timely treatment most survive and can be returned to a full and productive life. It is well established that without organised trauma care, some 20–35% of injured patients who reach hospital alive will die unnecessarily.[1,2] With 12 000 deaths from injuries annually in the UK, the magnitude of the challenge is clear and over the last 10 years several modifications to trauma services have been made in order to improve services.

Pre-hospital care

Some 50% of all deaths occur at the scene, mostly from catastrophic injuries to the brain and great vessels. The creation of a paramedic service ensures that highly trained individuals reach injured patients swiftly. Vital interventions to secure the airway and staunch haemorrhage can be effected but field interventions are limited and given that the speed of adequate resuscitation and definitive treatment determine outcome, it is perhaps not surprising that a clear advantage over a 'scoop and run' rescue policy has not yet been identified. The means of transport does not itself determine outcome – there is no global benefit associated with helicopter rescue although its advantage in certain cases is self evident.

Trauma teams

The outcome from major injury is often determined by events during the Golden Hour – the first hour where the opportunity exists to control matters before the onset of multisystem complications. The reception of injured patients should therefore be by a multidisciplinary trauma team comprising appropriately trained senior surgeons, anaesthetists and emergency staff. The team should be alerted before the patient arrives and the equipment necessary for immediate management of life threatening injuries prepared for use. The establishment of a team therefore requires planning, communication and training.

ATLS

The impact of the adoption of the Advanced Trauma Life Support System (ATLS) around the world cannot be underestimated.[3] This system has provided staff from all disciplines with a common consensus and plan for immediate management, thereby improving immediate outcome.[4] Priorities are clearly defined and the likelihood of significant management errors or omissions reduced. Interspecialty conflict is diminished and resuscitation and definitive treatment are achieved more rapidly.[5] Not only will deaths during the Golden Hour (usually from missed injuries or haemorrhage) be reduced but likewise, later deaths will be prevented. These occur usually on the Intensive Care Unit from multi-organ failure and are contributed to by slow initial resuscitation.[6]

Trauma centres

The system whereby seriously injured patients are directed to major hospitals with full 24-hour facilities for their care (trauma centres) has been used extensively in America with remarkable improvements in standards of care,[7] and avoidable deaths can be almost completely prevented. Limited British experience suggests that within the NHS at present, the trauma centre approach makes less of an impact.[8]

Notwithstanding this, the importance of getting the injured patient to a team of surgeons who are familiar with and who can care adequately for their injuries is a basic requirement. The value of these modern approaches has been well illustrated by experience from Edinburgh, where with centralisation of trauma services, immediate senior input and early involvement of specialists, the former peak of deaths during the Golden Hour has been largely abolished.[4] The challenge remains for later stages of care to be similarly improved and most importantly of all, for efficient means of injury prevention to be seen as a medical priority.

Immediate management

Immediate management of the injured patient is conducted in a systematic order which identifies and treats life-threatening injuries according to priority. Once immediately threatening injuries have been dealt with, further investigation and treatment can take place, but the importance of speedy and complete treatment must be emphasised as this determines outcome. Following a system of assessment such as ATLS permits a resuscitation team to achieve these aims most consistently. The degree of intervention necessary will vary enormously from patient to patient – some may require surgery in order to achieve even the first phase of stabilisation. In such cases the fatality of delay is clear, but even in less severe cases slow treatment predisposes the patient to later organ failure.

Table 9.1 *Securing an airway*

Chin lift/jaw thrust
Pharyngeal airway (oral/nasal)
Cuffed tracheal tube (oral/nasal)
Surgical airway: cricothyroidotomy (needle/surgical)

The first priority is to maintain and secure an open airway and the measures used to achieve this are shown in Table 9.1.

Through the patent airway, oxygen is delivered at high flow using a reservoir mask (12–15 l min^{-1}). The risk of causing harm to a severe chronic bronchitic with an hypoxic drive to ventilation by high flow oxygen therapy is exceedingly rare and should essentially be discounted at this stage except in the most obvious of cases. Injuries which result in airway compromise also predispose the patient to cervical spine injury and, given the catastrophic consequences of damage to the spinal cord, it is essential that the cervical spine is protected in every injured patient until the spine can be shown to be intact by adequate radiographs interpreted by a competent doctor. The cervical spine can be protected either by manual immobilisation, the use of a semi-rigid collar, or forehead tape and sandbags placed on either side of the head. Increasing numbers of injured patients are being managed on radiolucent full length spine boards which incorporate 'sand bags and tape' in their structure.

Surgeons should familiarise themselves with techniques of cricothyroidotomy. Temporary needle cricothyroidotomy, using a 14 gauge cannula, can maintain ventilation for modest periods (30 min), but limiting retention of carbon dioxide occurs. This limitation does not apply to surgical cricothyroidotomy, which is made through a transverse incision directly over the cricothyroid membrane. The airway is entered, the wound spread with a dilator, and a tracheostomy tube (size 6 in adults) inserted. These techniques can be learned and practised on appropriate courses (e.g. Advanced Trauma Life Support Courses).

Provision and maintenance of adequate ventilation is the next priority. This is assessed clinically and common life-threatening conditions treated directly. The commonest immediate problem is tension pneumothorax: this requires instant needle decompression through the second interspace and then formal chest drainage. Chest drainage is best performed through the third or fourth intercostal space in the anterior axillary line by a cut-down technique. This ensures entry to the chest and obviates the need for use of the trocar, thereby removing the patient from the risk of an iatrogenic impalement injury. Massive haemothorax, identified by the presence of a hemi-thorax which is dull to percussion, hypotension and reduced breath sounds, also requires chest drainage. It is advisable to obtain venous access before inserting the chest drain. If more than 1500 ml of blood emerges, or if haemorrhage continues apace (greater than 200 ml h^{-1}), then a thoracotomy will very likely be required. A sucking chest wound should be covered with an occlusive dressing taped down on three sides to act as a flap valve. A chest drain should be inserted at a remote site. Cardiac tamponade can be difficult to detect. The identification of Beck's Triad of elevated jugular venous pressure, muffled heart sounds, and pulsus paradoxus, is notoriously difficult in a busy Emergency Department but the presence of hypotension and an appropriate injury (penetrating injury, with entry wounds between the nipples or the scapulae) should raise suspicions. Treatment is by pericardiocentesis, followed by thoracotomy in all cases. Pericardiocentesis is performed by advancing a long cannula beside the xiphoid upwards and backwards each at 45° until blood is aspirated. The development of an injury pattern on the ECG indicates that penetration has been too deep. Aspiration of 20–30 ml of blood from the pericardial cavity is usually enough to bring about improvement. The cannula should be left in place while the patient is transferred to theatre for a thoracotomy. In dubious cases, an echocardiogram can help make this diagnosis. Flail chest can cause immediate and life-threatening compromise of ventilation. Immediate treatment is by the institution of positive pressure ventilation. The clinician should be alert to the possibility of a tension pneumothorax developing at any stage during the treatment of a patient who has sustained chest injury when positive pressure ventilation is introduced, either in the operating theatre or in the intensive care unit, or when the external air pressure falls, for example during air transfer. Immediate treatment by chest drainage is again required.

The third priority in the immediate management of the injured patient is to re-establish and maintain an adequate circulation. Injured patients lose clear fluid as oedema into injured tissues, but their principal loss is of blood. The priorities therefore, are first to stop any ongoing haemorrhage and, secondly, to replace the lost blood. The folly of continuing to pour large volumes of crystalloid and colloid into patients who are continuing to haemorrhage is obvious, but still occasionally happens. Adequacy of circulation is assessed clinically to begin with, but it should be remembered that, particularly in younger patients, blood pressure is maintained until the final phase of shock when a catastrophic and sometimes irretrievable fall suddenly occurs. Peripheral perfusion and the injury sustained give a better early indication of the likely replacement volume required. External haemorrhage should be controlled by pressure. Internal haemorrhage (usually into the thorax, abdomen or pelvis) should be diagnosed and treated, as necessary, by immediate surgery. Wherever possible, surgery should be carried out in the operating theatre as the results of operating in the emergency room are very poor indeed. Patients who have sustained penetrating injury to the chest who suffer a cardiac arrest, either immediately before arrival at hospital, or when in the emergency department, should undergo immediate thoracotomy. Performing this for other injuries is not consistently associated with survival. Very occasionally, laparotomy can be performed in the emergency room to pack and control haemorrhage, but again this is all too often a futile exercise. Perhaps more logically, the descending aorta can be cross-clamped through the left chest before transferring the patient to theatre. These dramatic interventions are seldom successful and it is much more profitable to identify the unstable patient who has not yet reached this terminal state and to ensure they are transferred promptly to theatre rather than undergoing ineffectual resuscitation elsewhere.

Fuel has recently been added to the controversy of the administration of intravenous fluids and the timing of surgical intervention by the publication of data showing that survival is worse among patients sustaining penetrating injury to the torso who receive intravenous fluids before reaching the operating theatre.[9] The probable reason for this is that expansion of the intravascular space and elevation of the blood pressure simply provokes further haemorrhage. More transfusion is then necessary, resulting in further hypothermia, coagulopathy and reduced survival. The importance of surgical control of haemorrhage is again clear.

More patients, however, present with blunt injuries and for these patients there is no doubt that the protocol of obtaining large bore (16 g or greater) vascular access at two peripheral sites with the rapid infusion of 1–2 litres of warm crystalloid fluid as an initial measure remains appropriate. The need for early surgery remains and this should particularly be the case in any patient who is hypotensive, or who shows signs of continuing shock or obvious haemorrhage. Blood should be drawn for cross-matching when the first cannula is inserted and in general terms blood should be administered when infusion requirements exceed 1.5–2 litres. Central venous line insertion should usually be reserved for a later stage for monitoring rather than as a prime infusion site: performing a cut down at the ankle is usually safer and faster than attempts to insert a central line in a hypotensive patient. Continuing observation is required to assess the patient's response to fluid resuscitation. If hypotension recurs, then further searches for the source of haemorrhage must be undertaken rapidly as surgery will often be necessary.

Rapid assessment of the neurological state of the patient and removal of clothing completes the immediate management of the injured patient. If the patient has not improved by this stage, they should be moved directly for therapy (usually surgery) to achieve this. More commonly, some improvement will be seen and time can now be taken to establish basic monitoring and obtain initial radiographs of the cervical spine, chest and pelvis. Unless specifically contraindicated by clinical suspicion of an anterior cranial fossa fracture or urethral trauma respectively, nasogastric tubes and urinary catheters should now be inserted. Thereafter, the patient is examined in detail and all injuries recorded. If the patient deteriorates at any time, then a further rapid survey of the airway, breathing and the circulation is undertaken and appropriate therapy immediately instituted. A history of the patient's comorbid state should be obtained and equally importantly, the history of the accident should be obtained from ambulance staff or witnesses, as this may often bring to light injuries that would otherwise be missed.

An injury pattern and plan of action should now be emerging. If stable, the patient is often now transferred to the Radiology Department for investigations. It is important that senior multidisciplinary involvement continues at this stage, such that appropriate management decisions can still be made rapidly. This early hospital phase of care beyond the 'golden hour' now represents a greater organisational and management challenge than the initial resuscitation.

Abdominal trauma

It will be evident from the above that injuries to the abdomen cannot be managed in isolation and that the general surgeon has an important role to play in the immediate resuscitation and decision-making process of injured patients. The abdomen itself harbours an enormous capacity for serious injury through the mechanisms of early haemorrhage or late sepsis. Diagnosis may be self-evident, but is often difficult as clinical signs are inaccurate.[10] Although a liberal policy of a laparotomy will confirm or refute the presence of abdominal injury, it should be remembered that unnecessary operations expose the patient to hypothermia, some degree of risk, and perhaps most importantly divert attention away from other injuries which should have received a higher priority. The early involvement of a senior surgeon is therefore necessary for all patients suspected of having abdominal trauma. Laparotomy is immediately indicated in certain patients and here, unnecessary investigation will simply result in hazardous delay, Table 9.2.

In most cases, the criteria shown in Table 9.2 are not present and re-assessment and investigation are necessary. Clinical re-assessment is an essential weapon in the armoury as this permits not only re-evaluation of the abdominal signs, but also of the patient's response to intravenous fluids. Time remains of the essence as all too often abdominal injuries are only diagnosed after some delay.[1] When examining the patient clinically, it should be remembered that the abdomen

Table 9.2 *Unequivocal indications for laparotomy*

Hypotension in the presence of obvious abdominal trauma
Gunshot wound of the abdomen
Obvious peritonitis
Gastrointestinal haemorrhage following abdominal injury
Evisceration through a wound (excluding omentum)

Table 9.3 *Techniques for investigating the injured abdomen*

Diagnostic peritoneal lavage
Computer tomography
Ultrasound scanning
Laparoscopy
Laparotomy

extends from the fourth intercostal space to the perineum, that missiles can follow almost any path through the body and that the abdomen is divided into compartments. The three principal compartments, the retroperitoneum, the pelvis and the peritoneum exhibit differing clinical signs and patterns of injury. Signs of peritoneal irritation carry a false positive rate of 40–60% following injury and a false negative rate of 30–50%.[11] Importantly, false negative examination is associated with a significant mortality.[12] Examination findings can be misleading for a number of reasons: abdominal and thoracic wall injury contribute to tenderness; free blood within the peritoneum may cause very little irritation; and the effects of alcohol, drugs or cerebral injury may mask clinical signs. Signs of abdominal wall injury (e.g. bruising, seat belt or tyre marks) are known as London's sign and are important pointers to the severity of injury and the risk of visceral damage. Consequently, when doubt exists, further investigation is essential. The five principal means of investigating the abdomen further are shown in Table 9.3. Each has its advantages and disadvantages and these will be considered in turn.

Diagnostic peritoneal lavage (DPL)

DPL has been in use for over thirty years.[13] Overall, DPL remains the best single test for diagnosing the presence of abdominal injuries. It is 97% accurate[14,15] and it can be performed rapidly and safely provided an appropriate technique is used. The accepted current technique is the mini-laparotomy method (Table 9.4). If objective criteria for assessing peritoneal lavage fluid are not followed, then the sensitivity of the test is diminished. The site of insertion may need to be modified on account of previous abdominal incisions or pregnancy, but the only absolute contraindication to performance of DPL is the established need for a laparotomy. In the presence of a pelvic fracture, lavage may be falsely positive on account of the haematoma and here it is advisable to perform a cut down above the level of the umbilicus and to look simply for the presence of free blood within the abdomen. The presence of a positive peritoneal lavage necessitates laparotomy.

Peritoneal lavage gives no indication of the source or volume of haemorrhage, nor whether that haemorrhage is continuing. A positive result will therefore result in a non-therapeutic laparotomy in up to 25% of cases. When conservative treatment of selected solid visceral

Table 9.4 *Technique of diagnostic peritoneal lavage (mini-laparotomy)*

Empty stomach and bladder
Clean and anaesthetise skin below umbilicus
5 cm vertical midline incision, just below umbilicus
Retract skin, dissect through linea alba
Pick up peritoneum and enter
Egress of free blood indicates need for laparotomy
Insert peritoneal dialysis catheter towards pelvis
Infuse 1 litre of warmed crystalloid fluid and roll patient gently from side to side
Syphon fluid from abdomen by placing bag on floor

Positive criteria
Egress of free blood on opening peritoneum
Presence of enteric content in abdomen
Greater than 100 000 red blood cells per mm^3
Greater than 500 white blood cells per mm^3

injuries is employed, this oversensitivity of DPL is made effectively greater. Finally, DPL fails to investigate the retroperitoneal organs.

Computer tomography (CT)

CT scanning can diagnose the presence of blood within the abdomen and also the presence of specific visceral injury, both within the peritoneum and among the retroperitoneal structures. In centres of excellence, high degrees of specificity and sensitivity have been recorded but this has not been the uniform experience. A significant proportion of serious injuries, particularly to the bowel, can still be missed. The principal limitation of CT scanning is the need to transfer the patient to the scanner and in many hospitals this is in a remote, and therefore dangerous, location. CT scanning is therefore contra-indicated in unstable patients and furthermore, a single CT scan is also unable to give an indication of the continuing rate of haemorrhage.

Ultrasound scanning

This is a popular approach and has the advantage of being safe, cheap and rapid. Scans can be performed in the resuscitation area, but the principal drawbacks are interobserver variability, incomplete imaging of visceral damage and consequently a small but highly significant rate of missed injury (10%), even when the end point is taken simply as the presence of free fluid within the abdomen.[16] Although expert centres have reported excellent results,[17] there is no doubt that it remains safest when it shows a positive finding in a stable patient.

When ultrasound scans are repeated, accuracy improves but circumstances may be too pressing for this to be carried out.

Laparoscopy

Inspection of the peritoneal cavity can be performed under general anaesthesia in theatre, or under sedation using a 5 mm cannula with an appropriate light source. The advantages of the technique are that continuing haemorrhage, for example from liver wounds can be seen, the presence of peritoneal penetration by a stab wound can be confirmed or refuted and, on occasion, diaphragmatic injuries have even been repaired. The persisting shortfall of the technique is the difficulty of examining the entire length of small bowel and also of examining adequately the retroperitoneal structures. The use of mini-laparoscopy has increased, slowly but steadily, since the initial report[18] but concerns remain about the limitations, except in the circumstances indicated above. Recent experience has however shown that laparoscopy has some role to play in stable patients with suspected abdominal injury, but it is fair to say that debate continues about whether it can be used safely to replace established diagnostic modalities.[19]

Laparotomy

On certain occasions and circumstances laparotomy will remain the most appropriate way of excluding the presence or absence of injury and dealing with it in a timely fashion[20] but a more selective yet safe approach should be practicable in well equipped centres which handle a significant volume of trauma.

The optimum diagnostic tool will clearly vary from patient to patient and each has its strengths and weaknesses. These investigations complement and do not replace careful and, if necessary, repeated clinical evaluation. DPL remains useful because of the ease and rapidity with which it can be performed in adverse circumstances. It is probably most used now in unstable victims of multiple injury to confirm the presence of haemoperitoneum and therefore the need for laparotomy as a high priority treatment. CT scanning is useful in stable patients in defining the anatomical pattern of injury. Follow-up scans can be conducted on the ward using ultrasound and this particularly applies when conservative management of stable patients with solid visceral injury is being employed (see below). In expert hands, ultrasound scanning can also achieve excellent results, but concern remains about its use as a prime modality to direct management in the multiply injured patient: it should certainly not be permitted to over-ride clinical suspicion and early recourse to other investigations as necessary. Where appropriate facilities and expertise exist, laparoscopy may emerge as a useful tool, but again for the moment, only in the stable patient.

Penetrating and blast injuries: special considerations

Penetrating abdominal injuries are less common in UK practice than in many countries but still account for some 20% of injuries. They present their own challenges in diagnosis and management. Management is often simpler than blunt injury – most are caused by knives which usually result in simple holes in a straight line which are very amenable to surgical repair, when required. Management will be discussed in the sections on specific visceral injury below, but it is worth stating that impaled weapons and other objects should not be removed until the patient is in the operating theatre. Abdominal gunshot wounds (and other missile injuries) cause visceral damage in more than 90% of cases and laparotomy is always necessary. The more common stabbing injury may not breach the abdominal wall and even if it does, will only cause significant damage in 50% of cases.[21] Overall, perhaps some 30% of stabbed patients (compared with 20% of patients with blunt injury) need laparotomy. Stabbed patients with hypotension, peritonism, gastrointestinal bleeding or evisceration (but not omental evisceration alone) require operation. In the absence of these signs, the first priority is to determine whether the peritoneum has been breached. This can be accomplished by local wound exploration (not probing) or alternatively by laparoscopy through a remote site. If the peritoneum has not been breached then no further action, apart from wound care, is needed. When the peritoneum has been breached and where it is not clear whether or not laparotomy is needed, DPL is, again, useful, being accurate in 91% of cases.[22] The alternative approach has been serial physical examination and this too, is highly effective at reducing the need for non-therapeutic operation without exposing the patient to an unduly high risk of missed injury (< 3%). Clearly, stab wounds to the flank or back may injure retroperitoneal structures without causing peritoneal signs or abnormalities on DPL. Here, the investigative choice lies between serial examination and contrast CT enema, the latter to look in particular for occult injury to retroperitoneal structures including ascending and descending colon.

The assessment and management of specific penetrating injuries will be discussed regionally but a few general comments about the mechanism and management of blast and gunshot injuries are appropriate. A missile, of whatever type, will cause tissue damage along the track it makes through the tissues. In a low energy transfer wound, damage is restricted to the track whereas in a high energy transfer wound, there is damage outside the track caused by the transfer of excess kinetic energy from the missile. With high velocity bullets in particular, the process of cavitation occurs. This denotes the formation of a destructive temporary cavity within the tissues into which dirt and debris may be sucked. If bone is struck, secondary fragments may cause even more extensive damage. This separation of wound types cannot be absolute and similarly, a certain weapon may not necessarily cause the same type of wound in all cases, depending on the bullet type, its flight and the angle and tissue of impact. Rifles and machine guns have a high initial velocity whereas hand guns and most bomb fragments cause low energy transfer wounds. It is worth emphasising that missiles may follow remarkably tortuous courses as they ricochet around the body and unusual combinations of injuries and entry points, many of which are survivable, have been reported. During explosions, injuries may be caused by blast waves, burns from hot gases, from missiles propelled by the blast or by casualties being thrown through the air. Thus, a spectrum of injuries may be present.

Surgical management follows the basic principles whereby dead tissue is excised, foreign materials removed and wounds left open until healing free from sepsis is likely. Delayed primary closure is often appropriate at or around the fifth day following injury. It can be difficult to determine the extent of tissue damage caused by any missile and experienced military surgeons stress that one should treat the wound and not the weapon. It is relatively straightforward to re-examine or re-explore wounds in civilian practice, if necessary with repeated debridements as non-viable tissue declares itself. During conflict, delay, gross contamination and multiple casualties are likely and undue reliance on antibiotics without adequate early excision will lead to a high mortality from wound sepsis. The retrieval of missile fragments must be kept in perspective: some will be located in dangerous territory where they are best left alone.[23]

Specific abdominal injuries: assessment and investigation

Even with experience, clinical examination of the potentially injured abdomen is difficult and apart from the investigations discussed above, repeated clinical assessment both of the abdomen and of the patient as a whole is the principal mechanism whereby injuries are detected and disaster avoided. The history of the injury may provide useful clues. Left-sided rib fractures may suggest injury to the spleen or left kidney, right-sided lower rib fractures injury to the liver. Upper lumber spinal fractures are associated with trauma to the pancreas and duodenum, whereas a deceleration injury with a seat belt sign indicates the patient exposed to the risk of duodenal rupture, mesenteric haematoma, laceration of the bowel at points of fixity (i.e. duodeno-jejunal flexure or terminal ileum) in addition to liver trauma. Pelvic injuries are associated with bladder and urethral or rectal damage, in addition to significant vascular injury. Furthermore patients with, for example, major injuries to the right leg, right arm, right side of chest and head will very likely have injured right sided abdominal viscera, but it is surprising how often this can be overlooked.

In some cases of abdominal injury the need for operation, usually to control haemorrhage, is obvious, but in many more cases more detailed clinical assessment may be necessary to identify the need for operation. During periodic re-assessment it may become clear that an established indication for laparotomy has arisen or that further specific tests such as peritoneal lavage, are now needed. Alternatively, during systematic examination certain signs may warrant further investigation. The presence of blood in the nasogastric aspirate suggests upper gastrointestinal injury and indicates the need for an urgent contrast swallow to be performed. An elevated serum amylase suggests pancreatic or pancreaticoduodenal trauma and unless other indications for operation may exist (as is often the case) contrast CT scanning should be carried out in an appropriately stable patient. Stab wounds to the back and flank may cause obvious intraperitoneal injury but may also cause occult damage to vascular structures or to the retroperitoneal portions of the gut. Rectal examination may show the presence of colonic haemorrhage in these cases but further information may be obtained, again in stable patients, by CT scanning with rectally and orally administered contrast.[24] Rectal examination may also indicate injury to the spinal cord (flaccid sphincters) or penetration of the rectal wall by pelvic bony fragments in addition to evidence of direct injury to the prostate, urethra or anal sphincter complex. Rectal examination should be performed before urethral catheterisation in order to look for potential urethral trauma, as on occasions catheterisation may convert a partial urethral tear into a complete one, which is considerably more difficult to treat. Other signs of urethral injury include blood at the external meatus and perineal bruising. Possible urethral injuries should be investigated by urethrography. The presence or absence of bowel sounds adds little to the assessment of the injured patient and abdominal girth is mentioned only to be discarded. Large volumes of blood can be lost into the abdomen with little change in its girth: a constant girth offers no reassurance whatsoever and many other reasons for abdominal distension following injury exist.[25]

Laparotomy for abdominal trauma

In undertaking an operation for abdominal injury the surgeon should be mentally prepared for the unexpected but it is well worth bearing in mind that almost all haemorrhage can be controlled with either modest digital pressure or the judicious placement of packs. The patient is usually placed supine and the skin prepared from nipples to groins. A long midline incision provides rapid access and adequate exposure of all viscera. Blood should be aspirated and packs placed carefully in each quadrant of the abdomen before a systematic search is made for sources of haemorrhage and sites of injury by sequentially removing one pack after another. If exsanguinating haemorrhage continues and control has not been previously obtained through the left hemithorax by clamping the descending aorta, control can now be obtained by compressing the aorta at the diaphragmatic hiatus by manual pressure or with a long bladed retractor protected with a large swab. Aortic inflow control can also be obtained with a vascular clamp or by passing a large Foley catheter retrogradely through a distal aortotomy. As the exploration and treatment of identified injuries usually provokes further haemorrhage it is worth checking with the anaesthetist at this stage to see whether or not they wish a short period of time during which to catch up with blood loss.

Attention is then turned to specific injuries as detailed below. When no injuries are found or once identified injuries have been dealt with, it is essential that a full examination of all other viscera is carried out. This always includes opening the lesser sac and adequate exposure of the other areas of retroperitoneum by mobilisation of the fourth part of duodenum to expose the aorta, the right hemicolon and duodenum to expose the vena cava and posterior surface of the pancreas, and occasionally by mobilisation of the left hemicolon to gain access to the left renal pedicle. In general terms, expanding haematomas should be explored once vascular control has been obtained. Haematomas associated with pelvic fractures are best left undisturbed unless there is continuing expansion despite the application of pressure packs and after fixation of unstable bony fragments. In contrast, upper abdominal central retroperitoneal haematomas should almost always be explored (these are associated with damage to larger vessels) and repair effected although this may be challenging and require specialist help.

It has long been recognised that speedy surgery carries benefits to the patients. Long operations, often with major blood loss, result in hypothermia, acidosis and coagulopathy and a point of organ failure and diminishing surgical return can soon be reached. In the last few years, the concept of 'damage control surgery' has emerged.[26] Here the least possible is done surgically at a first operation in a patient with multiple injuries. Haemorrhage will be controlled by packing or perhaps temporary vascular shunting, and injured areas of bowel may simply be stapled closed rather than formally resected. The skin is closed with staples or towel clips and the patient returned to the intensive care unit for correction of hypothermia, acidosis and coagulopathy. Staged definitive surgery can then be performed within 36 h. Experience with this technique is now considerable and was applied in one series to 9% of patients undergoing laparotomy for trauma.[27] In this study 54% of patents survived to undergo reconstructive surgery but further emergency operation will be necessary in any normothermic patient with unabated bleeding (greater than 2 units packed cells per hour). This degree of further haemorrhage might be expected in some 10–20% patients following packing as may an abdominal compartment syndrome where a progressive rise in intra-abdominal pressure results in difficulty in ventilation, CO_2 retention and oliguria. An alternative therapeutic strategy is the non-operative management of blunt injuries to solid viscera, particularly the liver and spleen, and this will be considered more in detail below.

Liver injuries

Liver injuries are common and range from the essentially trivial to the inevitably fatal. Many patients sustain minor lacerations to the peripheral hepatic parenchyma which cause a small amount of haemoperitoneum and which stop bleeding spontaneously (grade I injury). These injuries require no treatment and account for many of the 'false positive' peritoneal lavages. Superficial lacerations which continue to bleed (grade II injury) can be simply closed with lightly opposing sutures. In deeper lacerations (grade III) with continuing haemorrhage, the source vessels and associated biliary radicles should be identified and ligated or clipped. This may require extension of the laceration by standard techniques of liver surgery such as finger fracture or its contemporary equivalents. Appropriate hepatic mobilisation should be performed. Executing the 'Pringle manoeuvre' can reduce blood loss while assessment or surgery is undertaken. This involves clamping the hepatic artery and portal vein (together with the bile duct) with a soft clamp at the free edge of the lesser omentum. The manoeuvre causes hepatic ischaemia and should not be extended beyond 30 minutes or so. Very occasionally the degree of liver damage (lobar destruction, grade IV) will be such that it is simpler to resect a portion but in general, formal liver resection following injury simply increases blood loss and morbidity. Liver surgery should be kept to the necessary minimum. The omentum can usefully be deployed to pack a wound in the liver or to cover raw surfaces following liver surgery for trauma. The use of drains has been debated for some years – the risk of introducing infection must be weighed against the benefit of draining further accumulation of bile or blood.

Bleeding liver lacerations which are particularly complex or burst types (type IV), are best treated by perihepatic packing. Large abdominal packs are placed over non-adherent sheets in order to tamponade the lacerations. Packs can then be removed a day or two later following a period of stabilisation, correction of coagulopathy and hypothermia and transfer to a specialist centre. By this stage, haemorrhage will often have stopped. Patients referred to a hepatobiliary unit, often following placement of perihepatic packs, can be investigated by angiography. This will permit bleeding vessels to be embolised if necessary before further surgery is carried out to remove the packing, or can occasionally be used in a stable patient as the sole intervention. Packing is increasingly seen as appropriate initial treatment for lesser injuries in non-specialised units.

Two further patterns of injury merit specific comment. A large central intrahepatic haematoma should not be explored immediately but should be referred for specialist investigation and treatment as indicated above as late rupture may occur. The most severe form of liver injury involves simultaneous damage to the hepatic veins or vena cava (grade V). Pringle's manoeuvre will clearly not control haemorrhage and usually every manoeuvre to inspect the site of injury results in the loss of several units of blood. The patient's ability to withstand this is limited and if haemostasis can be obtained by packing then this should be employed. If haemostasis cannot be obtained then one technique is to insert a caval atrial bypass before attempting repair. The vena cava is isolated below the liver and a large shunt passed up through the retro-hepatic cava into the right atrium. This is secured within the fibrous pericardium and ideally, just above the level of the renal vein. Even with these dramatic interventions, survival is uncommon, being recorded in perhaps 10% of cases.[28,29]

Many stable patients will have liver injury identified on CT scanning and it is now well established that these patients are best managed conservatively in a specialist centre. It should be emphasised that conservative management of all solid abdominal visceral injury is an active and not a passive process. The surgical team should be immediately prepared to undertake surgery for potentially exsanguinating haemorrhage and if adequate surgical and support facilities are not available for this then the patient should be transferred. In a large recent North American series[30] 11% of patients went on to require laparotomy, half of these for previously non-identified non-hepatic injuries. Modest daily transfusion (up to 2 units) is acceptable but if this continues or is exceeded then recourse to operation is necessary. The study by Croce et al.[30] showed that patients with major injuries (grades III–V) could also be treated successfully by the non-operative approach with a reduced requirement for blood transfusion and fewer abdominal complications compared with patients requiring operation for conventional indications. Importantly, these authors showed that admission characteristics and CT findings could not predict patients who would fail non-operative treatment and therefore intensive care unit monitoring is considered mandatory. Overall some 34–51% of adult blunt hepatic injuries can be treated non-operatively.[31] Perhaps not surprisingly, grade V injuries seem to behave differently with fewer than one in ten being stable enough to undergo conservative treatment.[32]

Patients sustaining gunshot injuries of the liver will obviously undergo laparotomy in all circumstances and various specific liver injuries can be managed along similar lines to blunt trauma. In a large series from South Africa, perihepatic packing was again useful for the more severe injuries whereas all less severe injuries (grades I–II) and most moderate injuries (grade III) were managed with simple operative techniques without mortality.[33]

Splenic injury

Emergency splenectomy can be performed relatively simply and expeditiously by mobilising the spleen upwards out of its bed by the division of the lienorenal ligament. Care is taken to avoid damage to the tail of the pancreas and to the greater curvature of the stomach where it often encroaches close to the upper pole of the spleen. Such a procedure has saved many lives but it is now accepted that splenectomy is not necessary for all injuries and that splenectomy may very occasionally be associated with overwhelming post-splenectomy sepsis (OPSS). A variety of lesser operations on the spleen have now been described including partial resection, ligation of specific feeding vessels, packing and enveloping the spleen in an absorbable mesh bag.[21] In reported series, on average some 50% of injured spleens can be repaired instead of removed but this depends on the severity of injury. If haemostasis is obtained, further haemorrhage from the spleen is highly unlikely (<2%). With major ruptures of the splenic substance, however, splenectomy probably remains the best option as this will be necessary in any event in more than 85% of patients.

The advantage of conserving all or some of the splenic substance is that it removes the risk of postoperative overwhelming post-splenectomy sepsis, a condition where the patient becomes liable to rapidly fulminating infection particularly with encapsulated organisms. This risk is most marked in children but is also considered to be significant in adults.[34] Individuals who have undergone splenectomy should be protected by the administration of oral penicillin on a daily basis for life and should be immunised against the likely causative organisms, particularly *Pneumococcus* and *Haemophilus*.

An alternative in stable patients is to treat the patient non-operatively in a manner similar to the non-operative management of hepatic injury. This has been pursued successively in adults and in children but careful patient selection is required. Patients with haemodynamic instability, signs of peritonism at any time and those who require more than two units of blood may be better treated by operation. Published series have generally employed less selective criteria and consequently the incidence of operation ranges from 20 to 80%. Once again observation must be maintained on the intensive care unit with continual readiness for emergency operation. In addition to the risk of missed injuries to other viscera, particularly the gastrointestinal tract, there is concern about the incidence of delayed splenic rupture in these patients. The precise frequency of this is unknown but occasional catastrophes have occurred. It seems prudent to advise patients to continue a period of rest at home and certainly to avoid contact sports for at least two months.

Gastric, duodenal and pancreatic injuries

Gastric injury usually occurs as a result of penetrating trauma, although blunt trauma in the presence of a distended stomach can result in a 'blow-out injury'. The principal danger is to miss a wound on the posterior surface of the stomach because of failure to open the lesser sac. Occasionally wounds at the margin of either curvature can be overlooked as they are hidden in the omentum. Careful search at operation can be complemented by the installation of methylene blue down the nasogastric tube to show occult leakage. The stomach should be repaired in two layers and decompressed nasogastrically after operation.

The duodenum and pancreas are often injured together. They tend to be injured by seat belts compressing these fixed viscera against the lumbar vertebrae simultaneously with spinal flexion during sudden deceleration. The duodenum may rupture, usually on the lateral convexity of its second part, and in children a sizeable haematoma may occlude the lumen without rupture occurring. Duodenal rupture should be particularly suspected when there is blood seen on insertion of a gastric tube. Further pointers include the loss of psoas shadow on a plain abdominal radiograph or the presence of retroperitoneal air. Further investigation and treatment is needed. Simple haematomas can generally be treated conservatively but perforations must obviously be repaired. As ever, devitalised tissue will have to be excised but usually simple, interrupted closure is possible. It is advisable to lead large drains down to the area of the repair and to decompress the stomach postoperatively in order to minimise the impact of the principal complication of fistulation. Suppression of gastric acid output is advisable. More complex injuries, usually associated with pancreatic trauma, are discussed below.

Injuries to the pancreas are usually associated with multiple injuries to other viscera. The diagnosis is usually suspected by an elevation of the serum amylase level and this should be measured in every patient suspected of having sustained abdominal injury. Hyper-amylasaemia is not specific, however, and further investigation will be necessary unless laparotomy is otherwise indicated. Imaging of the injured pancreas is fraught with pitfalls and CT scanning of the injured pancreas can significantly underestimate the severity of injury even when carried out 2–3 days after the injury has been sustained. The crucial management decisions at operation hinge around whether or not the main pancreatic duct is intact and while endoscopic retrograde pancreatography would provide this information this is seldom feasible in these patients. A recent review indicated that the outcome from isolated pancreatic injury is improving but, of course, most injuries to the pancreas are associated with multivisceral damage.[35] In the absence of ductal injury simple suture haemostasis, omental plugging and pancreatic drainage should suffice. The same holds true of any pancreatic injury in an unstable coagulopathic or hypothermic patient where it may be better to limit the initial procedure and return for a definitive procedure some 36 hours later. If the tail of the pancreas is injured, external drainage alone may be adequate. The alternative is to resect the tail of the pancreas with or without the spleen and this is a particularly attractive option in patients who have transected their pancreas across the vertebral column and in whom a sizeable part of the left portion of the pancreas is separated from its physiological route of ductal drainage. Severe injuries to the head of the pancreas can be managed by simple drainage in the acute phase. Definitive treatment depends on the presence or absence of ductal damage and one option involves suturing the opened end of a Roux loop of small intestine to the area of injury. Occasionally resection of the pancreatic head will be necessary but this is a formidable undertaking in an injured patient. Complex repairs should be supported by diversion of the food stream away from the area. This can be achieved by the triple tube technique where the stomach is drained by a gastrostomy, a proximal jejunostomy drains the duodenum and a more distal jejunostomy is used for feeding. This is particularly applicable to duodenal injuries. Alternatively, the pylorus can be temporarily closed with an internal suture of absorbable material and a formal gastro-jejunostomy created.

Patients sustaining upper gastrointestinal injuries, including those who undergo laparotomy for liver or splenic injury are suitable candidates for enteral nutrition. This has been shown to significantly reduce the incidence of septic complications following laparotomy for abdominal trauma when compared with parenteral nutrition. The feeds are well tolerated from an early phase (1–3 days after operation) and this affords the patient the greatest advantage.[36]

Injury to the small intestine

Injuries to the small intestine are simply managed by repair or by resection as necessary. Pitfalls include small perforations hidden along the mesenteric border and areas of devascularisation caused by parallel laceration to the mesentery. Mesenteric haematomas should not be explored unless they are expanding.

Colonic injuries

Different management strategies have been advocated for blunt and penetrating colonic injuries although these strategies are in fact based around traditional principles of excision of dead tissue and avoidance of repair when there has been delay in undertaking operation or adverse systemic factors such as hypotension or coagulopathy. Minor colonic contusions in the absence of tissue compromise can be left alone or protected by a proximal diverting loop stoma as the severity of the case dictates. More significant areas of colonic contusion should be resected. In stable patients undergoing prompt operation and in the absence of significant contamination few would argue with the creation of an immediate ileocolic anastomosis. The creation of a stoma would generally be a more advisable procedure than the creation of a primary colocolic anastomosis for blunt injury. Double-barrelled stomas are easier to close than separated end stomata.

Debate continues about the optimal means of treating penetrating colonic injury. In the past the traditional treatment of exteriorising repaired colon within a stoma bag as a type of unopened loop stoma has been superseded by polarisation towards primary repair or the creation of formal opened stomas. With mounting experience in specialised centres, there is a growing movement towards primary repair, particularly in patients without the adverse features outlined above for blunt colonic injuries. A small randomised study has recently reported that primary repair or resection with anastomosis is the choice method of treatment of all penetrating colonic injuries[37] whereas others consider that there is not yet sufficient evidence to support this approach.[38] Certainly, it is appropriate to close any colostomy 2–3 weeks after injury providing that the distal bowel has healed on contrast study and postoperative instability and sepsis have been dealt with.[39]

Rectal injuries

Injuries to the extraperitoneal portion of the rectum present their own problems of difficulty of diagnosis and spreading infection. Commonly these injuries are caused by the insertion of foreign bodies, knife or gunshot wounds but pelvic fracture may also be responsible. Where doubt exists as to their presence, a water-soluble contrast study may help. Traditional treatment has been to defunction the rectum by means of a sigmoid colostomy, lavage the rectum clean and achieve adequate presacral drainage. When accessible the rectal wound should be repaired. Treatment with appropriate antibiotics will obviously be necessary. Similar considerations apply when the anal sphincters are injured. Initial management should include colostomy, antibiotics and bowel cleansing. Early repair can then be undertaken by a specialist surgeon.

Renal injuries

Injury to the kidneys is common and often trivial. It is, however, important to identify the patient with continuing blood loss and in particular to be alert to the possibility of injury occurring to a solitary kidney either on account of previous surgery or congenital absence. Many patients present with haematuria only on dipstick testing and provided this resolves promptly further investigation is not necessary.[40] Patients with more severe degrees of haematuria require investigation either by intravenous urography or more commonly nowadays, by contrast enhanced CT scanning. The severity of haematuria, however, does not always reflect the severity of injury and it is salutary to note that the kidney can be completely avulsed from its vascular pedicle without haematuria occurring, although hypotension, local loin tenderness or other signs of injury would usually be present. The role of investigation is to confirm not only the nature and the extent of the injury but also the presence of a functioning kidney on the other side. Ultrasound examination will confirm the presence of two kidneys but not their function and the traditional method of immediate assessment is the single shot intravenous urogram. This investigation can be performed in the resuscitation room or operating theatre: a bolus of intravenous contrast is followed by a single film five minutes later.

In major renal damage requiring urgent laparotomy the kidney has often been completely avulsed and nephrectomy and vascular control is required. With lesser degrees of injury it is advisable to obtain specialist urological help and initial control of the vascular pedicle as salvage of all or part of the kidney may be possible. Most renal injuries can, however, be treated with conservative measures and follow-up ultrasound scans can be used to monitor the progress of any perinephric haematoma or urine collection. An expanding haematoma will require contrast CT scanning (if this has not already been done) as a forerunner to intervention. Likewise, persisting or recurrent pain or enlargement of a perirenal mass or the development of sepsis will require intervention. This might be by the percutaneous route for an infected urine collection or by conventional operative means. For any delayed intervention the opinion of a specialist urologist should be sought. Penetrating injury to the renal substance requires management only to control haemorrhage and to afford drainage for any subsequent temporary leakage of urine.

Bladder

The bladder is prone to rupture particularly when full and this may occur either into the peritoneal cavity or extraperitoneally among the tissue planes of the pelvis and lower abdominal wall. Either type of rupture may be associated with very little in the way of clinical signs particularly initially, but subsequent infection is common. Rupture is diagnosed by cystography (300 ml contrast via catheter) and repair is effected by suturing using a two-layer absorbable technique. This is supported by postoperative drainage for at least 10 days and a trans-catheter cystogram should be performed before the catheter is removed.

Urethral injury

Urethral injury was alluded to earlier in relation to the insertion of a urinary catheter. When signs of urethral injury are present, a preliminary urethrogram should be obtained and a specialist opinion sought. The suprapubic route offers an alternative means of catheterisation in the interim. There are two common sites of urethral injury. First, the bulbous urethra may be injured by a direct blow to the perineum. The membranous or posterior urethra is usually injured in association with major pelvic fractures and it is in these cases that the prostate may be felt to be high-riding (i.e. separate) on rectal examination. Posterior injuries and complete disruptions of the urethra prove more difficult to treat but either can be compounded by injudicious attempts at urethral catheterisation or extravasation of urine on attempted micturition.

Pelvic fractures

The general surgeon will be involved with the management of pelvic fractures as co-existing abdominal injury is common in these patients and to begin with the source of haemorrhage may not be clear. Pelvic fractures range from relatively minor isolated fractures of a pubic ramus to major disruptions, often accompanied by considerable associated haemorrhage. The surgeon may be called upon to coordinate the management of these patients and to exclude the presence of intraperitoneal haemorrhage from associated injuries. He should try and refrain from breaching any associated pelvic haematoma either by diagnostic peritoneal lavage (see above) or at operation. If haemorrhage is continuing from the tissues disrupted by the fracture then management options include the application of an external fixator or the angiographic embolisation of feeding vessels.

Summary In the management of all patients with abdominal trauma it is important to treat the whole patient rather than possible isolated abdominal injuries. A patient with multiple trauma may have life-threatening injuries to many systems and it is essential that in the early resuscitation, assessment and investigation of these patients, priorities of management are clearly understood. This will often involve close cooperation and coordination between different specialists, sometimes in different hospitals, and input from senior clinicians at an early stage is essential in order to prioritise injuries and subsequent management. Failure to identify significant injuries at the outset may have disastrous consequences. The ATLS system of initial assessment and treatment of injured patients has a proven track record and protocols such as this should be encouraged by all specialists involved in trauma care.

References

1. Anderson ID, Woodford M, de Dombal T, Irving MH. A retrospective study of 1000 deaths from injury in England and Wales. Br Med J 1988; 296: 1305–8.
2. West JG, Trunkey DD, Lim RC. Systems of trauma care. Study of two counties. Arch Surg 1979; 114: 455–60.
3. Committee on Trauma, American College of Surgeons, Advanced Trauma Life Support Programme. Provider's manual. Chicago, American College of Surgeons, 1993.
4. Wyatt J, Beard D, Gray A, Busuttil A, Robertson C. The time of death after trauma. Br Med J 1995; 310: 1502.
5. Driscoll PA, Vincent CA. Organizing an efficient trauma team. Injury 1992; 23: 107–10.
6 Dunham CM, Damiano AM, Wiles CE, Cushing BM. Post-traumatic multiple organ dysfunction syndrome – infection is an uncommon risk factor. Injury 1995; 26: 373–8.
7. Shackford SR, Hollingworth-Fridlund P, Cooper RN, Eastman AB. The effect of regionalisation upon the quality of trauma care as assessed by concurrent audit before and after institution of a trauma system: a preliminary report. J Trauma 1986; 26: 812–20.
8. Cost effectiveness of the regional trauma

system in the North West Midlands. London, Department of Health, 1996.

9. Bickell WH, Wall MJ, Pepe PE, *et al.* Immediate versus delayed fluid resuscitation for hypotensive patients with penetrating torso injuries. N Engl J Med 1994; 331: 1105–9.

10. Anderson ID, Irving MH. The investigation of abdominal trauma. Arch Emerg Med 1990; 7: 1–8.

11. Bivins BA, Sachatello CR, Daugherty MR, Earnst GB, Griffen WO Jr. Diagnostic peritoneal lavage is superior to a clinical evaluation and blunt abdominal trauma. Am Surg 1978; 44: 637–41.

12. Federle MP. Computer tomography of blunt abdominal trauma. Radiol Clin North Am 1983; 21: 461–725.

13. Root HD, Hauser CW, McKinley CR, Le Fave JW, Mendiola RP. Diagnostic perineal lavage. Surgery 1965; 57: 633–7.

14. Fisher RP, Beverlin BC, Engrav LH, Benjamin CI, Perry JF. Diagnostic peritoneal lavage: 14 yrs and 2586 patients later. Am J Surg 1978; 136: 701–4.

15. DuPriest RW, Rodrigues A, Khaneja SC *et al.* Open diagnostic peritoneal lavage and blunt abdominal trauma. Surg Gynecol Obstet 1979; 148: 890–4.

16. Gruessner R, Mentges B, Dueber CH, Rueckeret K, Rothmand M. Sonography versus peritoneal lavage in blunt abdominal trauma. J Trauma 1989; 29: 242–4.

17. Bean IM, Braithwaite M, Oakley P, Kirby RM. Use of abdominal ultrasound for the diagnosis of intra-abdominal injury in severely injured patients. Br J Surg 1996; 83 Suppl. 1: 62.

18. Berci G, Dunkelman D, Michel SL, Sanders G, Whalstrom E, Morganstern L. Emergency mini laparoscopy in abdominal trauma. Am J Surg 1983; 146: 261–5.

19. Smith RS, Fry WR, Morabeto DJ, Koehler RH, Organ CH Jr. Therapeutic laparoscopy in trauma. Am J Surg 1995; 170: 632–7.

20. Hill AC, Schecter WP, Trunkey DD. Abdominal trauma and indications for laparotomy. In: Mattox KL, Moore EE, Feliciano DV (eds) Trauma, Norwalk, CT: Appleton and Lange, 1988.

21 Feliciano DV. Abdominal trauma. In: Schwartz SI, Ellis H (eds): Maingot's abdominal operations, 9th edn. Norwalk; Appleton and Lange, 1990.

22. Feliciano DV, Bitondo PA, Steed G, Mattox KC, Burch JM, Jordan GL. 500 open taps or lavages in patients with abdominal stab wounds. Am J Surg 1984; 148: 772–7.

23. Ryan JM, Cooper GJ, Haywood IR, Milner SM. Field surgery on a future conventional battlefield: strategy and wound management. Ann R Coll Surg Engl 1991; 73: 13–20.

24. Phillips T, Sclafani SJA, Goldstein A, Scalea T, Panetta T, Shaftan G. Use of the contrast enhanced CT enema in the management of penetrating trauma to the flank and back. J Trauma 1986; 26: 593–601.

25. Collicott PE. Initial assessment of the trauma patient. In: Mattox KL, Moore EE, Feliciano DV (eds) Trauma. Norwalk: Appleton and Lange, 1988.

26. Hirshberg A, Mattox KL. 'Damage control' in trauma surgery. Br J Surg 1993; 80: 1501–2.

27. Morris JA Jr, Eddy VA, Blinman TA, Rutherford J, Sharp KW. The staged celiotomy for trauma. Issues in unpacking and reconstruction. Ann Surg 1993; 217: 576–84.

28. Baumgartner F, Scudamore C, Neir C, Karusseit O, Hemming A. Venovenous bypass for major hepatic and caval trauma. J Trauma 1995; 39: 671–3.

29. Chen RJ, Fang JF, Lim BT, Jeng LB, Cheng MS. Surgical management of juxtahepatic venous injury in blunt hepatic trauma. J Trauma 1995; 38: 86–90.

30. Croce MA, Fabian TC, Menke PG *et al.* Non-operative management of blunt hepatic trauma is the treatment of choice for haemodynamically stable patients. Results of a prospective trial. Ann Surg 1995; 221: 744–53.

31. Pachter HL, Hofstetter SR. The current status of non-operative management of adult blunt hepatic injuries. Am J Surg 1995; 169: 442–54.

32. Boone EC, Federle M, Billiar TR, Udekwu AO, Peitzman, AB. The evolution of management of major hepatic trauma: identification of patterns of injury. J Trauma 1995; 39: 344–50.

33. Degiannis E, Levy RD, Velnahos GC *et al.* Gunshot injuries of the liver: the Baragwanath experience. Surgery 1995; 117: 359–64.

34. Holdsworth RJ, Irving AD, Cuschieri A. Postsplenectomy sepsis and its mortality rate: actual versus perceived risks. Br J Surg 1991; 78: 1031–8.

35. Johnson CD. Pancreatic trauma. Br J Surg 1995; 82: 1153–4.

36. Moore FA, Moore EE, Jones TN, McCroskey BL, Peterson VM. TEN versus TPN following major abdominal trauma – reduced septic morbidity. J Trauma 1989; 29: 916–23.

37. Sasaki LS, Allaben RD, Golwala R, Mittal VK. Primary repair of colon injuries: a prospective randomized study. J Trauma 1995; 39: 895–901.

38. Ryan M, Dutta S, Masri L *et al*. Faecal diversion for penetrating colon injuries – still the established treatment. Dis Colon Rectum 1995; 38: 264–7.

39. Velmahos GC, Degiannis E, Wells M, Souter I, Saadia R. Early closure of colostomies in trauma patients – a prospective randomized trial. Surgery 1995; 118: 815–20.

40. Kisa E, Schenk WG. Indications for emergency intravenous pyelography in blunt abdominal trauma: a reappraisal. J Trauma 1986; 26: 1086–9.

10 Abdominal emergencies in children

Lewis Spitz

Abdominal emergencies in children should be considered in regard to the age of the child. Three age periods will be considered separately:

1. Neonatal period (up to 1 month old)[1-3]
2. Infancy (1 month–2 years)[4]
3. Child 2 years and upwards.[5,6]

Neonatal abdominal emergencies[1-3]

Intestinal obstruction is the common presentation of almost all abdominal emergencies in the neonatal period. The cardinal sign of intestinal obstruction is bile-stained vomiting. In high obstructions the vomitus is clear green in colour whereas in obstructions affecting the lower intestine, although green initially, the vomitus becomes more faeculent with increasing delay in establishing the diagnosis. Where the obstruction is above the ampulla of Vater, the vomitus will be non-bilious but will be persistent and forceful. The degree of abdominal distension (Fig. 10.1) will depend on the level of the obstruction, affecting only the upper abdomen in high obstruction. There will be gross abdominal distension occasionally severe enough to cause respiratory embarrassment, in low obstructions or where there has been a significant pneumoperitoneum. In complete obstructions, the infant either fails to pass any meconium or may pass small quantities of mucus. A minority of infants with intestinal atresia may pass a small amount of normal meconium which entered the distal bowel prior to the development of the atresia. Oedema of the anterior abdominal wall and/or periumbilical erythema signifies the presence of perforation, peritonitis or impending or established intestinal necrosis.

A plain abdominal radiograph is often diagnostic and the only radiological investigation required. It may indicate the level of the obstruction as well as providing additional information such as

Figure 10.1
*Neonate with
abdominal distension*

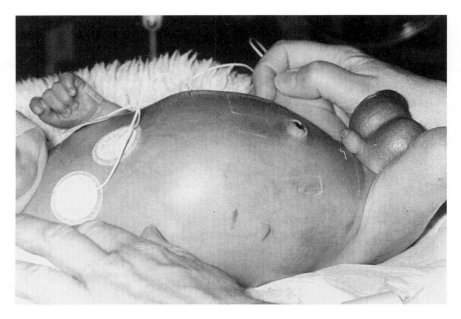

pneumoperitoneum in the event of perforation, calcification from antenatal perforation or pneumatosis intestinalis in necrotising enterocolitis.

In doubtful cases of incomplete high obstruction such as malrotation, an upper gastrointestinal contrast study is the investigation of choice whereas in suspected low obstructions, a contrast enema will define whether the colorectum is involved or whether the obstruction involves the distal small intestine. It is impossible on a plain radiograph to distinguish between small and large intestine.

Prenatal diagnosis

The diagnosis of intestinal obstruction may be suspected on antenatal scan by the presence of distended loops of fluid-filled bowel, double-bubble in the case of a duodenal atresia and multiple loops in small intestinal atresia. The presence of hyperechogenic bowel may signify meconium peritonitis and cystic lesions may be due to mesenteric or omental cysts.

Aetiology

The cause of the intestinal obstruction may be broadly classified into two main categories: mechanical and paralytic conditions (Table 10.1).

Table 10.1 *Classification of neonatal intestinal obstruction*

Mechanical
(a)   intraluminal
            meconium ileus
(b)   intramural
            atresia/stenosis
            Hirschsprung's disease
            anorectal anomalies
(c)   extrinsic
            malrotation ± volvulus
            duplications
            inguinal hernia

Paralytic ileus
Septicaemia
Necrotising enterocolitis

General principles

Infants with suspected intestinal obstruction should be transferred in a portable incubator to a specialised paediatric surgical unit for definitive management. A large-calibre nasogastric tube (size 8–10 F.G.) should be aspirated at frequent intervals and kept on free drainage at all other times. Intravenous fluid resuscitation may be necessary in the base hospital prior to transfer. An initial bolus of 20 ml kg^{-1} of plasma or human albumin solution should be administered if hypovolaemia is present. In other circumstances, a maintenance solution of 0.18% saline in 10% glucose at 3–6 ml kg^{-1} h^{-1} should be given.

Meconium ileus

Cystic fibrosis is the most common inherited defect affecting the Caucasian population. It is transmitted as an autosomal recessive condition affecting 1:2500 live births with a carrier rate of 5%. The cystic fibrosis transmembrane conductance regulator gene is located on the long arm of chromosome 7 and the delta F508 mutation is mainly responsible. Around 10–15% of affected infants present at birth with meconium ileus which may be uncomplicated or complicated by volvulus, atresia or perforation with meconium peritonitis.

In uncomplicated meconium ileus, the obstruction is caused by the thick, sticky, tenacious meconium intraluminally in the distal ileum. The colon and terminal ileum are filled with greyish inspissated pellets. The diagnosis may be suspected on the plain abdominal radiograph which shows dilated loops of intestine of varying calibre, an absence of air-fluid levels and a 'soap bubble' appearance in the right lower quadrant of the abdomen. A contrast enema will reveal a 'micro colon' containing meconium pellets. In the absence of complicated meconium ileus, the obstruction may be relieved by a therapeutic enema using Gastrografin (diatrizoate meglumine) which is hyperosmolar and contains an emulsifying agent. The enema is performed by an experienced paediatric radiologist following satisfactory rehydration of the infant with intravenous fluids. The Gastrografin is carefully infused into the colon under fluoroscopic control until the contrast is seen to enter into the dilated loops of ileum. If the infant remains obstructed after the initial enema and is otherwise stable, the procedure can be repeated once or even twice. The success rate is around 55% with unsuccessful cases requiring simple enterotomy and mechanical washout of the obstructing meconium.

Infants with complicated meconium ileus present at birth with gross abdominal distension. An abdominal mass may be palpable. The plain abdominal radiograph shows clear evidence of intestinal obstruction while the presence of calcification denotes the presence of meconium peritonitis. These infants require vigorous resuscitation followed by prompt laparotomy. In the presence of a volvulus or atresia, the grossly affected bowel is resected, the proximal and distal intestine cleared of meconium and primary end-to-end anastomosis performed. Blood loss in meconium peritonitis may be considerable due to vascular adhesions. All necrotic intestine should be resected and the small and large bowel mobilised and inspected before a primary anastomosis is fashioned. Ileostomies, double-barrelled or Bishop–Koop, are reserved for the occasional unstable infant.

The definitive diagnosis of cystic fibrosis should be confirmed by gene probe (ΔF508) and sweat test (minimum 100 g sweat) showing a sweat sodium and chloride in excess of 60 mEq l^{-1}.

Intestinal atresia/stenosis

(a) Duodenum

The occurrence of associated anomalies in over 50% of patients with duodenal atresia is indication that the aetiology of the abnormality is developmental rather than acquired *in utero*. Down's syndrome and malrotation occur in 30%, congenital cardiac malformations in 20% and oesophageal atresia and anorectal anomalies in 8% of cases. The diagnosis is confirmed by a 'double-bubble' appearance on abdominal radiograph (Fig. 10.2). Contrast studies are only required in cases of incomplete obstruction where it is important to differentiate intrinsic from extrinsic causes such as malrotation with volvulus or duplications. Treatment is by side-to-side duodeno-duodenostomy.

Small intestinal atresia

These atresias are usually isolated anomalies which caused by intra-uterine interference with the blood supply to the affected segment.

Figure 10.2
Abdominal radiograph showing the typical 'double-bubble' appearance of duodenal atresia.

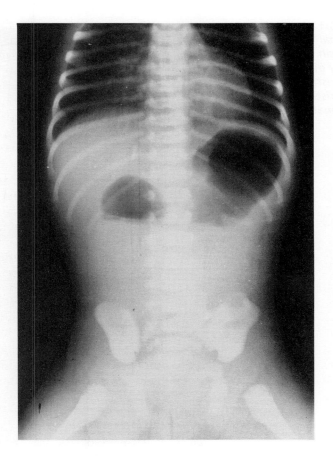

The lesions are classified into four types as follows: Type I – membrane or web between the proximal and distal intestine which are in continuity with an intact mesentery; Type II – blind ends joined by a band; Type IIIa – disconnected blind ends with a V-shaped gap in the mesentery; Type IIIb – 'apple peel', 'Christmas tree' deformity as in Type IIIa but with an extensive mesenteric defect, the distal ileum receiving its blood supply from a collateral vessel from the ileocolic artery and Type IV – multiple atresias. The proximal bowel is grossly dilated and hypertrophied and displays defective peristalsis for some distance from its blind end. The diagnosis is generally made on plain abdominal radiograph (Fig. 10.3) with contrast enema being reserved to distinguish large from small bowel obstruction. Treatment consists of resection of grossly distended proximal bowel (Fig 10.4) and a limited length of distal intestine with the fashioning of an end-to-end seromuscular anastomosis. In high jejunal atresias, the extent of proximal resection is restricted and a tapering jejunoplasty may be necessary in order to achieve an end-to-end anastomosis.

Figure 10.3
Abdominal radiograph showing massively dilated small intestinal loops characteristic of a high jejunal atresia

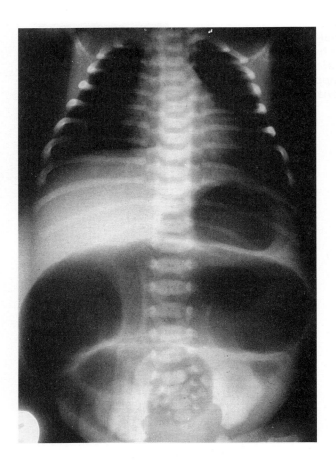

Hirschsprung's disease

Hirschsprung's disease results from an absence of ganglion cells within the wall of the intestine, commencing at the internal sphincter of the rectum and extending for a varying distance proximally. The disease is confined to the rectosigmoid in 75% of cases whereas in 10% of patients there is total colonic involvement. The incidence is estimated to be 1 per 5000 live births. An autosomal dominant gene responsible for certain cases of Hirschsprung's disease has recently been mapped to chromosomes 10 and 13. The region concerned contains the RET proto-oncogene.

Over 80% of cases of Hirschsprung's disease present in the neonatal period with delayed passage of meconium which is defined as failure to pass meconium during the first 24 hours after birth. A few cases progress to complete intestinal obstruction, but in the majority the passage of meconium is stimulated by a digital rectal examination or a saline rectal washout – only for the problem to recur within a few days. Around 25% of infants may present initially with entero-colitis – profuse diarrhoea often accompanied by blood in the stool,

Figure 10.4
Operative view of an intestinal atresia showing the proximally dilated and hypertrophied intestine and the collapsed distal bowel.

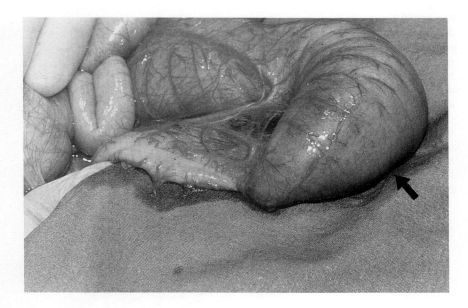

abdominal distension, bilious vomiting and dehydration. This is a life-threatening complication which demands vigorous resuscitation, gentle distal bowel washouts followed by the establishment of a proximal defunctioning stoma.

The diagnosis may be substantiated by a carefully performed barium enema and/or anorectal manometry. The barium may show a contracted rectum with cone-shaped transitional zone above before contrast enters a dilated colon proximally. Confirmation of the diagnosis is achieved on rectal suction biopsy which typically shows an absence of ganglion cells in the submucosa, the presence of large nerve trunks and an increase in acetylcholinesterase-stained nerve fibres in the muscularis mucosa and in the lamina propria (Fig. 10.5).

Definitive treatment consists of bypassing (Duhamel, Soave) or excising (Swenson, Rehbein) the aganglionic intestine and restoring intestinal continuity in a one-, two- or three-stage procedure.

Anorectal anomalies

Anorectal malformations cover a wide spectrum of abnormalities which occur in 1 in 5000 births. Of crucial importance is the precise determination of the level of the defect. A translevator or low anomaly can be diagnosed clinically by evidence of the passage of meconium on the perineum (Fig. 10.6). These lesions are amenable to immediate local reconstructive surgery in the expectation of the acquisition of normal continence. All other anomalies, supralevator, high and intermediate lesions, require the fashioning of a defunctioning colostomy in the neonatal period followed by meticulous reconstruction of the

Figure 10.5
Acetylcholinesterase stain of a rectal suction biopsy in Hirschsprung's disease showing an absence of ganglion cells, hypertrophied nerve trunks in the submucosa (a) and increased nerve fibres in the lamina propria (b)

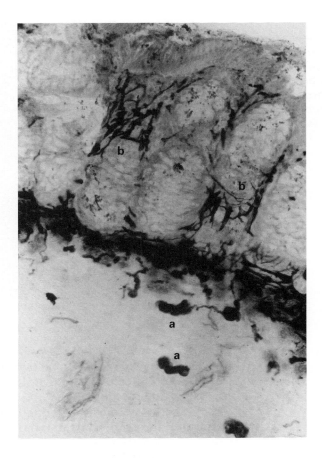

anorectal muscular complex after mobilising the distal end of the rectum and fashioning a new anal orifice.

Malrotation

Failure to complete the normal process of intestinal rotation and fixation by the twelfth week of intrauterine development leads to the potentially lethal condition of malrotation. The duodenojejunal flexure lies to the right of the midline and caecum and appendix are located in the right hypochondrium or upper midline of the abdomen. The result is a narrow-based mesentery of the midgut which is prone to undergo volvulus.

The infant presents with intermittent bile-stained vomiting. This may be the only clinical indication of the presence of a malrotation until volvulus occurs when the infant rapidly becomes shocked and passes blood per rectum and develops abdominal tenderness. In the older child presentation varies from intermittent vomiting, failure to thrive and anorexia to colicky abdominal pain and malabsorption.

Figure 10.6 *Infant with a low anorectal anomaly. Note the spot of meconium (arrow) just anterior to the covered anus.*

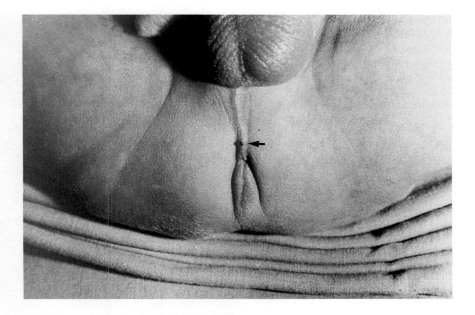

The plain abdominal radiograph in the infant with volvulus typically shows a 'gasless' appearance (Fig. 10.7). If time permits, an upper gastrointestinal contrast study is the investigation of choice. It will show an abnormally placed duodenojejunal flexure with small intestinal loops located on the right side of the abdomen in uncomplicated cases or a 'corkscrew' of 'twisted ribbon' appearance in the presence of a volvulus.

Treatment consists of urgent resuscitation and emergency laparotomy to untwist the volvulus and reposition the bowel after widening the mesentery of the midgut (Ladd's procedure).

Duplications

These are rare anomalies which may be cystic or tubular and may affect any part of the alimentary tract. Cystic lesions present clinically with intestinal obstruction and a palpable or ultrasonographically detected mass, whereas tubular duplication causes intestinal bleeding due to the presence of ectopic gastric mucosa within the duplication.

Inguinal hernia

Inguinal hernia is the most common condition treated by paediatric surgeons. It occurs in 2% of full-term infants and in 10% of preterm infants. There is a male preponderance of 5–10:1 and the right side is affected twice as often as the left. Bilateral hernia occurs in 10% of cases. The hernias most commonly present with an intermittent bulge in the groin which increases with crying and reduces spontaneously

Figure 10.7
Abdominal radiograph showing a relatively gasless abdomen suspicious of malrotation with midgut volvulus.

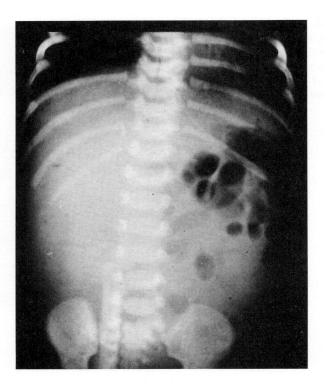

when the infant is relaxed. The hernia, not infrequently, presents initially with irreducibility. The vast majority of these irreducible herniae can be manually reduced by 'taxis' once the infant has been sedated. Treatment consists of simple herniotomy which in infancy should be taken as soon as possible after diagnosis as the chances of incarceration (Fig. 10.8) are very high (30–40%).

Necrotising enterocolitis (NEC)

A disease process which predominantly affects preterm infants, NEC is one of the most common surgical emergencies encountered in the neonatal period. The pathogenesis involves three processes: (a) intestinal ischaemia, (b) bacterial colonisation, and (c) the presence of a substrate, milk formula, in the lumen of the intestine. It most commonly affects the terminal ileum and colon but no part of the intestine is immune.

The infant displays lethargy, abdominal distension, bilious vomiting or nasogastric bile-stained aspirate, refusal of feed and bleeding per rectum. Early signs may be indistinguishable from neonatal septi-caemia. The pathognomonic radiological finding is the presence of pneumatosis intestinalis (Fig. 10.9) while pneumoperitoneum indicates a perforation and portal venous gas extensive, but not necessarily lethal, intestinal involvement.

Figure 10.8 *Infant with an incarcerated left inguinal hernia*

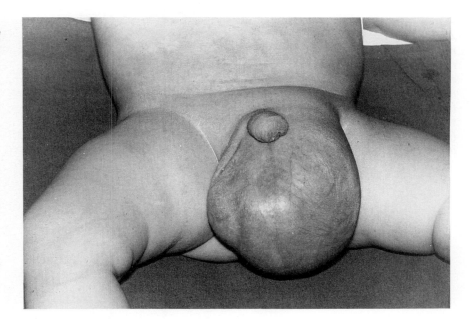

Early institution of medical treatment including nasogastric decompression, broadspectrum antibiotics, fluid and electrolyte resuscitation and parenteral nutrition for 7–10 days, results in resolution of the process in 70–80% of cases. Indications for surgery include intestinal perforation and failure to respond to conservative treatment indicating advanced intestinal disease. At surgery, frankly necrotic bowel is resected and either a primary anastomosis is fashioned or stomas are constructed. About 10–15% of cases develop late postoperative strictures which require surgical resection.

Infancy   Intussusception[4]

Intussusception is the most common cause for an abdominal emergency in infants between the ages of 3 months and 2 years. The peak incidence is from 6 to 9 months and there appears to be a seasonal incidence with the peaks in spring and in mid-winter. Most cases of intussusception at this age are 'idiopathic' with the leading point being an enlarged Peyer's patch which develops secondary to a viral infection. Only around 5% of intussusceptions in infants are due to a recognisable lesion such as a polyp, Meckel's diverticulum, duplication or tumour. The site of intestine most frequently involved is the ileocaecal region, although any part of the intestine may be affected.

The pathophysiology of the intussusception commences with the invagination of one part of the intestine (intussusceptum) into the adjacent part (intussuscipiens) causing a subacute incomplete intestinal obstruction and venous compression of the intussusceptum

Figure 10.9
Abdominal radiograph in necrotising enterocolitis showing intramural gas (arrow) on the right side of the abdomen (pneumatosis intestinalis).

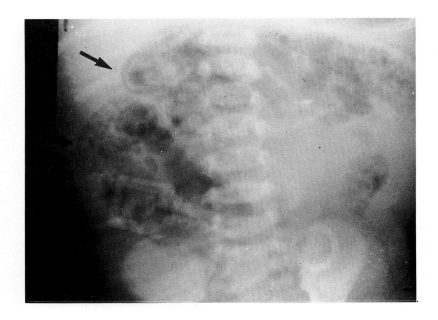

which if uncorrected will eventually result in arterial insufficiency and bowel necrosis.

The clinical features of an intussusception include colicky abdominal pain and vomiting secondary to the incomplete obstruction and the passage of blood and mucus per rectum as a result of the venous engorgement. In addition, a sausage-shaped mass may be palpable on abdominal examination. The episodes of abdominal pain are classically intermittent recurrent attacks of screaming and of the infant drawing up its knees accompanied by pallor. The attacks last about 1–2 minutes and recur every 10–15 minutes.

The diagnosis may be made solely on the clinical findings. A plain abdominal radiograph may show air outlining the head of the intussusception which appears as a soft tissue mass and an absence of gas in the right iliac fossa (Fig. 10.10). Where the diagnosis remains doubtful, a contrast enema or an ultrasound scan will establish the pathology.

Treatment of an intussusception commences with initial resuscitation with correction of any fluid and electrolyte imbalance and nasogastric decompression. In the uncomplicated case, the treatment of choice is reduction by means of either an air or contrast enema under fluoroscopic or ultrasound control. Where complications have developed such as perforation or where there is clinical evidence for bowel necrosis and when reduction has failed, an operative approach is adopted. At surgery (Fig. 10.11) the intussusception is either reduced manually or if non-viable or in the presence of a recognised leading point a limited resection and primary anastomosis is undertaken.

Figure 10.10
Abdominal radiograph showing the soft tissue mass (arrow) of an intussusception in the upper abdomen.

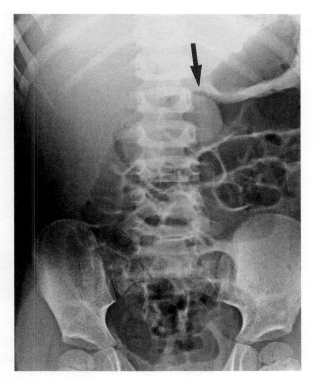

Children   Appendicitis[5]

The diagnosis of acute appendicitis should be considered at all ages but is most common between the ages of 5 and 15 years.

The pathological process of appendicitis commences with a luminal obstruction as a result of a fecolith or secondary to mucosal or sub-mucosal lymphoid hyperplasia. The mucosa distal to the obstruction continues to secrete and with increased peristalsis in an attempt to overcome the obstruction, pressure within the lumen of the appendix increases. Bacteria within the lumen proliferate in the presence of stasis and, together with the increased intraluminal pressure, invade the wall of the appendix. The process may progress to full-thickness necrosis with perforation and local or generalised peritonitis.

The classical presentation of acute appendicitis is of vague non-specific periumbilical pain which rapidly radiates and localises in the right iliac fossa. There is almost invariably loss of appetite and vomiting and a low-grade pyrexia of 38°C. Palpation of the abdomen reveals tenderness and guarding in the right iliac fossa with rigidity when perforation has occurred. There is no need to attempt to elicit rebound pain which is an unreliable sign in young children and only increases the distress and the discomfort. A rectal examination may be helpful in doubtful cases but is unnecessary if the diagnosis has already been made. The rectal examination may reveal a mass in the presence of a perforated pelvic appendicitis.

Figure 10.11
*Operative view of
an ileocolic
intussusception.*

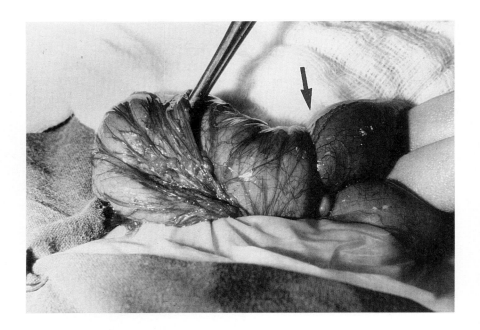

The diagnosis of acute appendicitis is generally made on clinical findings. Laboratory investigations are less helpful but a leucocytosis of 10 000–15 000 mm^{-3} supports the diagnosis. Radiological investigations are not often required but a plain abdominal radiograph may show a calcified fecolith and more recently ultrasonography has been found to be useful in doubtful cases particularly in teenage girls. The ultrasound may reveal other gynaecological causes such as an ovarian cyst or may be suggestive of the diagnosis of appendicitis when the diameter of the appendix is greater than 6 mm and there is surrounding fluid in the vicinity. Diagnostic laparoscopy has also been advocated and is again most helpful in the teenage girl.

The differential diagnosis of acute appendicitis is extensive and it is particularly difficult to establish the diagnosis in very young children who usually present late with perforation and peritonitis, teenage girls and in children suffering from other medical conditions such as urinary tract infections, sickle-cell disease, diabetes and leukaemia.

Treatment of appendicitis falls into four categories. In early uncomplicated appendicitis, the patients should undergo appendicectomy as soon as possible. Patients with perforated appendicitis with signs of peritonitis require intensive resuscitation and antibiotic administration prior to being subjected to appendicectomy. The presence of an abdominal mass indicates a localised perforation which generally will respond to antibiotic therapy with appendicectomy delayed electively for 6–8 weeks. In patients where the diagnosis is in doubt, a period of active observation in hospital is strongly recommended. It is extremely rare for such an appendix to rupture during observation and the diagnosis will usually become apparent within 12–24 hours.

Torsion of the testis[3]

There are two types of testicular torsion, extravaginal torsion which occurs in the perinatal period, and intravaginal torsion related to an abnormal suspension of the testis ('bell-clapper' anomaly) which affects the older child. The onset of torsion is heralded by sudden severe scrotal pain. The testis is swollen and tender and lies within the upper scrotum. The diagnosis is made on clinical examination and the condition should be distinguished from torsion of a testicular appendage which can be treated conservatively and epididymo-orchitis. If there is any doubt it is preferable to proceed to an emergency exploration of the scrotum. The testis is detorted and its viability assessed. If the testis is clearly necrotic it should be removed, if viable, it should be fixed with three or four non-absorbable sutures to prevent a recurrence. It is mandatory to fix the contralateral testis in a similar fashion to protect it from torsion as the abnormal lie of the testis is commonly bilateral.

Urinary tract infections

Urinary tract infections can occur at any age and the symptoms produced vary according to the age period at which the infection occurs. In the neonatal period the common presenting features are irritability, temperature, instability, lethargy, anorexia, vomiting and jaundice. In infancy failure to thrive is a common presentation. Screaming and irritability are frequent symptoms and may be associated with vomiting and diarrhoea. Malodorous or cloudy urine, haematuria and frequency are more specific features of urinary tract infections. Older children tend to present with frequency and dysuria associated with pyrexia and abdominal pain. Confirmation of the diagnosis is obtained on urinalysis and culture. All patients with a documented urinary tract infection merit full investigation which should include renal ultrasonography and ultrasound scanning of the ureters and bladder. In addition, a voiding cystourethrogram should be performed. The most common underlying abnormalities associated with urinary tract infections include vesicoureteric reflux and voiding dysfunction and pelviureteric junction obstruction which classically presents with pain, a mass, haematuria, nausea and vomiting and hypertension.

References

1. Freeman NV, Burge DM, Griffiths DM, Malone PSJ. Surgery of the newborn. Edinburgh: Churchill Livingstone, 1994.

2. Lister J, Irving IM. (eds) Neonatal surgery, 3rd edn. London: Butterworths, 1990.

3. Rowe MI, O'Neill JA, Grosfeld JL, Fonkalsrud EW, Coran AG (eds) Essentials of pediatric surgery. St Louis: Mosby, 1995.

4. Nixon HH, O'Donnell B. (eds) Essentials of paediatric surgery, 4th edn. Oxford: Butterworth–Heinemann, 1992.

5. Apley J. The child with abdominal pains. 2nd edn. Oxford: Blackwell Scientific Publications, 1975.

6. Hutson JM, Beasley SW, Woodward AA (eds) Jones' clinical paediatric surgery; 4th edn. Oxford: Blackwell Scientific, 1992.

11 Management of severe sepsis and intensive care

Brian J. Rowlands

Introduction Infection continues to be a major cause of postoperative and post-injury morbidity and mortality in surgical practice. Sepsis can be caused by infection with Gram-negative bacteria, Gram-positive bacteria, fungi and viruses. Sepsis may also occur in the absence of detectable bacterial invasion and in these cases microbial toxins, particularly Gram-negative bacterial endotoxin (lipopolysaccharide) and endogenous cytokine production have been implicated as initiators and mediators of the inflammatory response. A characteristic of sepsis and infection is a generalised inflammatory condition featuring fever, leucocytosis, hypermetabolism and hypoperfusion of organs. The generalised inflammatory response is the result of complex interactions of host homeostatic systems involving complement, coagulation and arachadonic cascades; cytokine production; neuroendocrine reflexes; and microvascular, endothelial and leucocyte activation. The interactions of these systems produces a microvascular injury that leads to organ ischaemia and organ failure.

Over the past 20 years, many advances have been made in the diagnosis and therapy of surgical infection, notably the introduction of new chemotherapeutic agents, radiological innovations such as computed axial tomography, nuclear scanning and magnetic resonance imaging, together with better management of patients in the intensive care unit, utilising advances in fluid resuscitation, nutritional support, and the treatment of respiratory, hepatic and renal failure. Sequential failure of vital organs often precedes death from sepsis and infection. Successful reversal of this deterioration of metabolic and immune function requires its early diagnosis and aggressive management. The assessment of innovative methods of diagnosis and treatment has often been difficult due to the heterogeneity of the patient population studied, and the spectrum of diseases producing septic complications.

Several diseases are complicated by a high incidence of sepsis syndrome, systemic inflammatory response syndrome (SIRS) and multiple organ dysfunction syndrome (MODS). These diseases include multiple trauma, obstructive jaundice, inflammatory bowel disease, acute pancreatitis and major intra-abdominal sepsis. These clinical conditions and their septic complications are characterised by a state of 'hypermetabolism' which leads to rapid consumption of endogenous stores of energy and protein, immunological dysfunction and deterioration of organ function. These changes which affect the liver, kidney, gastrointestinal tract, heart and lungs are orchestrated by a series of neuroendocrine events and the release of cytokines, activators and mediators of the systemic metabolic response. The 'gut–liver axis' appears to have a central role in these responses, altered gastrointestinal structure and function and associated changes in hepatic Kupffer cell function contribute to metabolic dysfunction. These changes may be modified by pharmacological, nutritional and immunological therapies which produce beneficial effects in several ways, e.g. support of generalised immune function, modification of hepatic Kupffer cell function, cytokine release and acute phase protein production by the liver. Improved understanding of the pathophysiology of sepsis syndrome, SIRS and MODS may lead to better therapeutic strategies to reduce mortality and morbidity in septic patients. This chapter describes the clinical presentation of severe sepsis, its evaluation and treatment, and the identification of an appropriate level of clinical care. It will also assess conventional and novel strategies of management designed to prevent and treat sequential organ dysfunction and failure, which hopefully will lead to improvements in outcome in these surgical diseases.

The patho-physiology of sepsis

Sepsis and related conditions are not well-defined entities. In the continuum of surgical care there is a gradation of severity of illness. At one end of the spectrum there is minimal derangement of normal physiology with rapid return to normal metabolic homeostasis following therapeutic intervention. At the other extreme is a massive disruption of normal organ function which leads to progressive deterioration and death despite treatment. Central to our understanding of these events is an appreciation that initially there is a localised response to any insult. This may lead subsequently to systemic manifestations if the local host defence mechanisms are inadequate or overwhelmed.[1] Localised infections due to bacteria, viruses, fungi and parasites stimulate the release of various mediators, e.g. cytokines, prostaglandins, thromboxanes, platelet-activating factors and the complement system. These help to combat infection by activating neutrophils with consequent degranulation and release of oxygen radicals which increase local blood flow and vascular permeability allowing the influx of phagocytic cells. They also activate white blood cells and induce chemotaxis. These local responses are beneficial to the host. If the severity of the infection is sufficient that these mediators spill over into the systemic circulation, a septic cascade is initiated which may lead to septic shock, SIRS and MODS. Superoxide radicals now damage host cells. Endotoxin and various cytokines, activators and mediators, e.g. tumour necrosis factor, the interleukins, transforming growth factor beta and prostaglandin E_2 all contribute to the initiation and maintenance of this cascade which may be beneficial or detrimental, depending on the clinical setting.

Some patients are more susceptible to septic complications than others and the risk factors associated with a poor outcome have been defined initially in retrospective studies of patient outcome and subsequently in prospective studies that have assessed changes in patient outcome following therapeutic intervention.[2] Age is a variable that cannot be changed by therapy, but extremes of age, particularly old age, are prone to infectious complications due to a number of interrelated variables such as impaired immunity, cardiovascular and respiratory disease and malnutrition. Concurrent diseases such as diabetes, malignancy, cirrhosis and renal failure also increase complications. Protein-calorie malnutrition often accompanies these conditions and may be present in up to 50% of surgical patients.[3] Assessment of anthropometric, biochemical and immunological measurements may define patients with impaired nutritional status who have a poorer outcome than those who are normally nourished.[4] Other factors such as medications that depress immunity (steroids), malignancy (chemotherapy and radiation therapy), or lead to other complications (anticoagulants) may all impact on the incidence of sepsis. Good aseptic technique, excellent pre- and postoperative care and elective rather than emergency treatment of most conditions have a positive effect on outcome. The classification of surgical procedures into clean, clean contaminated, contaminated and dirty cases accurately predicts the incidence of infective complications, from less than 2% in clean cases to 40% in dirty cases.[5] More complex cases are now being undertaken as surgical techniques and anaesthetic practice become more sophisticated, but these advances often involve more invasive monitoring and diagnostic procedures which invariably increase the risk of infection.[6] The factors that predispose to the development of sepsis in the surgical patient are summarised in Table 11.1 and in some patients several factors may be present simultaneously.

Definitions

In 1992, the following list of terms and definitions emerged from a consensus conference, between the American College of Chest Physicians and the Society of Critical Care Medicine, to agree terminology by which sepsis could be discussed.[7]

Infection – an inflammatory response to microorganisms or their invasion of normal sterile host tissue.

Table 11.1 *Factors that predispose to the development of sepsis*

Extremes of age
Malignancy
Burns, wounds, multiple trauma
Hepatic failure
Renal failure
Diabetes mellitus
Post-splenectomy
HIV infection
Organ transplantation
Immunosuppressive drugs
Urinary catheter
Arterial and venous access
Tubes and drains
Malnutrition
Radiation therapy
Anticoagulants

Bacteraemia – the presence of viable bacteria in the blood. This definition may be extended to include viruses (viraemia), fungi (fungaemia), parasites (parasitaemia) and other microorganisms which may cause infection.

Sepsis – the systemic response to infection

Severe sepsis – sepsis associated with organ dysfunction that persists despite adequate fluid resuscitation.

Systemic inflammatory response syndrome (SIRS) – a systemic inflammatory response that is characterised by well-defined clinical parameters and which may or may not result from infection. When due to the presence of bacteria, sepsis and SIRS are synonymous. (Table 11.2).

Multiple organ dysfunction syndrome (MODS) – organ dysfunction caused by SIRS induced damage in which homeostasis cannot be maintained without supportive measures. This may take the form of a primary insult such as an aspiration injury to the lung or a secondary phenomenon such as cytokine induced adult respiratory distress syndrome (ARDS) in severe acute pancreatitis. The development of MODS is the penultimate stage of the sepsis continuum that may lead to death.

Multiple organ dysfunction syndrome (MODS)

In the 1970s it was recognised that death following a septic complication involved the sequential deterioration of organ function, most notably cardiovascular, respiratory, hepatic and renal.[8] In 1980, a study of 553 patients undergoing emergency surgical procedures found that failure of two or more organ systems in 30 patients was associated

Table 11.2 *Systemic inflammatory response syndrome (SIRS)[a]*

The response is characterised by two or more of the following:

- Temperature   greater than 38°C
  or less than 36°C

- Heart rate   greater than 90 beats per minute

- Respiratory rate   greater than 20 breaths per minute
  or $Paco_2$ less than 32 mmHg

- White blood cell count   greater than 12 000 cell ml^{-1}
  or less than 4000 cells ml^{-1}
  or 10% immature (band) forms

[a]In the presence of bacteria, SIRS is synonymous with sepsis.

with a 74% mortality.[9] Stress, ulceration, gastrointestinal haemorrhage, disseminated intravascular coagulopathy, coma, malnutrition and abnormalities of substrate metabolism all contributed to significant morbidity and mortality. The most important factor relating to death was the development of acute renal failure. Other factors contributing to the development of MODS are hypovolaemic shock, massive resuscitation, use of blood products, specific organ injury and clinical sepsis.[10] Organ failure usually occurs sequentially commencing in sepsis and pulmonary failure and progressing to hepatic, gastrointestinal and renal failure. The longer organ failure is present, the less likely is recovery. The ability of an organ system to withstand failures of perfusion and oxygenation depend on the functional reserve of the organ, emphasising the attributes of youth for survival. Patients who already have chronic organ dysfunction, e.g. chronic obstructive airways disease, cirrhosis, are more likely to develop acute deterioration of organ function as a result of their disease, injury, or infection. A number of scoring systems (such as APACHE Score, Sepsis Score, Injury Severity Score and Revised Trauma Score) in common usage are capable of identifying such patients and accurately predicting the outcome of their illness.[11] Discussion of these scoring systems is beyond the scope of this chapter but a number of clinical conditions predispose to the development of MODS (Table 11.3) and dysfunction/failure of each organ system (Table 11.4) can be defined by a number of clinical, biochemical and haematological parameters.

Cardiovascular – one or more of the following:

- Mean arterial pressure less than 49 mmHg
- Ventricular tachychardia/fibrillation
- Serum pH less than 7.24 (perfusion related)
- Acute complete heart block
- Use of vasoactive drugs to support arterial pressure

Respiratory – one or more of the following:

- Respiratory rate greater than 49 min^{-1}
- $PaCO_2$ greater than 50 mmHg in the absence of opioid drugs or metabolic alkalosis
- Dependence on mechanical ventilation for more than 12 h

Renal – one or more of the following:

- Oliguria (less than 0.5 ml kg^{-1} h^{-1} urine output) with rising or elevated creatinine despite adequate fluids
- Serum urea greater than 35 mmol l^{-1}
- Serum creatinine greater than 300 umol l^{-1}

Hepatic – either

- Clinical hepatic failure causing other organ failures (e.g. renal) or complications (bleeding/encephalopathy)
  or
- Prothrombin time prolonged 3 s over control and biochemical LFTs twice upper limit of normal

Gastrointestinal – one or more of the following:

- Prolonged ileus or uncontrolled diarrhoea
- Gastrointestinal haemorrhage requiring transfusion
- Pancreatitis

Haematological – one or more of the following:

- WBC less than 1000 mm^{-3}
- Platelets less than 20 000 mm^{-3}
- Haematocrit less than 20% in the absence of bleeding

Neurological – either

- Best Glasgow Coma Scale (GCS) less than 8 in the absence of sedative drugs or metabolic cause
  or
- Neuropathy, myopathy or cord lesion limiting respiratory reserve or mobility

Metabolic – endocrine or metabolic failure causing coma (e.g. diabetes, myxoedema)

Skin – loss of skin integrity affecting greater than 15% of body surface area

Muscoloskeletal – Injury Severity Score of greater than 25.

All these clinical, biochemical and haematological parameters are clear indications that there has been deterioration in the overall clinical condition of the patient. It is important that the early signs and symptoms of sepsis are identified so that therapeutic intervention is initiated at the earliest opportunity.

Table 11.3 *Surgical conditions that commonly are associated with the development of sepsis, SIRS, MODS*

Multiple trauma
Acute pancreatitis
Intra-abdominal sepsis
Obstructive jaundice
Major hepatopancreaticobiliary surgery
Inflammatory bowel disease
Abdominal aortic aneurysm
Bowel ischaemia
Splanchnic hypoperfusion

Table 11.4 *Systems that may develop progressive deterioration of function and failure associated with sepsis, SIRS, MODS*

Cardiovascular
Respiratory
Hepatic
Gastrointestinal
Haematological
Neurological
Metabolic
Skin
Musculoskeletal

Table 11.5 *Presenting features of sepsis and SIRS*

Hyperthermia, hypothermia
Tachypnoea
Tachycardia
Hyperdynamic state
Hypotension
Impaired organ perfusion
Circulatory shock
Dehydration
Metabolic abnormalities (diabetes)
Acid–base imbalance, especially lactic acidosis
Multiple organ dysfunction syndrome
      ARDS
      Renal failure
      Hepatobiliary dysfunction
      CNS dysfunction
Haemorrhage and bruising
Decreased conscious level

Clinical features of sepsis

The clinical presentation of sepsis and SIRS varies widely due to the features already discussed with regard to patients, underlying cause, and the local and systemic manifestations of the sepsis syndrome. The patient may present at various times in the natural history of the development of a septic complication and signs of local infection may or may not be present. There are no characteristic symptoms of sepsis but patients may complain of chills, sweats, and rigors, breathlessness, nausea, headache, vomiting or diarrhoea. Confusion may occur especially in the elderly. Typical signs that suggest sepsis are fever or hypothermia, hypoxia and breathlessness, and hypotension not due to hypovolaemia or cardiac causes. There may be significant metabolic acidosis as a reflection of poor tissue perfusion. There may already be evidence of organ dysfunction or failure (e.g. clinical jaundice, poor renal output) at the time of presentation (Table 11.5). In making a diagnosis of sepsis a high index of suspicion is required when confronted by a patient whose overall condition is deteriorating.

Initial assessment and monitoring

Because of the diversity of presentation of the patient with sepsis it is important that a systematic approach to initial assessment and resuscitation is adopted. The two should proceed simultaneously using a format similar to that advocated for the trauma patient using the Advanced Trauma Life Support (ATLS) system of the American College of Surgeons. This aims to establish assessment and management priorities which can be divided into four main phases – primary survey, resuscitation, secondary survey and definitive care. During the primary survey and resuscitation which involves assessment of airway, breathing, circulation and neurological status, no attempt is made to ascertain the exact aetiology of the patient's deteriorating condition.[12] Once resuscitation has been initiated and the primary survey completed, the next phase involves a secondary survey to include routine assessment by means of a complete history and physical examination, systemic review of the patient's notes and charts and initiation of routine investigations. If the patient responds to initial resuscitation and remains stable a definitive plan for further investigation and treatment can be formulated including specific laboratory or radiological investigations to establish the underlying pathology. If, however, the response to resuscitation is transient or the patient continues to deteriorate this should mandate a reassessment of airway, breathing and circulation together with the involvement of specialist senior help in the continuing resuscitation and monitoring of the patient. At this stage in an unstable septic patient it may be necessary to transfer the patient from the ward to a higher level of care in a high dependency unit (HDU) or intensive care unit (ICU).

The goals in the initial management of sepsis should be to restore tissue perfusion and oxygen transportation together with metabolic support and control of the source of the sepsis. This means that assessment, evaluation, diagnostic tests and definitive therapy all have to proceed in a logical sequence. Initial signs of decreased tissue perfusion are restlessness or decreased conscious level, cool peripheries, reduced urinary output, prolonged capillary refill, decreased oxygen saturation by pulse oximetry and metabolic acidosis. Priorities in clinical management and monitoring are to establish peripheral venous access with a large bore peripheral cannula, insert a bladder catheter either per urethram or suprapubically, ECG monitoring, pulse oximetry and measurement of core and peripheral temperature. Insertion of a central venous line via the subclavian or internal jugular vein may be difficult or hazardous in a hypovolaemic patient, but provides useful information following initial fluid and oxygen administration of adequacy of resuscitation and myocardial function. Initial haematological assessment of venous blood should include haemoglobin concentration, haematocrit and white blood cell count, together with blood grouping and cross-matching of blood if indicated and assessment of clotting status. Blood urea and electrolytes, blood glucose, liver function tests and blood lactate should be evaluated to establish a base line. Arterial blood should be taken for blood gas analysis and repeated at regular intervals to assess response to therapy. Blood, urine, sputum, drainage fluid, wound swabs and any obvious septic lesion should all be cultured when sepsis is suspected so that this information can be used to guide subsequent antibiotic therapy. Obvious sources of sepsis such as wound infection, an undrained abscess or necrotic tissue, or contributing factors such as gastrointestinal haemorrhage resulting in hypovolaemia may require surgical intervention after initial resuscitation and transient stabilisation of the patient. In this situation, definitive drainage, excision or haemostasis may produce a dramatic improvement in the overall general condition of the patient as the surgical intervention facilitates the restoration of tissue perfusion and oxygenation. In other situations, the source of the infection will be less obvious but physical examination may point to a pulmonary source (breathlessness, productive cough), abdominal problem (pain, ileus, diarrhoea) or complication in the urinary tract (dysuria, frequency, haematuria). The site of recent operative procedures especially within the abdominal cavity should always be high on the list of possible sources of infection together with sites of vascular access, invasive monitoring, urinary catheterisation and invasive diagnostic procedures. A chest radiograph is mandatory in all cases of suspected sepsis. Other radiological investigations that may prove useful in localising the source of infection within the chest, abdomen or pelvis are ultrasound, CT scanning and radionuclear imaging. Patients should only be transported to the radiology department for these investigations if they are haemodynamically stable and if there is a plan to intervene radiologically or surgically if a localised abscess or source of infection is defined. All patients with possible intra-abdominal or pelvic abscess should have a rectal and pelvic examination as part of their routine assessment prior to more sophisticated modalities of evaluation.

Definitive management of sepsis

Patients with sepsis or SIRS may be cared for in a variety of locations depending on the level of medical/nursing care required and the need for monitoring or ventilation. During the continuum of surgical care from onset of illness to rehabilitation a patient may be accommodated in a surgical ward, postoperative recovery unit, high dependency unit (HDU) or intensive care unit (ICU). The highest level of care in the ICU provides a comprehensive diagnostic and therapeutic service for patients with, or at risk from, potentially reversible organ failure in two or more systems or in need of ventilator support for greater than 12 h. There is optimum nurse to patient ratio (1:1), 24 h consultant specialist cover and dedicated 24 h resident ICU cover by trainees with advanced life support (ALS) skills. In a HDU there is a lower nurse to patient ratio, usually not capable of respiratory support, has less monitoring and immediate availability of medical staff. Patients in HDU usually have single organ failure. At ward level, there may be a special area within the general ward set aside for more dependent patients who need close observation, monitoring and intensive nursing. Surgeons are usually responsible for the care of their patients on the ward and in HDU and although primary responsibility for care in the ICU may be assumed by the specialist team it is essential that surgeons participate in the assessment and decision making for ICU patients. An understanding of the capabilities of each level of care enables the patient with sepsis, SIRS and MODS to be assigned to the appropriate level of care throughout the continuum of surgical care with a smooth transition between resuscitation, definitive care, recovery, convalescence and rehabilitation. Patients who spend a significant period of their acute illness in the ICU or HDU will inevitably have a prolonged period of care in the normal surgical ward, and they will benefit from continuous involvement in their care by the surgical staff.

Respiratory support

Specific clinical signs may indicate respiratory insufficiency. These may include increasing rate and diminishing depth of respiration, dyspnoea, cyanosis and unexplained confusion due to hypoxia. A number of factors predispose to respiratory insufficiency and many of them may be exacerbated by sepsis or SIRS (Table 11.6). Arterial blood gas (ABG) measurement gives information about arterial oxygen tension (PaO_2), carbon dioxide tension ($PaCO_2$) and acid–base balance. From these figures and the inspired oxygen concentration (FiO_2) we can derive information on the oxygen delivery to the tissues and the degree of shunting due to ventilation/perfusion mismatch in the lung. Serial ABG measurements allow us to follow the response to respiratory management which may include airway management, oxygen therapy, physiotherapy and mechanical ventilation.[13] During active resuscitation the airway may be maintained by lifting the jaw forward or the use of an oropharyngeal airway but long-term airway control usually

Table 11.6 *Contributing factors to the development of respiratory insufficiency in sepsis and SIRS*

Preoperative	Pre-existing lung disease
	Smoking
	Aspiration
	Trauma to chest wall, lung, diaphragm
Operative	Thoracoabdominal incisions
	Anaesthetic – CNS depression
	Neuromuscular blockade
Postoperative	Pain inhibiting respiration
	Drugs depressing respiration
	Fluid overload
	Abdominal distension
	Supine position
	Cough suppression = pain, sedation, NG tube
	Respiratory tract infection
	Pulmonary embolus
	Fat embolus
	ARDS

mandates the use of nasotracheal or endotracheal intubation. Humidified oxygen may be administered by face mask or nasal catheters and is an important first step in restoring normal tissue oxygenation. Frequent and effective physiotherapy to the chest and lungs is essential to remove secretions and sputum, maintain optimal ventilation of the lungs by reducing airway collapse and plugging of bronchi and bronchioles by mucus. If, despite the institution of these therapies, the patient's clinical signs continue to deteriorate and the PaO_2 falls, mechanical ventilation may be required. A number of techniques are available to ensure adequate alveolar ventilation and oxygenation are achieved by precisely controlling FiO_2, tidal volume, inspiratory minute volume, inspiratory/expiratory ratio and inflation pressure. Detailed knowledge of the modifications of positive pressure mechanical ventilation are beyond the scope of this chapter. Suffice it to say, however, that the delivery of adequate ventilation and oxygenation is only one aspect of respiratory therapy and it is important to address the underlying cause of respiratory failure.

Adult respiratory distress syndrome (ARDS) may develop despite early introduction of mechanical ventilation in sepsis. The fundamental problem is interstitial and alveolar oedema due to increased alveolar/capillary permeability. This results in a reduction in lung compliance and functional residual capacity with consequent fall in arterial oxygen tension. ARDS should be suspected if arterial hypoxaemia persists despite increases in FiO_2 and bilateral diffuse pulmonary infiltrates appear on chest radiograph. Treatment consists of ventilation with PEEP (positive end expiratory pressure), sedation, oxygen therapy, careful fluid and electrolyte management and maintenance of plasma protein concentrations to minimise oedema formation. Successful management of ARDS depends on the skilful interpretation of results and manipulation of support techniques. Even with optimal management there is a high mortality (50%).

Cardiovascular support

Support of the cardiovascular system consists of fluid resuscitation to restore normovolaemia, blood replacement and inotropic support if indicated. These measures are essential to restore adequate tissue perfusion and oxygenation in the presence of adequate respiratory function. The haemodynamic response to sepsis is well characterised. Initially there is a fall in systemic vascular resistance (SVR) due to vasodilatation and loss of vascular tone. The healthy myocardium responds by a reflex increase in cardiac output maintaining blood pressure in the early phase of sepsis. Later the myocardium may be unable to sustain adequate output so that blood pressure falls. Increased capillary permeability causing fluid loss from the intravascular compartment may contribute to hypotension.

Initial resuscitation requires the placement of two large-bore intravenous cannulae and the rapid infusion of fluid, together with oxygen administration by mask, to improve cardiac output and oxygen transport. The type of fluid used is not important as most patients tolerate anaemia better than they tolerate hypovolaemia. In the past there has been debate about the relative merits of crystalloid and colloid fluid for resuscitation. Initial management consists of the use of 2–3 litres of crystalloid followed by the use of colloid and blood, depending on initial response and assessment of haemoglobin and blood gas measurements. Synthetic colloids increase the circulating volume by a greater degree per volume infused initially but are then redistributed in the same way as crystalloids. Colloids also carry the risk of anaphylaxis and coagulopathy. Large volumes of resuscitation fluid may cause dilution of clotting factors and coagulopathy so that early use of blood, fresh frozen plasma, platelets, factor VIII and administration of vitamin K may also be necessary. Failure of the patient to respond to resuscitation should prompt a reappraisal of the patient's clinical condition and may dictate the use of more invasive monitoring devices (central venous pressure and pulmonary artery wedge pressure monitoring) to ascertain the reason.[13] Patients with sepsis and SIRS may have large fluid requirements in the first 24 h and close monitoring of volume status, urinary output (at least 30 ml h^{-1}) and capillary refill is essential to avoid fluid overload. If possible crystalloid fluids should be warmed to 39°C prior to infusion to avoid hypothermia and associated coagulopathy. Fluid management should be reassessed at regular intervals and adjusted according to the patient's response to therapy.

The use of inotropes

If cardiac output remains poor despite careful resuscitation and monitoring, it may be necessary to use inotropic drugs to improve myocardial contractability and regional perfusion. The inotropes include naturally occurring catecholamines, dopamine, noradrenaline and adrenaline and synthetic substances such as isoprenaline and dobutamine. Ideally an inotrope should improve cardiac output with a minimal increase in heart rate and vasoconstriction and a low incidence of dysrhythmias. Low-dose dopamine (3–5 μg kg^{-1} min^{-1}) improves renal and hepatic blood flow and is often used empirically in sepsis although there are few data to support its efficacy in preventing renal failure. Higher doses of dopamine improve stroke volume and are less likely to cause tachycardia or arrhythmias than other inotropes. Adrenaline and dobutamine have potent central effects but are more likely to produce vasoconstriction. Combinations of drugs may be indicated in severe sepsis to achieve the dual aim of improving myocardial contractility and enhancing tissue perfusion. The use of other pharmacological agents to support cardiac function and to enhance tissue perfusion are occasionally indicated, but discussion is beyond the scope of this chapter. At all times it should be remembered that the inotropes are no substitute for adequate fluid replacement and their use in a hypovolaemic septic patient will further decrease splanchnic blood flow and increase risk of sepsis.

Renal support

The mortality from acute renal failure following sepsis and SIRS is high (60%) despite advances in diagnosis and treatment. The causes of renal dysfunction and failure are multifactorial but most commonly a combination of prerenal hypovolaemia, and the presence of nephrotoxic agents such as bacterial toxins, cytokines, hyperbilirubinaemia and drugs have an additive effect. The importance of maintaining tissue oxygenation and perfusion have been emphasised and the kidney is particularly sensitive to hypovolaemia. Acute renal failure should be suspected in the septic patient when serum urea and creatinine rise and urinary output falls on serial assessment. Any acute or chronic impairment of renal function will limit the ability to concentrate the urine and confirmation of renal dysfunction may be obtained by measuring urinary sodium and potassium excretion and urinary osmolarity. Complete anuria may be due to lower renal and urinary tract obstruction but once this cause is eliminated anuria and oliguria are usually due to a combination of sepsis, hypovolaemia and drug toxicity. Restoration of normal cardiac output and normovolaemia should be achieved by using a combination of volume expansion, inotropic and pressor agents. A number of drugs impair renal function in a dose-dependent manner, e.g. aminoglycoside antibiotics, non-steroidal anti-inflammatory agents, opioids, beta-blockers, and their use in the septic patient should be avoided or closely monitored. Drug dosages of all drugs eliminated by the kidney should be adjusted to avoid further nephrotoxicity once renal impairment is established. Management of renal failure consists of control of hyperkalaemia, correction of the underlying septic condition and fluid and electrolyte management to avoid overhydration and fluid retention. Dopamine, diuretics and mannitol will all increase salt and water excretion but there is no evidence that they alter the natural history of acute renal failure once it is established. Peritoneal haemodialysis or haemofiltration are required if the above measures are unsuccessful and are indicated when there is persistent uraemia, uncontrollable hyperkalaemia, and severe salt and water overload often with pulmonary oedema. Vascular access is via venous or arterial cannulation and treatment is intermittent or continuous until renal function is sufficient to allow adequate clearance of nitrogenous waste products. In sepsis and SIRS, the breakdown of endogenous protein stores will be high so that adequate nutritional support is essential. Exogenous protein and calories should be provided to the patient with acute renal failure in amounts that satisfy their requirements even if this dictates more frequent haemodialysis or haemoperfusion. There is no place in acute renal failure for restricting nutrient intake.

Hepatobiliary impairment

Hyperbilirubinaemia is a common accompaniment to sepsis and SIRS. It usually occurs due to a direct toxic effect on liver parenchymal cells causing inflammation in the portal triads and intrahepatic cholestasis. It may be exacerbated by hypovolaemia, the use of intravenous nutrition, drugs and excessive haemolysis. The combination of fever, rigors and obstructive jaundice should always be investigated quickly as ascending biliary sepsis can lead to rapid deterioration of the patient with onset of MODS, especially acute renal failure. Abdominal ultrasound may indicate extrahepatic biliary obstruction due to stone or stricture and this should be dealt with swiftly by endoscopic or radiological drainage and stenting or surgical intervention. Acute acalculous cholecystitis may also be diagnosed by abdominal ultrasound and this should be treated with cholecystectomy or cholecystostomy prior to the onset of gall bladder necrosis and biliary peritonitis. Unrecognised and untreated, this condition has a very high mortality. In the absence of extrahepatic pathology which is treatable, sepsis and hyperbilirubinaemia usually indicates severe parenchymal liver disease and/or intrahepatic cholestasis which carries a bad prognosis.

Gastrointestinal tract

In the past 10 years the gastrointestinal tract has assumed more importance in the management of the septic patient in the intensive care unit.[14] Previously the gastrointestinal tract was regarded as an organ that contributed little to the pathophysiology of sepsis but it is now recognised that the small intestine and colon make important contributions to the maintenance of hypermetabolism in sepsis, SIRS and MODS.[15] This is due to changes in gastrointestinal structure and function that promotes loss of intestinal barrier function. When taken in conjunction with abnormal colonisation by luminal microorganisms, bacterial translocation and absorption of toxins due to increased intestinal permeability, there is a constant trigger to the widespread activation of proinflammatory cells and the release of cytokines and other mediators of the metabolic response to sepsis. These problems appear to be enhanced by malnutrition.[16]

Gastrointestinal haemorrhage used to be a major problem in septic patients requiring ICU management but improvements in overall patient management has diminished the problem to an extent that prophylaxis with antacids, H_2 receptor antagonists or sucralfate are only occasionally required. The use of selective digestive decontamination (SDD) of the gastrointestinal tract has its advocates but a meta-analysis of the randomised controlled trials of SDD showed that it was an effective technique for reducing infection related morbidity in ICU patients but there was no convincing reduction in mortality.[17] The data suggested that to prevent one respiratory tract infection you would need to treat six patients and to prevent one death you would need to treat 23 patients. Although SDD continues to be evaluated in specific groups of patients admitted to ICU, it has not been universally adopted due to doubts about efficacy in the general ICU population and concerns about the development of multiresistant organisms if its use became widespread.

The use of nutritional support techniques (see Chapter 3) has improved the outcome of patients with sepsis and SIRS.[18] Recently there have been two major trends in the use of nutritional support. First there is a major shift from intravenous administration of nutrients to enteral feedings and second the quantity of nutrients being administered is decreasing and the quality of nutrient mix is improving. In sepsis a number of studies have demonstrated that enteral feeding has a major advantage over parenteral nutrition.[19,20] The beneficial effects of nutrition are its support of generalised immune function, enhancement of mucosal barrier function, reduction of bacterial translocation, modification of hepatic Kupffer cell function, cytokine release and acute phase protein production by the liver. Additional benefits of enteral nutrition are the maintenance of the structural and functional integrity of the gastrointestinal tract by stimulation of 'gut' hormone release, 'gut' motility and mucous production and maintenance of luminal milieu of nutrients, microorganisms and trophic factors that are important for normal digestion and barrier function. The theoretical advantages of enteral nutrition are sometimes undermined by an inability to deliver sufficient nutrients into the gastrointestinal tract due to prolonged ileus, bloating, abdominal distension or diarrhoea. The latter may have a small additional benefit in reducing numbers of luminal bacteria and toxins which are potentially deleterious. If diarrhoea persists it may lead to dehydration and electrolyte imbalance.

Antibiotic therapy

It has been emphasised that the main difference between sepsis and SIRS is the demonstration of microorganisms in the former. When therapy is initiated it may not be possible to distinguish them apart. The initial empiric antibiotic therapy should be directed against the suspected predominant causative microorganisms, should have the lowest toxicity and have the smallest likelihood of inducing multi-resistant organisms.[21] If the gastrointestinal tract is the origin of the sepsis, broad spectrum therapy against anaerobes and Gram-negative aerobes is recommended. Following trauma, exogenous contamination occurs with pyogenic cocci and clostridia requiring beta lactamase stable penicillins or cephalosporins. Catheter-related sepsis is usually due to skin contaminants such as *Staphylococcus* but the potential for candidal infection should be remembered. In sepsis the normal relationship between drug dosages and tissue antibiotic levels may be altered due to expanded volumes of distribution of antibiotic and changes of rates of breakdown and elimination. High tissue levels are required for successful therapy, but beware of toxicity. The antibiotic regimen should be adjusted promptly when information from cultures demonstrates the causative microorganisms and antibiotic sensitivities. The patient should be given a defined course of antibiotic therapy and then reassessed with further microbiological surveillance. Therapy should continue if there is clinical improvement because cessation of therapy prematurely can result in relapse. A prolonged ICU stay and the use of multiple antibiotic regimen may encourage the development of multiresistant strains of bacteria or infection with unusual organisms, viruses or fungi.

Steroids

In the past corticosteroids have been recommended for patients with septic shock but a number of randomised controlled clinical trials have now been published showing no benefit and potentially detrimental effects in some patients.[22]

Newer therapies

Despite the application of the above treatment strategies, sepsis continues to be the leading cause of death in surgical ICU. Over the past decade a number of new therapies have been developed based on three important theories about the sepsis syndrome namely: oxygen debt causes organ injury; endotoxin is a critical mediator; the host inflammatory response is harmful.[23] A number of clinical trials employing new therapeutic strategies have now been published and most have failed to show convincing evidence of an improved outcome for patients with sepsis or septic shock and some agents have caused harm.[24] A possible explanation of this lack of therapeutic success is that our concept of the pathophysiology of sepsis is too simplistic or incorrect and has failed to take into consideration the compensatory anti-inflammatory response of the body. The importance of this response in predicting mortality and organ failure in sepsis syndrome has recently been demonstrated by Goldie *et al*.[25] More studies are required of specific diseases to document their pro-inflammatory and anti-inflammatory responses before we will be able to embrace this new information to develop new therapeutic strategies that benefit our patients with sepsis.

Surgical intervention

Throughout this chapter reference has been made to the need for controlling the underlying source of infection. In some circumstances this may be comparatively easy if the patient presents with an obvious wound infection, an abscess or soft tissue infection or a necrotic limb. In other situations the source of the sepsis or SIRS may not be readily apparent and diagnostic radiological investigations may be required in a stable patient to identify the exact anatomical location of the problem. Intrathoracic or intra-abdominal sepsis may be particularly difficult to diagnose. Treatment may require thoracotomy or laparotomy. When surgical exploration is required it should be carried out by a senior member of the surgical team after appropriate resuscitation of the patient. The extent of the surgical procedure will depend on the location and extent of the septic lesion but adequate drainage and debridement should be carried out. In abdominal sepsis it may be necessary to consider the use of stomas, tubes or drains and in certain circumstances planned relaparotomy or laparostomy may be a treatment option.[26] The chances of survival are enhanced by the early eradication of the source of sepsis or SIRS. The surgical approach is dictated by the condition of the patient and the experience of the surgeon. The survival rate for patients requiring laparotomy for abdominal sepsis in an ICU setting is approximately 40% and multiple operations are associated with diminishing returns and increasing mortality.

Summary   Each year in the United States there are 400 000 cases of sepsis, 200 000 cases of septic shock and 100 000 deaths. The incidence of sepsis is increasing and despite advances in treatment the mortality rate is unchanged. Death from sepsis is usually preceded by MODS and a similar fate may await the patient with SIRS. Successful therapy on the surgical ward, HDU or ICU demands an early recognition of the problem, aggressive resuscitation to improve oxygen delivery and tissue perfusion and definitive treatment to eliminate the underlying cause. Adjunctive therapy with surgical intervention, antibiotics, nutritional support and prevention of additional complications enhances the prospect of a successful outcome. Nonetheless mortality remains high at 50% and more research and a better understanding of the pathophysiology of sepsis are required to improve mortality and morbidity in these critically ill patients. They represent a major clinical challenge and their management demands a multidisciplinary approach.

References

1. McCrory DC, Rowlands BJ. Septic syndrome and multiple system organ failure. Curr Pract Surg 1993; 5: 211–15.
2. Dominioni K, Bianchi M, Dionigi R. Factors predisposing to surgical infections and identification of patients at risk. Surg Res Commun 1990; 9: 1–7.
3. Hill GL, Blackett RL, Pickford I *et al.* Malnutrition in surgical patients: an unrecognised problem. Lancet 1977; i: 689–92.
4. Dionigi R, Cremashi R, Jemos V. Nutritional assessment and severity of illness classification systems: a critical review of their clinical relevance. World J Surg 1986; 10: 2–11.
5. Cruse PJE, Foord R. The epidemiology of wound infection, a 10-year prospective study of 62,939 wounds. Surg Clin North Am 1980; 60: 27–40.
6. Ericsson CD, Rowlands BJ. Surgical infection: principles of management and antibiotic usage. In: Miller TA, Rowlands BJ (eds) Physiological basis of modern surgical care. St Louis, Mosby: 1988; pp. 113–35.
7. The ACCP/SCCM Consensus Conference Committee. Definitions for sepsis and organ failure and guidelines for the use of innovative therapies in sepsis. Chest 1992; 101: 1644–55.
8. Baue AE. Multiple progressive and sequential systems failure, a syndrome of the 1970's, Arch Surg 1975; 110: 779–81.
9. Fry DE, Pearlstein L, Fulton RL *et al.* Multiple system organ failure. Arch Surg 1980; 115: 136–40.
10. Fry DE. Multiple system organ failure. Surg Clin North Am 1988; 68: 107–22.
11. Rowlands BJ, Blair PHB. Infection scoring systems. In: Taylor EW (ed.) Infection in surgical practice. Oxford: Oxford University Press: 1992; pp. 101–8.
12. Diamond T, Rowlands BJ. Resuscitation of the critically ill (including trauma). In: Taylor I, Karran S (eds) Surgical principles. London: Arnold 1990; pp. 105–13.
13. Blair PHB, Rowlands BJ. Postoperative intensive care. In O'Higgins N, Chisholm G, Williamson R (eds) Surgical management. Oxford: Butterworth Heinemann, 1991, pp. 14–29.
14. Cerra FB. Hypermetabolism; organ failure and metabolic support. Surgery 1987; 101: 1–14.
15. Deitch EA. Multiple organ failure. Pathophysiology and potential future therapy. Ann Surg 1992; 216: 117–34.
16. Reynolds JV, O'Farrelly C, Feighery C. *et al.* Impaired gut barrier function in malnourished patients. Br J Surg 1996; 83: 1288–91.
17. Selective Decontamination of the Digestive Tract Trialists Collaborative Group. Meta-analysis of randomized controlled trials of selective decontamination of the digestive tract. Br Med J 1993; 307: 525–32.
18. Wilmore DW. Catabolic illness; strategies for enhancing recovery. N Engl J Med 1991; 325: 695–702.
19. Kudsk KA, Groce MA, Fabian TC *et al.* Enteral vs. parenteral feeding: effects on

septic morbidity after blunt and penetrating abdominal trauma. Ann Surg 1992; 215; 503–13.

20. Moore FA, Feliciano DV, Andrassy RJ *et al*. Early enteral feeding, compared with parenteral reduces postoperative septic complications – the result of a meta analysis. Ann Surg 1992; 216: 172–83.

21. Reed RL. Antibiotic choices in surgical intensive care unit patients. Surg Clin North Am 1991; 71: 765–89.

22. Veterans Administration Systemic Sepsis Cooperative Study Group. Effect of high-dose glucocorticoid therapy on mortality in patients with clinical signs of systemic sepsis. N Engl J Med 1987; 317: 659–65.

23. Freeman BD, Natanson C. Clinical trials in sepsis and septic shock in 1994 and 1995. Curr Opin Crit Care 1995; 1: 349–57.

24. Bone RC. Sir Isaac Newton, sepsis, SIRS, CARS. Crit Care Med 1996; 24: 1125–8.

25. Goldie AS, Fearon KCH, Ross JA *et al*. Natural cytokine antagonists and endogenous anti-endotoxin core antibodies in sepsis syndrome. JAMA 1995; 274: 172–7.

26. Anderson ID, Fearon KCH, Grant IS. Laparotomy for abdominal sepsis in the critically ill. Br J Surg 1996; 83: 535–9.

Index

Page numbers in *italic* refer to illustrations and tables; **bold** page numbers indicate a main discussion.